VISION AND AGING

Crossroads for Service Delivery

Edited by Alberta L. Orr

AFB

PRESS

New York

VISION AND AGING: CROSSROADS FOR SERVICE DELIVERY

is copyright © 1992 by

10001

·k may be reproduced or transmitted in any
mechanical, including photocopying and
age or retrieval system, except as may be
·ight Act, or in writing from the publisher.
·essed in writing to the American Foundation
for the Blind, 11 Penn Plaza, Suite 300, New York, NY 10001.

Printed in the United States of America
Reprinted 1997

Library of Congress Cataloging-in-Publication Data

Vision and aging: crossroads for service delivery / edited by Alberta
    L. Orr.
        p.   cm.
    Includes bibliographical references.
    ISBN 0-89128-216-5 (acid-free)
    1. Blind aged–Services for–United States. 2 Blind aged–United
    States. I. Orr, Alberta L., 1950-   . II. American Foundation for
    the Blind.
    HV1597.5.V57 1992
    362.4 '1' 0846—dc20

                                                                    92-5088
                                                                      CIP

Photo credits: Photographs in Chapter 12, "Orientation and Mobility Services for Older Persons," taken by Ann G. Hubbard.

For updated information on the programs and organizations listed in the Resources section of this publication, readers may contact the American Foundation for the Blind's hotline at (800) 232-5463 or consult its web site at http://www.afb.org.

To
Sandra M. Maskell
Lee Crespi
Kathleen M. Huebner

TABLE OF CONTENTS

FOREWORD

Increasing numbers of older persons will experience vision loss each year through at least the first three decades of the 21st century. Older blind and visually impaired persons will number nearly 6 million by the year 2030, doubling the number documented in 1990. We can only imagine the gravity of their life circumstances if enormous changes in policy and service delivery do not take place to prepare to meet this population's needs now and during the next 40 years. We do not know the specific developments in the areas of funding, technology, legislation, and services that will occur during this period to benefit older visually impaired persons. But we do know that they will not just happen. Needed change will not take place without efforts in every political and service arena to transform an unsatisfactory status quo into an environment characterized by innovative and effective programs.

Vision and Aging: Crossroads for Service Delivery focuses on the impact of visual impairment on older persons and their families. It also discusses the extent of that impact when services in the aging and blindness fields theoretically designed to enable older visually impaired persons to function independently are not available or accessible. The picture that it presents suggests that service providers in every arena touching on the lives of older blind and visually impaired persons need to become knowledgeable advocates for positive change.

What older visually impaired people need is not that difficult and not that costly to provide. But without it, independence and quality of life are seriously threatened when they could so easily be enhanced. Because we at the American Foundation for the Blind believe that the growing numbers of older persons who are visually impaired demand the immediate attention of all of us, we hope that the message of *Vision and Aging* will encourage the blindness field to seize the opportunity to work on behalf of older persons with visual impairments.

Carl R. Augusto
President and Executive Director
American Foundation for the Blind

SECTION I

Setting the Framework

CHAPTER 1

Aging and Blindness: Toward a Systems Approach to Service Delivery

Alberta L. Orr

This book is about older persons, the process of aging, and the vision loss many older persons experience. This introductory chapter has several purposes. It describes the blind and visually impaired elderly population, examines the professionals and service delivery systems responsible for providing services to this population, presents the challenges and opportunities facing both older visually impaired persons and service providers, and suggests how professionals in the fields of aging and blindness can meet the growing and changing demands for service.

The purpose of this book is to help professionals in the blindness and aging fields reach out more effectively to older visually impaired persons in order to assist them in remaining as independent as they wish to be and are capable of being. It attempts to promote a new knowledge base for professionals and to encourage a dialogue between the two vitally important service delivery networks represented by the aging and the blindness fields. It is intended to be valuable to those who provide direct services to older visually impaired clients. However, this book should also be useful to any professional who wishes to become acquainted more closely with the issues and trends in the fields of aging and blindness and the services designed to meet the needs of older visually impaired persons.

Effective services begin with an understanding of the needs of the people to be served. The material presented in this book on aging and vision loss is designed to help professionals who provide services learn to recognize the special needs of visually impaired older persons and, consequently, to respond to these needs with greater knowledge, understanding, and insight. The first step in improved service delivery is to develop outreach strategies to identify more clients, particularly clients with special needs who are hard to reach. These hard-to-reach groups include older persons who live in rural areas or who are members of minority groups experiencing language and cultural barriers to services. The next step is to include these clients in service delivery systems. The third step is to adapt services and the environment in such a way that older visually impaired clients have access to programs. In addition to needing the skills and knowledge to accomplish these efforts, practitioners need to know how to refer clients to services that complement each other and thus satisfy clients' needs. They also need to know how to network and work collaboratively across fields and disciplines. The fruitful consequences of increased knowledge and skills can be the meaningful design of services and programs under the joint auspices of blindness and aging agencies.

For visually impaired elderly clients to receive effective, well-coordinated services, both the blindness and aging delivery systems must assume responsibility for providing services and must work together cooperatively to enhance clients' independence and to improve their quality of life. As a start, this chapter will provide essential information of relevance to professionals in both fields. This introduction therefore includes the following:

- a brief overview of the demographics of aging and of aging and visual impairment,
- a description of the older visually impaired population,
- a review of the service delivery system in the aging and the blindness fields,
- an outline of the key issues in the fields of aging and blindness, and
- the rationale for collaborative planning and networking between these fields.

Demographics of Aging and Blindness

It is impossible to pick up a newspaper today without seeing a reminder that the population in this country is aging rapidly. According to the

U.S. Bureau of the Census, there were only 3 million persons 65 years of age or over in the United States at the turn of the century. Today there are 31 million persons in this category. This means that 12.5 percent, or approximately one in every eight Americans, are age 65 or over; 18.3 million are women; 12.5 million are men. The ratio of women to men in the 65-69 age group is 120 to 100, increasing dramatically to 258 women to every 100 men in the 85-and-over category, with an overall ratio of 145 to 100 for the entire 65-plus population (American Association of Retired Persons, 1990).

In the population of those 65 and over, gerontologists have described three cohorts—those 65 to 74, the young-old; those 75 to 84, the middle-old; and those 85 and over, the old-old. A fourth, younger cohort, those 55 to 64, may also need services from the aging and blindness systems. Many older persons begin to experience vision problems while in this age group, and many older people in general need help during these years to plan financially for long-term care, to carry out preretirement planning, and to focus on employment and other issues. Although all the cohorts are expanding, the 85-plus category is the fastest growing segment. Members of this group number 2.9 million, a figure 23 times larger than that prevailing at the turn of the century. At 9.3 million, the 75-to-84 cohort is 12 times larger than it was, and those 65 to 74, at 17.7 million, are 8 times larger (American Association of Retired Persons, 1990).

By the year 2000, the 65-plus group will represent 13 percent of the people in the United States. An astoundingly rapid rise in the percentage of the population age 65-and-over is projected for the years 2010 to 2030, when the baby boom generation reaches age 65. By 2030, 66 million people will be 65 or older, more than double the number today (American Association of Retired Persons, 1990).

These statistics and projections are critical, for policymakers and service providers need to plan effectively for the present and the future. A coordinated effort of service delivery systems, such as in the areas of health care, social services, and rehabilitation, must now be directed toward working creatively to meet this growing population's changing and diverse needs. With 10 to 12 percent of the age 65-and-over population currently visually impaired, the number of visually impaired older persons in the decades to come is also projected to expand at a rapid rate.

Many older persons of all ages experience good health and physical functioning. However, as the elderly population becomes a greater proportion of the overall population, this country can anticipate an even greater demand for health care services than is already being experienced. The population is living longer as a result of tremendous achievements in the fields of medicine and technology, but two-thirds of those 65 and over have more than one chronic condition that can decrease independent mobility. The primary conditions that disable America's elderly population today are arthritis, hypertension, hearing impairment, heart disease, visual impairment, and stroke (Blake, 1984). This situation creates great challenges for the health care and allied fields in helping older persons reach the levels of independent functioning they seek and are capable of achieving. Currently, two out of three Americans will die with a disability, but they do not have to be totally disabled as a result of an impairment if the necessary supports and services are available (Williams, 1986). It is therefore important for anyone involved with older persons to know about the kinds of services and programs available to enhance the quality of life for elderly individuals, whatever the disability. For the older visually impaired person, rehabilitation services for blind and visually impaired persons and assistance from agencies serving the elderly population can have a tremendous impact on psychological and physical functioning and overall well-being.

The exact number of visually impaired persons 65 years of age and over in this country is not known because of the difficulty in gathering such data and the reliance on self-reporting of visual impairment. It is safe to assume, then, that the data we do have represent a considerable undercount of the total number of older persons experiencing severe enough vision loss to interfere with their daily functioning. The questions related to vision loss on data collection instruments have generally been misworded (Nelson, 1988). For example, if a question asks, "Are you blind?" as it does in the U. S. census, older persons with gradually deteriorating vision tend to answer "no." They are correct. They are visually impaired, not blind; they still have usable vision. An older person who has lived 60, 70, or 80 years as a sighted person and has carried all the stereotypic thinking about blindness and blind persons throughout life will not want to be counted in this statistic. A more appropriate and accurately worded inquiry, such as "Do you have difficulty reading newspaper print?" will help researchers gather more accurate data.

The first sign of improvement in the wording of questions targeted for the older population occurred in 1984, when the National Center for Health Statistics (NCHS) Health Interview Survey (HIS) developed a Supplement on Aging. At that time, the survey was designed to document the number of older persons who were "severely visually impaired." This term had the functional definition of "difficulty reading newspaper print," one to which older persons could respond more freely. Although vision is a multidimensional function and this definition represents only one way to measure vision, the definition is significant because it documents the number of older persons who have difficulty with various aspects of daily functioning. The results of this survey concluded that at the time the survey was conducted in 1984, there were 2,038,000 older visually impaired persons, a remarkable 106 percent increase over the documented 990,000 reported just seven years prior (Nelson, 1988).

The search for accurate numbers is critical to document the burgeoning need for more service dollars for a population that is expanding both through increased numbers of aging persons and increased numbers of persons with visual impairment. According to the 1990 census, there are already 2,578,000 severely visually impaired persons 65 and over. Reflecting the graying of America, this means that between 1960 and 1990, the number of older visually impaired persons more than doubled. By 2030, the number will more than double again, to reach just under 6 million (Nelson, 1988).

By the year 2000, it is projected that there will be 3,203,000 older visually impaired persons, which will climb to 3,727,000 in 2010 and 4,549,000 in 2020. As the baby boom generation enters its senior years, the number increases dramatically, because in 2020, the oldest members of this generation will be in their early seventies. Just 10 years later, in 2030, nearly all the members of the baby boom generation will be 65 and over, accounting for the almost 6 million older visually impaired persons projected for that year (Nelson, 1991). Although 10 to 12 percent of the 65-plus population is severely visually impaired, as many as one in four is visually impaired in the 85-plus category, the fastest growing segment of the visually impaired population. In fact, in 20 years, it is projected that the 85-plus group will include 1.6 million severely visually impaired persons.

Additional factors account for the difficulties in measuring the number of older visually impaired persons. Because the process of losing vision among older persons is usually gradual, many older persons barely notice changes in vision, or they accept the decline as a normal part of aging. This can be a problem because these persons neither seek eye care nor learn about rehabilitation or other services for blind and visually impaired persons. As a result, they are not counted, treated, or served.

The incidence of visual impairment is high among the 55-and-over population because of four leading eye conditions associated with aging. Age-related maculopathy, or macular degeneration, along with cataracts, glaucoma, and diabetic retinopathy, largely accounts for blindness and visual impairment among the elderly population. Age 55 is often used as a base to describe the older visually impaired population because of the onset at this age of some of these eye conditions and the beginning of eligibility for some services for the older visually impaired population.

A majority of older visually impaired persons (66 percent), in spite of complications related to disability or multiple disabilities, continue to live in their own communities and their own homes. Approximately 26 percent live in nursing homes. The remainder live with adult children, other family, or in other housing arrangements. Of the nursing home population, only 3 percent are totally blind, but studies indicate that between 30 and 50 percent of residents of nursing homes are visually impaired. This country currently spends $6.9 billion to institutionalize the nation's older blind and visually impaired population, a cost that will continue to rise (Crews, 1988). However, nursing home placement is usually unnecessary for the older visually impaired person, unless he or she has other disabling health conditions. Community-based services can be less expensive and can meet the needs of many older persons outside the institutional setting. Community-based resources for the older blind person are important, therefore, to avoid premature and unnecessary institutionalization and to enable older persons to "age in place," that is, remain in their own homes.

Definitions of Vision Loss

Terms such as "visual impairment," "blindness," "legal blindness," and "low vision" are often used in the literature and in practice. Sometimes, they are used interchangeably. Without an understanding of these terms, it can be extremely confusing to hear someone who has vision referred to as legally blind.

"Legal blindness" is a term used to define conditions that make individuals eligible for government and agency benefits and services. An individual who is legally blind has a visual acuity of 20/200 or less in the better eye with the best correction or a visual field of no more than 20 degrees. (See Chapters 3 and 10 for discussions about visual acuity.) The "normal" visual field is 175 to 180 degrees, and normal visual acuity is represented by 20/20. This degree of vision loss is used as the baseline to determine eligibility for rehabilitation services from a public or private agency providing services to blind and visually impaired persons of all ages. (See Chapter 3 for a more extensive discussion of the physiological and functional aspects of vision.)

There are, however, many older persons who experience vision loss significant enough to interfere with their independent functioning and activities of daily living but who do not meet the criteria for legal blindness. Many agencies are becoming more responsive to this segment of the population, referred to as those who have "low vision" or who are "severely visually impaired." This important development in the blindness field allows a greater number of older persons with vision problems to have access to services and to learn adaptive techniques for carrying out daily tasks.

As mentioned above, as a data-gathering baseline, "severe visual impairment" is defined as an impairment resulting in difficulty in reading newspaper print, even with the use of the best possible corrective lenses. This definition obviously encompasses a much larger pool of older persons than that meeting the legal blindness criteria. Similarly, "low vision" describes a loss of vision severe enough to hinder the performance of activities of daily living but still allowing some useful visual discrimination. Low vision cannot be corrected to normal by regular eyeglasses or contact lenses. The range may extend from mild to severe vision loss, with a visual acuity of 20/70 or less. (As visual acuity decreases, the second or bottom number in the fraction increases. See Chapter 10 for a discussion of visual acuity tests.)

The terms "partially sighted" and "visually impaired" loosely differentiate those with some vision from those who are totally blind. These terms do not have technical definitions. They are heard or seen in print to differentiate needs for services. Some of the people they describe still have vision but need various forms of assistance and can benefit from rehabilitation teaching, from orientation and mobility (O&M) services, or from the use of a low vision device (a piece of adaptive equipment that maximizes remaining vision.) Some examples of low vision devices are magnifiers, telescopic lenses, and high-intensity lamps.

Older Visually Impaired Minority Populations

As in the general elderly population, the older visually impaired population is primarily female because women outlive men by seven years. Many older persons live on limited incomes, and many are poor. Many live alone. The older visually impaired person may be even poorer. Large numbers of the visually impaired elderly population represent minority groups, particularly Hispanics, blacks, and Native Americans. These groups are at the highest risk of developing visual impairments late in life. The major reason for the higher proportion of visual impairment in these minority populations, particularly Native Americans, is the high incidence of diabetes and diabetic retinopathy, the eye condition associated with diabetes. Unfortunately, for reasons related to language and culture, these older persons are more difficult to reach.

Reaching these minority populations is an important issue in the fields of blindness and aging. They continue to grow and require services but have little or no access to rehabilitation services for blind and visually impaired persons.

Agencies for blind persons located in high-density minority areas are developing nontraditional outreach strategies to identify people needing independent living skills training. Some examples of effective strategies are public service radio announcements in Spanish, the use of bilingual-bicultural community outreach workers who can speak directly to Hispanic community organizations and civic groups, and collaboration with clergy who know congregants and their needs.

Bilingual-bicultural staff are the key to service delivery and the learning of skills for many non-English-speaking clients. Stronger efforts to recruit minority persons into the blindness field are essential to effective service delivery in the field. The training of indigenous paraprofessionals can also be effective, as has been demonstrated in a national project to train Native American health care service providers to teach independent living skills to elderly blind and visually impaired Native Americans (Orr, 1990b). For the practitioner in general, acquisition of knowledge about culture and tradition and community functioning can be the key to enhanced service delivery methods.

Because of the heterogeneity of the population of older persons who are blind or visually impaired, programs and services must be designed to respond to a diversity of needs and capabilities. Particularly at the local level, services must respond to the composition of the population needing help. A closer look at the population of older visually impaired persons sheds further light on this special group and its growing and changing needs.

The Older Visually Impaired Person

For many older persons, gradually deteriorating vision may be the first sign of aging. For others, vision loss may come quickly on the heels of another disabling condition or loss in physical functioning. The impact of vision loss depends on an array of concomitant circumstances. These can include individual personal patterns of adjustment to change;

the extent of existing support from spouse, adult children, peers, or neighbors; and awareness of how to get professional help. Some older persons with deteriorating vision continue to live independently. Others are able to live at home because their spouses are still alive, in good health, and functioning well physically. Still others require the assistance of a family caregiver or a service provider to remain at home.

An older person whose only disability is blindness or visual impairment should not require nursing home placement. Frequently the first thoughts of the older person who is losing vision and of family members are: "I will never be able to manage by myself" and "My mother will never be able to live safely on her own." Few people are aware of rehabilitation agencies for blind and visually impaired people, which can help clients learn to continue to function independently by acquiring adaptive techniques for activities of daily living.

Newly visually impaired older persons experience an array of challenges in daily functioning. They need skills to perform activities in familiar or adapted ways. These activities include specific tasks, such as becoming oriented to the environment; preparing and eating food; reading mail and other material; writing letters, lists, and notes; and dialing the telephone. Often, the older visually impaired person will need to reorganize entire components of his or her household or life so that items, such as clothes in a closet, can easily be found or tasks, such as managing a checking account, can continue to be done. While learning ways of continuing necessary or favorite activities, the older person may need to learn how to use new technology, adaptive devices, and specialized techniques, for example, O&M techniques for moving safely indoors and venturing outside.

In addition, a host of other adjustments and behaviors may be required of the older visually impaired person. The following list outlines a sampling of these:

- facing the reality of vision loss,
- overcoming some of the myths and stereotypic thinking the person has about blindness and blind people,
- discovering new talents and opportunities for personal self-fulfillment,

- explaining one's current life situation and needs to others, including family members, a peer group, the community, clergy, social networks, and professionals who have never worked with a blind person,
- educating others along the way rather than withdrawing and retreating from them,
- continuing to live independently to preserve lifetime savings, prevent unnecesary and premature institutionalization, and maintain self-esteem,
- coping with the demands of retirement or of early retirement brought about by social values and pressures or by vision loss,
- coping with losses associated with aging, such as the loss of opportunities for productive activity; of significant others, such as spouse, siblings, and peers; of familiar social networks; of geographic proximity to adult children and to grandchildren; of self-worth, self-esteem, self-confidence, and self-reliance,
- being interdependent within the family and social context and continuing to be involved, and to retain valued roles,
- participating in activities with other newly visually impaired older persons,
- not only participating in the psychologically safe segregated programming of a blindness agency but becoming successfully integrated into activities and programs at a local senior citizens center.

Psychosocial Aspects of Aging and Vision Loss

At the onset of vision loss, many older visually impaired persons find themselves having two opposing desires—to retreat from everything and to continue participating in ongoing activities in and outside the home. Anxiety, fear, and depression may come into play. After being introduced to the possibility of working with an agency for blind and visually impaired persons, the older visually impaired individual may once again experience two contrasting desires—to remain in a safe environment with other visually impaired persons in similar circumstances and to reenter the sighted world, such as the senior citizens center, although fearing not being accepted or not fitting in. The following sections describe the range of ways in which newly visually impaired elderly persons might benefit from services by blindness and aging agencies.

CASE 1

Mrs. J is one of over 2 million noninstitutionalized Americans age 65 and over who has suffered severe vision loss. She considers the decline in her visual capacities a natural and perhaps inevitable consequence of aging. She is also reluctant to admit to herself and to others that she is increasingly aware of her failing eyesight. Initially she did not know what services might be available to her and made the assumption that there were no services in her community to help her solve, or at least ameliorate, her difficulties in being independent in her daily life.

As her eyesight deteriorated and interfered with daily activities, Mrs. J found it more difficult to get around her house and too difficult to go outdoors and to maintain her own strong sense of independence. She began having problems finding items in the supermarket, finding the curb at the street corner, knowing when the crossing signals changed, and even being sure which doorways on the block were the entrances to particular stores.

She had been active at a senior citizens center, serving on two committees. But more and more embarrassments and discomforts occurred there. Spilling food and drinks at the lunch table, having difficulty recognizing faces, not being able to read the monthly calendar and program and trip announcements, and missing special events created an uncomfortable situation for Mrs. J. She stopped attending the center. Leaving the house became intimidating. Mrs. J also felt it was unsafe to cook for herself. She had lost her husband over two years before and had put most of her energies into keeping busy at the center. Her only daughter lived across the country and therefore was not available for routine daily assistance. The daughter felt her mother's living arrangement was unsafe and asked her if she thought about moving to a nursing home. Mrs. J was uncertain and hesitated whenever she thought about life in a "home for old people."

The director of Mrs. J's senior citizens center had been on leave for three months during these most recent dramatic changes. On her return, she was told that Mrs. J had stopped coming to the center and called Mrs. J, thereby learning the sequence of events that had occurred.

The center director had experienced a similar situation with another center member a year before. At that time she knew nothing about resources in the field of blindness, but she was able to make contacts within the blindness system through a woman she heard speak at a local gerontology conference. Since that time she had helped her own mother gain access to services from an agency for blind people. She was well prepared to assist Mrs. J.

First, the senior center director arranged for Meals-on-Wheels for Mrs. J until Mrs. J could learn to cook safely for herself. Then she contacted the state agency for blind and visually impaired people located in the city. Mrs. J was put in touch with two professionals from the agency for the blind—a rehabilitation teacher who came to her home and taught her adapted methods for daily activities and an O&M instructor who taught her safety techniques for orientation and moving freely in her own environment. Mrs. J was not yet ready to learn to use a white cane in the street; she felt she would be embarrassed. But she was so excited about her new independence that the use of the cane seemed almost a certainty for the future. Meanwhile, the center director arranged for door-to-door transportation to the senior center through the local accessible paratransit system available to frail elderly and disabled people in the community.

The director of the center was committed to Mrs. J's success, and she spoke regularly to the social worker at the agency for blind persons. She also designated the center's social worker as the case manager for Mrs. J. She arranged for in-service training for staff and other members at the center to learn more about blindness and visual impairment and make Mrs. J's transition back to the center a little easier for all. This training was also helpful to other members having vision problems and to the center's clientele and staff in general.

Mrs. J visited an ophthalmologist, who then referred her to a low vision specialist who was an optometrist. She had a low vision evaluation and was able to get low vision devices (a high-intensity lamp and a hand-held magnifier) to read print larger than newspaper print.

Mrs. J's case is a success story. Her primary advantage was her linkage to the aging system and its services. She benefited enormously from the involvement of a professional who was knowledgeable about rehabilitation services available from the blindness system.

CASE 2

Contrast Mrs. J with Mrs. F, who was diagnosed as having macular degeneration, an eye disease associated with aging. Like Mrs. J's, Mrs. F's vision loss progressed over several years. Mrs. F had recently retired at age 70 and hoped to continue to be active in community volunteer activities. She began experiencing difficulties doing ordinary household tasks, managing her checking account, and paying bills and could no longer read comfortably. She began to feel devastated by her experiences, fearing that her opportunities for being productive and making a contribution to the community would be limited. She knew that younger people received vocational rehabilitation services from agencies for blind persons but had no idea what help older people could receive. She mustered up enough emotional energy to make a call to the local agency for blind and visually impaired persons, but only after almost 12 months had passed.

A social worker came to Mrs. F's home to assess her skills and adjustment to her circumstances. She assured Mrs. F that her feelings of helplessness and frustration were normal and encouraged her by describing some of the services available to her and some of the adaptive techniques she could learn. Mrs. F began a rehabilitation program and learned independent living skills—organizing her kitchen and closets and finding items easily, paying bills and keeping track of money, improving the lighting in her home, and using contrasting colors and other environmental modifications. She also learned O&M techniques to enable her to move about safely in her home and her community.

Mrs. F also applied to receive Talking Books, available free to all people with visual impairments from the National Library Service for the Blind and Physically Handicapped. She received a radio receiver to listen to a radio reading service for blind and visually impaired persons. She learned about devices and appliances, such as talking clocks and Hi-marks, a liquid used to mark dials and nontactile visual displays.

Mrs. F joined a self-help group to be with others with similar problems and to share experiences and tips. The social worker provided her with individual counseling as well. Mrs. F learned that several members of the peer support group attended a local senior center that offered an array of cultural and educational programs. The other visually impaired peer group members had no difficulty participating in the center's activities in spite of varying degrees of vision loss.

The senior center was unique in the community. The head of the local private agency for blind persons and the director of the senior center recognized the difficulties that visually impaired seniors had participating in some of the center's activities and agreed that adaptive techniques needed to be learned and understood by staff and by sighted and visually impaired center members.

A representative from the agency for blind persons and the center director began a series of in-service training sessions in the center and at the agency. Many staff members had found it difficult to work with older clients; their orientation had always been toward providing vocational rehabilitation services to younger clients.

The in-service training made a significant difference at both the center and the agency in work with older clients who were losing vision. But the surrounding community, a great number of whose residents were elderly, went one step further. Recognizing the numbers of older persons in the county and the concomitant number of older persons who were and would be experiencing vision loss, the state unit on aging, the public state agency for elderly people, designated special funds for innovations in senior citizens centers responsive to this population. Centers could receive funds to develop innovative, integrated programming for blind and visually impaired members if they submitted a proposal and planned jointly with the local agency for blind persons. Such expanded and collaborative programming helped integrate older visually impaired persons into senior citizens center life and into the mainstream of the community. These efforts were what Mrs. F needed. Eventually she attended the center two days a week and returned to work with her woman's organization, resuming her leadership role for three days of each week.

The hypothetical cases of Mrs. J and Mrs. F are intended to show how concurrent linkages to an agency for blind persons and to an agency for elderly individuals can have a significant impact on the life of the older visually impaired person. Cooperation and collaboration involving the blindness and the aging service systems can provide numerous opportunities for aging visually impaired people to learn new skills for physical and psychosocial independence and enhance self-esteem, self-worth, and self-confidence. The issue of collaboration among systems of service delivery is discussed in further detail in Chapter 15.

Blindness and Aging Service Delivery Systems Today

Two primary systems are responsible for services to blind and visually impaired older persons—the blindness system, with its categorical services targeted specifically for blind persons, and the generic aging system, mandated to serve all older people. The older person who is blind or visually impaired frequently requires services from both systems and has a right to services from both. Yet both fields—aging and blindness—have taken little time to fulfill this responsibility to the older person who is visually impaired and to respond to the needs of older blind and visually impaired persons. Service providers frequently have had little or no working knowledge of this special population and therefore have been slow to make claim to it.

Most service providers in the field of aging have no professional preparation in the area of vision loss; many of those in the field of blindness have a limited knowledge base in the issues of aging and vision loss. Few professionals have expertise in both blindness and aging. A service provider may ask, "To which system do blind and visually impaired elderly persons belong?" Those in the aging service system may believe that blind persons can best be served by professionals trained to work with blind and visually impaired people and should be referred to an agency for blind persons. But the service provider in a rehabilitation agency for blind persons may believe that older visually impaired clients belong to the aging network because they need so many services related to aging. As a result of such thinking and the shifting of responsibility that often accompanies it, clients are tossed from system to system and from referral to referral, frequently remaining on long waiting lists for services or leaving both systems without the services and supports that will enable them to function as independently as possible. Often, older visually impaired clients receive services from only one of the systems.

Under these circumstances, the older visually impaired person is not necessarily denied services by either service delivery system. But neither system, by tradition, has viewed the older person who is visually impaired as one of its target client groups. Service providers in both fields often believe it is best to make a referral. They frequently feel unprepared to face a client's compounded needs, which are different from the needs of their general population of clients.

The service provider in the field of aging who identifies a visually impaired client but does not know anything about community agencies for blind and visually impaired persons or how to access them is in a difficult position. So is his or her counterpart in the field of blindness. After making referrals between systems, service providers may feel that their job is done. Far too frequently there is no follow-up. If service providers fail to take this step, clients fall through the cracks or remain on waiting lists too long and become discouraged from seeking services.

Because of insufficient resources such as limited funds, time, and personnel, service providers in the field of aging frequently have difficulty responding to client populations with special needs. Some may believe that people with special needs take resources away from the general population, the well elderly; others may simply feel that someone without a visual impairment is easier to serve. For example, if visually impaired senior citizens are in a senior citizens center, they may require more assistance than the average member to participate fully. Because of the pressure of workloads and limited resources, service providers in both fields can often benefit from learning more about the older visually impaired population: Knowledge can facilitate more efficient service delivery and modify perceptions as well. A curriculum on issues related to aging and vision loss is needed in the professional preparation for both fields so that young professionals begin their careers with sound knowledge about both aging and vision loss. In-service training for service providers in both fields can help the practicing professional become attuned to special needs.

The need for professional knowledge is twofold. Content on aging and vision loss needs to be incorporated into the curriculum of gerontology programs and related human service areas, and content on aging needs to be integrated into professional preparation programs for blind rehabilitation across the country. The American Foundation for the Blind is developing guidelines for a model curriculum in aging and vision loss for gerontology programs throughout the country. However, in-service training for professionals and paraprofessionals in both fields, whether in community-based agencies or institutional settings such as nursing homes, is an especially important need. There are excellent in-service activities in many communities across the country, but these training models must be disseminated and replicated.

Accessibility to Services

A critical national issue is accessibility to services within the aging and blindness fields for older visually impaired persons. Accessibility in relation to disability means more than adaptations to the physical environment, such as building ramps and doorways accessible to people with physical disabilities. It means accessibility in terms of attitude and thinking about individuals with special needs and the elimination of nontangible barriers.

An even greater issue regarding accessibility to services exists for older persons from minority groups who encounter language and cultural barriers. Insufficient access is a critical problem for Hispanic, black, Native American, and rural elderly people. Within the field of aging, there is considerable recognition that services and printed materials must be available to persons whose first language is Spanish. Within the field of blindness, there is a critical need for black and Hispanic rehabilitation teachers and O&M specialists who are bilingual and bicultural. There is a need for minority group members to work as paraprofessionals in the field of aging as well. More members of minority groups in both fields would help eliminate barriers to service.

For Native Americans, who struggle for access to service in all areas, access to blind rehabilitation services has been almost nil, especially for the elderly population. Many elderly people fear working with Anglo service providers, whose cultural orientation is foreign and removed from their experience. Greater access to services is possible if service providers have a sufficient level of awareness about special client populations.

Rehabilitation and the Continuum of Care

It is helpful to view rehabilitation services for older blind and visually impaired persons as part of the continuum of community-based long-term care for elderly people. Long-term care should be seen as a range of services for the older person, from community-based services and supports within the community to institutional care, such as the nursing home. The idea of long-term care services as a continuum allows for the perception of the nursing home as part of the community's services to the elderly population.

It may be difficult for older clients to see services from this point of view because the notion of a continuum is a relatively recent concept, and various services seem unrelated. Nevertheless, receiving services concurrently from both the aging and the blindness systems enables older visually impaired clients to view agencies and service providers as working together on their behalf. Services from both systems help achieve comprehensive, holistic rehabilitation.

The rehabilitation process for the older person is more than learning adaptive techniques for daily living activities and the use of the long cane for orientation to indoor and outdoor environments. Rehabilitation encompasses the rehabilitation teaching of independent living skills, O&M instruction, concurrent social services, counseling by a social worker, family involvement to the fullest extent possible in the learning of adaptive techniques as well as in counseling components, participation in a peer support group, and involvement in programs and services for elderly persons, when desired. If rehabilitation provided by a blindness agency can take place while the older person continues attending a local senior citizens center, the learning of skills derived from the agency for blind persons can be put into practice in daily life. This is the ideal that is possible if professionals have familiarity across systems.

The key professional disciplines within the blind rehabilitation system are rehabilitation teaching and O&M. The term "rehabilitation" refers to all services enhancing the functioning of blind and visually impaired persons. Rehabilitation teaching refers to the instruction in adaptive techniques for carrying out activities of daily living. These skills are taught by a rehabilitation teacher. An O&M instructor teaches blind and visually impaired persons how to be oriented to the indoor and outdoor environments and how to travel safely outside the home. Instruction includes the use of the long cane. Low vision rehabilitation involves learning to use adaptive devices to make the best use of existing vision. When these specialized services are viewed as part of the continuum of community-based long-term care, a greater number of clients and professionals will make optimum use of both systems. The history of the two systems sheds light on why much work must go into collaborative efforts, networking, and planning together at the state and local levels.

History of the Aging and Blindness Systems

Many commonalities exist in the development of policy and practice in the fields of aging and blindness. In a sense, both areas of service were initially defined by the enactment of social security legislation in 1935. The Social Security Act represented the first big wave of social entitlement programs. For the first time, individuals were eligible for payments based on age or disability. Blindness was specifically targeted.

Both fields and professional disciplines share another common thread of history—they both became increasingly professionalized in the 1940s. Not until then did blind adults begin to receive help to improve independent functioning.

THE BLINDNESS SYSTEM

The blindness system in the United States dates back to the early 19th century, when the first residential schools for blind students were established. However, comprehensive rehabilitation services as they are known today developed after World War II, during which many thousands of soldiers were blinded in action. In the wake of the war, the blindness system focused on vocational rehabilitation to enable persons who were blind or losing their vision to remain in or reenter the work force. As a result, services for employable, preretirement-age persons were considered a priority. However, as the population of blind persons in this country became increasingly comprised of those age 55 and over, the need among this population for rehabilitation services, particularly for those related to independent living, also grew. Given the prevailing focus on rehabilitation based on the individual's potential for employment, rehabilitation services for older persons have not been treated as a priority. Included in vocational rehabilitation is the category of "homemaker," in which individuals not oriented toward a return to work outside the home can receive rehabilitation services to continue to function as independent homemakers. Although some older visually impaired persons receive rehabilitation through this category, elderly people have traditionally not been the prioritized group.

The most significant federal legislation related to rehabilitation services is the Rehabilitation Act passed in 1973 and its subsequent amendments. Funds from the Rehabilitation Act are administered at the federal level by the Rehabilitation Services Administration (RSA). These federal funds filter down to rehabilitation agencies at the state level. State agencies for blind persons are referred to as the state commission for the blind in some states; in others they are called the division of services for the blind. Thirty-seven states have a separate rehabilitation agency for blind persons; others have a generic vocational rehabilitation agency with a unit in blind rehabilitation. State funds are used at the local level through local offices of the state agency and through contracts with private agencies for blind and visually impaired persons, which provide rehabilitation services.

Where does the older visually impaired person fit into the blindness system? Not until 1978 did a special amendment to the Rehabilitation Act designate rehabilitation for independent living skills training for the elderly population through Title VII, Part C as part of the Independent Living stream of funding. Morever, funds were not available for Title VII, Part C until 1986. These funds are available only in half the states in the country, and each of these states receives only approximately $200,000. The goal of advocates for rehabilitation of older persons is that a baseline of $225,000 be available in each state, with an additional allocation based on the number of older visually impaired persons in the state. To a large measure, though, Title VII, Part C has revolutionized blind rehabilitation by setting a special priority for the rehabilitation of older persons. This legislation represents a landmark for visually impaired elderly persons.

A particularly significant result of Title VII, Part C is that many states have built-in collaboration among professional counterparts. Some states include a component in their Title VII, Part C services in which workers from the agency for blind persons provide community education and outreach efforts in senior citizens centers as well as in-service training. In this way, it is easier for both sighted and visually impaired members of senior centers to participate together. Others have built networking with service providers in the field of aging into the program so that the newly visually impaired person receives needed services from both systems. In a recent review of the field (Orr, 1990a), eight states were found to have used Title VII, Part C funds for special outreach to underserved and unserved minority and low-income clients. Twelve states used their funds to expand services, particularly to their more rural, hard-to-reach counties. Project funds improve family involvement in the rehabilitation process and provide services for severely visually impaired residents of nursing homes. Still other states have used their Title VII, Part C funds to establish self-help and peer support groups and volunteer networks. More funds are needed for Title VII, Part C so that every state can receive funds and not have to compete for them with other states.

In addition to their desire for rehabilitation training for independent living, a growing number of older persons who experience vision loss are interested in remaining in or reentering the work force. Only recently has society recognized that working beyond the standard social security retirement age of 65 may be a desirable option for many people. It has also only recently been recognized that even with a disability, such as vision loss, older persons may still wish to work and be capable of working. However, the system has not been primed to work in this direction. Employment-related services and training represent an area in which the aging and the blindness fields need to work closely together to create employment opportunities on behalf of older visually impaired persons.

THE AGING SYSTEM

Within the field of aging, two major professional leadership organizations were established in the 1940s. The American Geriatrics Society and the Gerontological Society of America were the first organizations of academics and professionals in the field of aging. The National Council on the Aging, comprised of practitioners in the field of aging, was created shortly thereafter. Not until 1965, with the enactment of the Older Americans Act (OAA) and its subsequent amendments, were services for the elderly population formally structured and funded through the creation of federal, state, and local program levels and networks of state and area agencies on aging (AAAs) along with community-based programs (see Chapter 7). The OAA established funds for nutrition sites, multipurpose senior centers, training for professionals, work opportunities for older workers, and special services for older Native Americans.

Funds from the OAA reach the community through the state. Each state has a state unit on aging known by such names as the office on aging, agency for the elderly, or department of aging. Within each state are AAAs representing a county or city office, such as the New York City Department for the Aging or the Philadelphia Corporation on Aging.

These levels of agencies for elderly persons have counterparts with which to network within the blindness system: the U.S. Administration on Aging (AOA) and RSA at the federal level, the state unit on aging and the state agency for the blind at the state level, and, at the local level, the AAA and the local office of the state agency as well as local private agencies for the blind. However, limited coordination exists at each level between the two service delivery fields. Public and private agencies for blind and visually impaired individuals need to work in collaboration with public and private agencies for elderly persons in order to bring about the most comprehensive system of serving older visually impaired persons. Joint projects and shared funding at the state and local levels can create this type of coordinated service delivery system.

Trends in the Field

The issues and trends in the fields of aging and blindness relate to the current needs of older visually impaired persons. Innovative service providers in both fields are attempting to create the services to meet this population's needs across the country. At a time of burgeoning needs, the creative use of existing resources and collaborative efforts are essential.

Times change, and trends toward a friendlier legislative environment for blind and visually impaired elderly persons and toward bringing services into the community and the home are sometimes observable. Movements to improve service accessibility for unserved and underserved people through innovative models of outreach and service delivery can also be seen. But professionals in both fields must continually evaluate what seem to be the best innovations, decide whether programs and services accomplish their goals, and redefine and redesign service delivery strategies and models.

There are many issues to address in the years to come. In summary, the following areas need professional attention and advocacy:

- increased funding for Title VII, Part C to ensure that each state has funds to offer rehabilitation services to the blind and visually impaired elderly population,
- improved professional preparation, including infusion of on content aging and vision loss into required curricula in blind rehabilitation and of material on aging and vision loss into gerontology programs and related disciplines,
- long-term care incorporating in-service training on aging and vision loss for all levels of nursing home staff (from administrators to housekeepers, including training in recognizing vision loss), low vision assessments, and low vision rehabilitation services,
- opportunities for older persons who are losing their vision to retain or acquire remunerative and nonremunerative employment, brought

about through the education of rehabilitation counselors about work opportunities for older visually impaired persons,

- access to blind rehabilitation service agencies for clients who are bilingual or bicultural,
- effective outreach strategies to rural visually impaired elderly persons (with special focus on rural minorities, particularly black individuals in rural areas),
- holistic rehabilitation, encompassing service within and outside the blindness system,
- increased integration and mainstreaming of older visually impaired persons into community resources and services, such as senior centers,
- a broader knowledge base about aging and vision loss issues as well as information on resources for caregivers of older visually impaired persons, particularly adult children and spouses,
- guaranteed access to entitlements and benefits based on income (Medicaid, Supplemental Security Income) for older visually impaired persons living below the poverty level,
- improved, accessible housing for disabled and visually impaired elderly persons,
- networking between the aging and blindness systems at the federal, state, and local levels to ensure collaborative planning and service provision to older blind and visually impaired clients,
- improved data collection strategies to increase knowledge of the demographics of aging,
- improved wording for questions on surveys regarding vision loss for older respondents, to ensure accurate demographic data for use in applying for increased service funding,
- recruitment of minority professionals for the blindness rehabilitation field, which is important for the successful rehabilitation of older visually impaired members of minority groups,
- opportunities for adult education and learning for retired older visually impaired persons who choose not to work,
- opportunities for volunteer work for older visually impaired persons, such as the Senior Companion Program, Retired Senior Volunteer

Program, Foster Grandparents Program, and seniors-serving-seniors programs,

- transportation and accessibility to public transportation for those who can no longer drive because of vision loss and the need for expanded O&M programs for elderly individuals,
- reimbursement of blindness rehabilitation professionals by Medicare and Medicaid, particularly for independent living,
- establishment of greater numbers of peer support, self-help, and mutual aid groups for older visually impaired persons as a response to isolation and depression,
- family involvement in rehabilitation of older visually impaired persons to ensure skill acquisition and retention,
- increased allocation of funds from the aging arena to be earmarked for programs aiding blind and visually impaired older persons.

Collaboration and Advocacy

The time is right for the fields of aging and blindness to come together—to advocate for services, plan and implement programs, develop collaborative efforts, and work for common goals. One promising collaboration between the national and state levels is a joint agreement between two national organizations—the National Association of State Units on Aging (NASUA) and the National Council of State Agencies for the Blind (NCSAB). NASUA is a national membership organization of directors of the state units on aging; NCSAB is an organization of the directors of the state departments (or offices) of services for blind and visually impaired people. Each organization represents the entrance point of public federal funds allocated to each state to serve blind and visually impaired persons and to serve the elderly population.

Legislative initiatives and interagency and interorganizational agreements can be a positive force at federal and state levels. The critical need for collaboration is, however, at the local level, the heart of activity and services for older visually impaired persons. Nevertheless, it is also true that if model collaborative efforts take place at the local level without collaborative thinking and activity at the state or federal level, local agencies may lack supportive legislation and administration. (Chapter 15 describes collaborative efforts in more detail.)

In addition to collaboration, advocacy is a key force that needs to be brought to bear to affect the aging and blindness fields. Since the 1980s, consumers have been advocates for their own causes in often dramatic ways. Greater numbers of older, disabled, and visually impaired persons also need to become their own best advocates and instruments of empowerment.

Consumer groups of blind and visually impaired persons have emerged to lobby effectively at the federal, state, and local levels. Groups of blind persons also lend support to groups representing other disabilities, for example, the Coalition for Citizens with Disabilities. These consumer groups share an interest in policies that promote independence, self-reliance, and equality. Peer counseling and self-help groups are also avenues for older visually impaired persons to learn their rights and develop advocacy skills. Although blind consumers have become increasingly effective as advocates, older visually impaired persons have not yet established themselves as a strong advocacy voice.

Current and Future Needs

Never before have we known as much about the size of the older visually impaired population. Never before could we project the volume of its needs as effectively. Given the growth rates in the size of this population projected over 40 years, we face many demands and challenges and increased opportunities as well. In a sense, we can say that the year 2000 has arrived; the number of older blind and visually impaired persons projected for that year was realized in the 1980s (Nelson, 1987).

From a certain vantage point, challenges and opportunities are the same. Tackling some of the challenges creates opportunities for the individual now and for the next cohort of older visually impaired persons.

Today, older visually impaired persons have greater opportunities than ever before to live active and productive lives. Advancements in technology for blind persons offer the older person a large array of assistive devices to aid independent functioning.

With the overall goal of collaborative planning between the two service delivery systems as a key concern, this book is intended to be a practical resource for practitioners who teach, counsel, or provide programs for older persons who are blind or visually impaired or who have responsibility for planning such programs and services. Its contents progress from theory and knowledge base to practice. It can be read in its entirety, or selected chapters can be used to fill in gaps in information. For example, persons working in the field of aging might focus attention on the chapters on blindness, and vice versa.

The book has three primary sections. Section I, "Setting the Framework," examines the environment of the older visually impaired person—its physical, psychological, and social dimensions. Section II, "Service Delivery," describes the services available from both the blindness and the aging fields. It contains a general overview and historical perspective of each professional network and reviews how the networks function at the federal, state, and local levels. Section III, "Meeting the Challenge," focuses on new, innovative approaches to service delivery in the areas of self-help and advocacy and collaborative planning and service delivery. This section also touches on trends and issues that will affect the fields of aging and blindness in their collaborative efforts.

The authors of the chapters in these sections represent broad experience and expertise. They include gerontologists and rehabilitation specialists, academics and practitioners, national experts and state and community leaders. We hope that this book offers new knowledge to those who have just begun work with older visually impaired persons or who have been without an opportunity to develop a knowledge base. This volume will also serve as a resource for those responsible for planning and implementing programs and services and for creating innovative service delivery models to meet the growing and changing needs of America's visually impaired elderly population now and in the decades to come.

References

American Association of Retired Persons. (1990). *A profile of older Americans.* Washington, DC: Author.

Blake, R. (1984). What disables America's elderly? *Generations, 7*(4): 6-9.

Crews, J. E. (1988). No one left to push: The public policy of aging and blindness. *Educational Gerontology, 14*(1): 339-409.

Nelson, K. A. (1988). Visual impairment among elderly Americans: Statistics in transition. In C. Kirchner (Ed.), *Data on blindness and visual impairment in the U.S.* (2nd ed., pp. 53-61). New York: American Foundation for the Blind.

Nelson, K. A. (1991). *Projected increases in the prevalence of severe visual impairment among elderly Americans.* Unpublished paper.

Orr, A.L. (1990a). *Innovative models of service delivery for older blind and visually impaired persons.* Unpublished paper.

Orr, A. L. (1990b). *A training model to teach community outreach workers to train older blind and visually impaired American Indians independent living skills: Focus on family rehabilitation.* Final report to the Administration on Aging. (Grant No. 90AM0261).

Williams, T. F. (1986). The aging process: Biological and psychological considerations. In S. Brodey & G. Ruff (Eds.), *Aging and rehabilitation.* New York: Springer.

CHAPTER 2

Physiological Aspects of Aging

Robert B. Mitchell

More than ever before, scientists are dedicating their lives to understanding the basic biological process of aging. The field that deals with the process of aging is known as "gerontology." It should not be confused with "geriatrics," which is the branch of medicine that focuses on the pathologies of old age. Growing numbers of physicians, referred to as geriatricians, are specializing in the care of elderly people. It is an essential specialty in medicine because people are living longer and therefore experiencing physical conditions and dysfunctions associated with aging. This chapter addresses the physical changes that occur naturally throughout the aging process and helps those who work with older persons understand the physiological aspects of aging that interact with the psychological and social aspects of the aging process.

The Nature of Aging

Strictly speaking, aging can be defined as an organism's change with time. This definition suggests that human aging begins at the time of conception and progresses through a series of stages—the embryonic and fetal development, birth and neonatal phases, infancy, childhood, adolescence, adulthood, and old age. The term "senescence," although often used interchangeably with aging, specifically refers to that period of old age that is characteristic of the latter part of life. Although gerontologists recognize that embryogenesis, differentiation, and growth play important roles in what happens during adulthood and old age, aging is often thought of and described as a deteriorative process beginning after maturity and resulting in decreased viability and increased vulnerability. It is important also to bear in mind the individual nature of the aging process. We age in our own unique ways, throughout our bodies' systems. With aging, an organism or one of its parts loses its ability to adapt to its environment and thereby has a reduced capacity to withstand the stresses to which it is constantly subjected.

One of the many problems confronting gerontologists is to determine which changes are indeed the result of basic biological aging. Strehler (1977) suggested four criteria that any age-associated change should meet before it can be considered part of the basic aging process:

1. Universality. A true age-related change must occur in all members of a species. It rules out hereditary aberrations and diseases as aging processes because they occur in only a fraction of the population. It also rules out environmentally induced changes because they also occur in subpopulations.

2. Intrinsicality. A true age-related change is intrinsic to the organism. This criterion excludes changes caused by external factors. It is possible, for example, for a change to be universal, such as damage resulting from cosmic radiation, but not intrinsic. Therefore, such radiation-induced changes would not be true age-related changes.

3. Progressiveness. True age-related changes generally occur gradually over time and are steadily progressive and cumulative. In contrast, developmental processes are not steadily progressive; they slow down or stop at about the time of maturity.

4. Deleteriousness. Most age-related changes are deleterious to the organism. The basis of this criterion is that the most characteristic change accompanying aging is the decline in functional capacity and the increase in rate of morbidity and mortality. Therefore, most age-related changes contribute to the increased probability of death. This criterion eliminates many changes occurring during development as age-related changes because they are not deleterious and they improve survival capacity.

These four criteria, along with the concept of aging just described, provide the gerontologist with a general but arbitrary basic framework for discussing the aging process and studying the mechanisms governing its control.

One way to measure the process of aging in a population is to construct and examine mortality or survivorship curves. If death were a random event, then the mortality rate would be constant with time and the proportion of survivors would decrease steadily. However, in a population with mortality rate increasing as a result of aging processes, the curve would be more rectangular. In this case, individuals would die from causes that would not have killed them earlier, and the shape of the curve would depend, to a large extent, on the rate of aging. Life expectancy at birth, or the average life span, is the length of time that an individual is likely to live from the moment of birth. For white American males, life expectancy is currently about 72 years; for white American females, it is 79 years. Life expectancy is not to be confused with "maximum" life span, the age at which the last individual in the population dies. For white Americans, the maximum life span is believed to be about 115 years (U.S. Department of Commerce, Bureau of the Census, 1985).

Genetics plays a primary role in determining life span, but environmental factors are important, too. Factors such as population density, sanitation, nutrition, and health standards play a major role in determining life expectancy. Survival is greatest from ages 5 to 14 years. Resistance to microbial disease is highest and deaths from accidents and stress are lowest at these ages. After maturity, there follows a period of slowly rising mortality up to age 60. It is within this period that the probability of dying doubles about every eight years. Some deaths are the result of disease, some of accidents, and others of aging. Between the ages of 60 and 80, the death rate increases rapidly until almost everyone dies by the age of 100. Although many people in this period still die from disease, it is the basic aging process that establishes the fertile ground for disease (Comfort, 1979).

Some claim that the goal of gerontology is and should be to investigate intervention procedures that will eventually result in an extension of the maximum life span. Most gerontologists believe, however, that the primary goal of gerontology should be to discover what is involved in normal aging. On the basis of this knowledge, the objective should then be to prevent abnormal or premature aging. Only through the accomplishment of this goal will individuals have the choice of how to live out their genetically determined life span and perhaps the opportunity to extend their working, productive years and combine vigor with wisdom.

Physiology of Human Aging

Human aging is the progressive loss of the individual's physiological adaptability to the environment. This decline in physiological competence inevitably increases the occurrence and effects of environmental stress, accidents, and disease and thereby results in increased probability of death with time. It should be emphasized, however, that the rate or pace of individual aging is extremely variable. More important, because this rate depends on such factors as genetic inheritance, nutrition, physical activity, and the psychosocial living environment, the process can be influenced to some measure by human control.

Over the years, many gerontology research centers have been collecting data from longitudinal studies on humans that show changes in physiological function with age. In measuring postprime declines in physiological function, several generalities become apparent:

1. The decline in physiological function is a gradual, silent process. People are generally unaware of the slow deterioration in their bodies. Indeed, it is often difficult to measure physiological decline in less than a five-year period and nearly impossible to define exactly when a specific functional decline begins. One probable explanation for this gradual loss of function with age is that the human body is endowed with a generous reserve capacity and redundancy in body tissues and organs.

2. Different body organs and systems decline at different rates (Shock, 1983). Such parameters as nerve conduction velocity and basal metabolic rate decrease at a much slower rate than do kidney function and maximum breathing capacity. In general, the more complex the physiological function, the more rapidly the performance drops with age. In other words, functions such as maximum breathing capacity, which involve many nerve-to-nerve and nerve-to-muscle connections and depend on several organ systems,

deteriorate at a faster rate than do simple functions, such as impulse transmission along a single nerve. But regardless of the function being measured, physiological decline is generally linear. This means that, excluding disease and accidents, functional loss in most systems is not greater between ages 50 and 60 years than it is between ages 30 and 40 years.

3. The rate of physiological decline varies greatly among individuals. At any one age, say, 50, for any one function, individuals might have losses ranging from 5 to 50 percent. This variation again illustrates that different people age at different rates, and thus older people are much more different from each other than they are alike. The important point is that one's physiological or biological age, which is based on the percentage of functional loss in body systems, is usually different from chronological age and much more meaningful in assessing fitness and the rate of aging.

4. One age-associated change in body function that is critical is the loss of homeostatic capacity. "Homeostasis" is defined as the state of equilibrium in the body with respect to various functions and the chemical composition of fluids and tissues. Many homeostatic systems (reflected in blood ph, blood sugar level, body temperature, and pulse rate) change little with age as long as the body is at rest. However, if the older body is stressed, either physically or emotionally, there is a decreased capacity to respond to this stress and maintain equilibrium. Homeostatic parameters, such as body temperature, are thereby displaced to a greater degree and return more slowly to prestress levels (Timiras, 1988).

In a single chapter it is impossible to discuss adequately all the specific physiological changes that occur with age; the changes are so many and so varied. Also, it is difficult to separate those changes that are a result of normal aging from those that are tied to disease or to the environment. What follows is a brief review of some of the more apparent functional and structural changes that eventually occur with aging in the ten body systems. A basic knowledge of these changes will help service providers understand the physical capabilities of their clients. A more complete description of these changes is found in Schneider and Rowe (1990).

THE INTEGUMENT

One body system that is often overlooked in discussions about physiology, but rarely missed when thoughts turn to aging, is the integument. Age changes in skin and hair are usually the first noticed and are most often used as indicators of chronological age. Old skin generally is pale, has pigmentation spots, and is more wrinkled, less elastic, and drier than younger skin. The alterations in collagen and elastin, important fibrous proteins of connective tissue, account for many of these changes. Also, the loss of subcutaneous fat and a weakening of tiny blood vessels can result in black and blue spots. Exposure to the ultraviolet radiation of sunlight accelerates the rate of aging in skin. Although some baldness is genetic and androgen related, the loss of scalp hair and the graying of hair are common occurrences in middle and late life.

MUSCULAR SYSTEM

The skeletal muscular system mainly expresses its age changes by a decrease in size and strength. Muscle fibers are made up of postmitotic, nondividing cells, and with age there is an apparent loss in the number and size of these cells. Muscle weight generally decreases after age 50, with much of the mass being replaced by fat and connective tissue. Age-associated drops in potassium and in the basal metabolic rate parallel this decline in muscle mass. Strength appears to peak between 20 and 30 years and then to decline slowly. The decline is more pronounced if measured by the cranking of an ergometer than by a static isometric pull. This is probably a reflection of the changes that occur at myoneural junctions in addition to intrinsic alterations in cells. Some decline in the size and function of muscles is undoubtedly a consequence of disuse, but it cannot be the entire answer. Muscles of the hand, eye, and larynx also show age changes. Whatever the cause of change in muscle functioning, physical activity within the older person's limits is certainly recommended for maintaining the health and slowing the aging of muscles.

SKELETAL SYSTEM

The reduction in height and limited mobility that come with aging are primarily a result of changes in the skeletal system. With age, there is a gradual modification of bone tissue characterized by decreased density of bones and degenerative changes in ligaments, cartilage, and articulations. The loss of bone density can account for the frequent fractures in weight-bearing areas, such as the hip joint, as well as changes in height and the narrowing of the chest and shoulders. There may even be some thinning (collagen loss) or collapse of intervertebral discs to exacerbate the loss of height.

The changes in ligaments, cartilage, and articulations lead to the characteristic stiffened joints of aged persons. Osteoporosis, the accelerated thinning of bone seen particularly in postmenopausal women, is primarily a result of the loss of bone minerals. The cause of this loss is not known, although diet (low calcium intake) and hormone levels (the drop in estrogen following menopause) are suspected as contributing factors. It has been found that physical activity can retard the rate of bone loss in adults and even restore bone in older individuals who participate in planned activity (Marx, 1978).

CIRCULATORY SYSTEM

The aging of the circulatory system leads to cardiovascular diseases, which are the primary health problems in the United States. More people die from cardiovascular complications than from all other causes of death combined. There is no doubt that cardiovascular diseases are age dependent. The presence and severity of atherosclerosis, heart degeneration, cerebral hemorrhage, coronary thrombosis, and hypertension increase exponentially with age and result in a decrease in organ perfusion with age.

It is difficult to distinguish the normal aging process of the circulatory system from cardiovascular diseases because the two become closely intertwined. For example, "arteriosclerosis" is a general term that refers to a thickening and hardening of the arterial walls. "Atherosclerosis" is a specific kind of arteriosclerosis characterized by the accumulation of fat in the innermost layers (intima) of the arterial wall. These fatty accumulations, along with changes in connective tissue, form white, scarlike rough areas called atheromas, or plaques. Such damage to a vessel's wall can eventually lead to the obstruction of the vessel, the formation of internal blood clots (thrombi), or the rupture of the vessel's wall (aneurysm), which then causes a heart attack or stroke.

RESPIRATORY SYSTEM

The respiratory system has one main function: to exchange oxygen and carbon dioxide between blood and environmental air. The efficiency of that process is partly determined by the volume of functional lung tissue (alveoli). Although there is no change in total lung capacity with age, there is a decrease in vital capacity (total amount of air that can be moved in and out of the lungs) and an increase in residual volume (air still left in the lungs after maximal expiratory effort). Obesity and changes within the bones, muscles, and connective tissues of the chest wall, including the diaphragm, are partly responsible for these volume changes. There is also some disintegration of the fibrous network (elastin and collagen) within the lung itself, which probably accounts for the decreased lung elasticity associated with age.

EXCRETORY SYSTEM

Kidneys, the central part of the excretory system, are the key organs in clearing blood of metabolic wastes, maintaining balance of water and electrolytes, and controlling acid-base balance. With age, there is deterioration of overall kidney function, attributed mostly to vascular insufficiency (nephrosclerosis) within the tissue and to a general loss in the number and functional capacity of filtering units (nephrons). The result can be age-associated disruptions in blood chemistry, especially when an individual is stressed.

Few studies have looked specifically at age changes in the bladder and urethra, although frequent urination is a common problem in elderly people. In men, frequent urination is usually caused by enlargement of the prostate (a secondary sexual gland located around the base of the urethra); in women, infections of the urethra and the bladder are often responsible.

DIGESTIVE SYSTEM

The digestive system, particularly the digestive tract, shows less dramatic changes than do other systems in the body, perhaps because the cellular turnover rate is so high in the gastrointestinal tract. Many digestive problems of older people are more nutritional than physiological. Most people experience dentition problems as they grow older, as well as more periodontal disease. Along with a decline in the senses of smell and taste, there is often an alteration of dietary patterns. Some changes that have been reported for the aging digestive tract are decreased acid secretion in the stomach, decreased motility in the stomach and intestines, and possible decreased calcium absorption. The decreased acidity of the stomach can interfere with specific enzyme activity and hence with the digestion of proteins. It is also possible that age-related changes in the stomach lining may be responsible for decreased vitamin B_{12} absorption, which can lead to anemia.

The decreased motility, or peristalsis, of the digestive tract simply means that digestion and absorption usually take longer, but it can also mean that constipation might result. If there is an age-associated decrease in calcium absorption, it could lead to a calcium imbalance and to the bone loss that is seen with aging. Another part of the digestive system, the liver, has received considerable attention in studies of aging and has been shown to function well into old age. There is a slight drop in blood flow through the liver of the aged individual and also fluctuations in enzyme activity and the response of enzymes to stimuli, but the tremendous reserve and regenerative capacity of a nondiseased liver preclude hypofunction.

REPRODUCTIVE SYSTEM

The effects of age on the reproductive system are of special interest to most people, not only because of the anatomical and physiological changes that result in the cessation of the reproductive function but also because of the concomitant psychological changes that influence self-image. In women, menopause, which occurs in middle age, is the cessation of the menstrual cycle, and it marks the end of the childbearing years. During and following menopause, the ovaries become inactive, the monthly follicular development eventually ceases, and estrogen and progesterone synthesis decreases. The mechanisms responsible for this ovarian shutdown are still a mystery. It is suspected that there is intrinsic aging within the ovary itself, but there is evidence that changes in the hypothalamus and pituitary alter the proportions of gonadotropin available for stimulating the ovary. With the drop in the levels of circulating estrogen and progesterone, there is a gradual atrophy of ovarian, uterine, and vaginal tissue and a decreased level of vaginal lubrication. Although estrogen-replacement therapy has, in some cases, been prescribed to alleviate some of these postmenopausal degenerative changes, it must be used with caution. Prolonged estrogen administration might increase the risk of some cancers.

In men, there is no set time of reproductive change such as menopause, but there are gradual changes in the structure and function of reproductive organs. Between ages 50 and 90, there is a slow decline in circulating levels of testosterone accompanied by a rise in the levels of gonadotropin. In contrast to the cells of the ovaries, the germ cells in the testes are constantly replenished, even in old age. However, the rate of spermatogenesis, as well as the number of viable sperm, declines in older men. The secondary sexual organs that are responsible for the production of semen also deteriorate, and the volume and viscosity of seminal fluid decrease. Particularly affected is the prostate gland, which after age 40 begins to show degenerative changes in the secretory glandular epithelium and a replacement of the muscle stroma with dense collagen. Also, the gland generally increases in size and becomes a frequent site of cancer in elderly men.

ENDOCRINE SYSTEM

It has long been known that hormones from the endocrine system play an important role early in life in differentiation and development, and so it is not surprising that many studies of aging have focused on endocrine glands and their hormones. Generalizing about endocrine changes with aging is complicated; the effects of aging can occur at many sites. The glands themselves may change in their responsiveness to stimuli, hormone production may be altered, the hormone clearance rate may change, and hormone action at target cells may decrease.

The master gland, the pituitary, shows histological changes, such as decreased vascularity, increased connective tissue, and a change in the distribution of types of cells. However, it does continue to secrete normal levels of growth, thyroid-stimulating, and adrenocorticotropic hormones. The posterior pituitary also secretes normal levels of antidiuretic hormone in aged persons, but the kidneys of older individuals respond at a lower rate than do those of younger people.

Thyroid function remains adequate into old age. Thyroids in elderly persons respond well to the thyroid-stimulating hormone (TSH) from the pituitary gland. There are some reports of decreased circulating levels of thyroid hormones with aging; such a change could be expected with concomitant age-related decrease in body mass.

One function of the pancreas is to release insulin in response to a blood glucose load, thereby lowering blood sugar levels. As early as the fifth decade, there is a reduction of glucose tolerance; when glucose is ingested by an older person, the blood sugar level increases to a higher point and takes longer to return to normal than it does in a younger person. According to Andres and Tobin (1975), the reason is the decreased sensitivity of beta cells in the aged pancreas to a given level of blood sugar. However, another possibility could be that less of the insulin secreted by the aged individual is biologically active. Also, it is possible that the peripheral utilization of insulin might change with age. Regardless of cause, this decline in glucose tolerance is likely related to the age-dependent increase in maturity-onset diabetes.

The adrenal cortex shows little change in the production of glucocorticoid and aldosterone with age. However, there is a significant decrease in adrenal androgens. One androgenic steroid, dehydroepiandrosterone, which decreases with aging, may protect against obesity and even cancer (Schwartz, Hard, Pashko, Abou-Gharbia, & Swerm, 1981). Adelman (1979) stated that hormones lose some of their effects (such as enzyme induction) on target tissues with age. In studies of rats, he showed that the initiation time for enzyme induction after hormone stimulation increases in direct proportion to the age of the animal. Even when the older animal is capable of producing as much enzyme as the younger, it takes longer to do so. The mechanisms of such impairment in adaptive response are not yet known, but they may affect the amount or quality of a hormone that is available for initiating response and hormone-hormone interactions and may alter the binding potential at the receptor site between the hormone and the target cell.

The thymus, now considered an endocrine gland, has long been a puzzle to biologists. Because it begins to involute and atrophy at about the time of maturity, many thought it was a vestigial organ like the appendix. However, it is now known that this small gland, located behind the breastbone, is a key organ in the development and probably in the aging of the body's immune system. Lymphocytes—the agents of the immune system—come in two varieties: T-cells, which are thymus derived and act as killer cells, and B-cells, which are bone marrow derived and produce antibodies. T-cells also play a role as regulators of B-cell activity. Soon after birth, the body's immune system goes through a mysterious process; it "learns" to recognize self from nonself. It is then the job of the T- and B-cells to attack invading organisms or antigens (foreign proteins). However, with aging, two phenomena occur. First, the protective efficiency of the system declines; second, autoimmune responses in the system increase (Walford, 1969). Autoimmunity refers to the destruction by the immune system of the body's own tissues.

NERVOUS SYSTEM

The nervous system, like the muscular system, is unique. Its cells (neurons) do not divide. One is born with all the nerve cells one will ever have, which means that the nerve cells remaining when you die are the same age as you are. It is generally reported that the weight of the brain decreases about 6 to 7 percent between the ages of 25 and 75 years. However, because of the inconsistency of sampling methods, the presence of disease in some individuals, and cohort-related problems, these figures are questionable. It is generally agreed that there is cell loss in the cerebral and cerebellar cortexes, but there are great differences between individuals and between different cortical areas, in addition to varying rates of loss during different periods of life. The hypothalamus and areas of the brain stem are conservative; there is no detectable loss of nerve cells. Glial cells, the small supportive elements of the brain, are reported to increase with age, which may be a compensatory response to the neuronal loss. In addition to changes in cell numbers, a loss of extracellular space in the brain has been reported.

Such structural degeneration, if widespread, could interfere with cognitive ability, memory, learning, creativity, and the control of sensory input and motor function. Information in this area is lacking, although there is at present a surge of interest in the activity of neurotransmitters in the aging brain and in how neurotransmitters may affect brain function and behavior. Some reports show the loss of monoamines with age in specific regions of the brain, accompanied by an increase in monoamine oxidase activity. This might be expected because this enzyme is involved in the degradation of monoamines. Finch (1973) found that in aged mice, norepinephrine turnover is slowed in some brain regions (such as the hypothalamus) and that dopamine content is decreased in other regions. The loss of dopamine in the basal ganglia of human brains causes Parkinson's disease. Alzheimer's disease, another age-related neuropathology, is now linked with a significant decrease in choline acetyltransferase, particularly in certain regions of the brain.

Perhaps the most significant neurological alteration concerning physiological efficiency later in life is the nervous system's overall loss of speed in receiving, processing, and sending signals. This loss of speed is apparent in its simplest form in the slight (about 10 percent) loss of nerve conduction velocity between ages 30 and 75. There is also a demonstrable loss in reflex and reaction times with age; the latter loss is greater because of the larger number of neuron-synapse-neuron connections. In general, elderly people have slower performance times on sensorimotor skills, which undoubtedly is related to their perceptual ability and response time. The specific causes of this general slowing down of the central nervous system are unknown, but they may be related to the decreased number of nerve cells, the loss of conduction velocity, the increased threshold of sensory receptors, physical-chemical changes at synapses or myoneural junctions, weakened excitation potentials, or the gradual failure of integrating ability at the higher brain centers. It also has been suggested that changes in neuronal function might be secondary to arteriosclerotic problems, which can lead to a decreased flow of blood to the brain.

Like other organs of the body, the eyes undergo progressive degenerative changes with age. Some of these age-related changes are intrinsic to tissues in the eye, and others are secondary to changes in other organ systems. Also, some changes are the results of accidents, whereas others are disease processes rather than results of aging. Regardless of cause, the effect of these deleterious changes in the structure and function of the eye is usually some degree of visual impairment. The physiological and functional aspects of vision are discussed in Chapter 3.

References

Adelman, R. C. (1979). Loss of adaptive mechanisms during aging. *Federation Proceedings, 38:* 1968-1971.

Andres, R., & Tobin, J. D. (1975). Aging and the disposition of glucose. *Advances in Experimental Medicine and Biology, 61:* 239.

Comfort, A. (1979). *The biology of senescence* (3rd ed.). New York: Elsevier North-Holland.

Finch, C. E. (1973). Catecholamine metabolism in the brains of aging, male mice. *Brain Research, 52:* 261-276.

Marx, J. L. (1978) Osteoporosis: New help for thinning bones. *Science, 207:* 628-630.

Schneider, E. L., & Rowe, J. W. (1990). *Handbook of the biology of aging.* New York: Academic Press.

Schwartz, A. G., Hard, G. C., Pashko, L. L., Abou-Gharbia, M., & Swerm, D. (1981). Dehydroepiandrosterone: An anti-obesity and anti-carcinogenic agent. *Nutrition and Cancer, 3*(1): 46-53.

Shock, N. W. (1983). Aging of physiological systems. *Journal of Chronic Diseases, 36:* 137-142.

Strehler, B. L. (1977). *Time, cells and aging* (2nd ed.). New York: Academic Press.

Timiras, P. S. (1988). *Physiological basis of aging and geriatrics.* New York: Macmillan.

U.S. Department of Commerce, Bureau of the Census. (1985). *1985 U.S. Census.* Washington, DC: Author.

Walford, R. L. (1969). *The immunological theory of aging.* Copenhagen: Munksgaard.

CHAPTER 3

Physiological and Functional Aspects of Aging, Vision, and Visual Impairment

Alfred A. Rosenbloom

Approximately 11.4 million people in the United States have some kind of visual impairment (Kirchner, 1988). This figure encompasses all people who have trouble seeing, including those who wear corrective lenses. Of these 11.4 million, about 3.1 million are severely visually impaired: Their impairment interferes with normal living. They cannot, for example, read newsprint. Out of this group, about 600,000 are registered as legally blind. In the age distribution of individuals who have severe visual impairment, about 70 percent (nearly 3 million visually impaired people) are age 65 and over; about 25 percent are 18 to 64 years old; and only about 5 percent are under age 18. That 70 percent of severe visual impairment occurs in people over age 65, even though this age group makes up only 12 percent of the total United States population, indicates that most eye problems are age related.

Visual impairment can be linked to basic aging processes, age-related diseases that indirectly affect vision, and the greater probability of accidents as people live longer. In addition to age, it is noteworthy that for the 65-and-over age group, more women are affected than are men. Low income and additional physical and sensory impairments, such as deafness, learning disability, and paralysis, are also often

The author greatly acknowledges the contribution of Dr. Robert B. Mitchell, Department of Biology, Pennsylvania State University, for his authorship of the material on the nature and physiology of aging appearing through page 53 of this chapter.

present in the older person experiencing visual impairment (Birren & Williams, 1982).

Visual impairment is quantified in terms of acuity and visual field. "Acuity" refers to the amount of detail a person sees compared to normal vision. For example, a person with 20/20 vision in an eye has normal vision, whereas a person with 20/70 has low vision. It means that the individual with 20/70 acuity must be at 20 feet to see what a person with normal vision sees at 70 feet. The larger the second number in the scale, the poorer the vision. A person with 20/200 vision in the better eye with the best possible correction is considered legally blind. "Visual field" describes the area that an eye can see and is measured, as an angle, in degrees. A person with normal vision who is looking straight ahead will be able to see all objects in a half-circle, 180-degree range. A person is considered to have low vision if he or she can see only a 20-degree field or less in the better eye. A deficit in visual field may result in either central or peripheral vision loss.

Physiology of Vision

Figure 1 is a diagram of the eye. As one ages, a number of normal and expected degenerative changes can be observed in the structure and, therefore, the function of the eye (Kasper, 1983). The transparent cornea, through which light rays enter the eye, tends to flatten, and often the corneal epithelium degenerates. Both changes can impair vision, the former through astigmatism and the latter through severe discomfort. Like many other tissues, the sclera, visible as the white of the eye, becomes less elastic with age and turns more yellow because of the accumulation of fat. The ciliary body, a circle of muscle tissue directly behind the iris, the colored part of the eye, thickens, and, also like other tissues during aging, its processes become hyalinized. Because of thickening and sclerosis of the trabecular meshwork in the angle of the eye's anterior chamber, there can be some obstruction in the canal of Schlemm, which drains aqueous fluid from the eye. Fortunately, a concomitant decrease in the production of aqueous fluid seems to take place, so that intraocular pressure is not normally elevated. Hyaline or colloid bodies develop in the layer of blood vessels known as the choroid and show up as rounded, yellowish spots in the retina, the special tissue containing the specialized nerve cells called rods and cones that respond to light.

During aging, the blood vessels of the choroid are usually narrowed and sclerotic. Similar vascular changes, believed to be a result of fibrosis of the vessel wall, also occur in the retina. With age, some loss of retinal photoreceptor cells, particularly rods in the peripheral region and cones in the fovea, the part of the eye that responds to the finest detail, can reduce the size of the visual field and adversely affect acuity.

The crystalline lens of the eye continues to grow with age and enlarges, becomes stiffer, and tends to turn yellow. The result is increased opacity of the lens, possibly increased intraocular pressure, and decreased focusing ability or accommodation, especially when viewing nearby objects. The speed of accommodation is also slower. This age-related loss of accommodation for close vision is called "presbyopia" and starts in most people during their forties. Fortunately, this condition is readily corrected with reading glasses or bifocals.

In addition to increased opacity of the lens with aging, the iris becomes more rigid and the diameter of the pupil, the aperture at its center, is lessened. The combined result is that less light gets to the photoreceptor cells of the retina. Because of cone sensitivity, the ability to adapt to a dark environment after being in a light environment, and

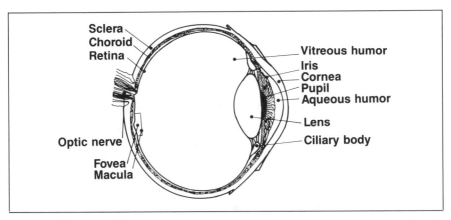

Figure 1: Diagram of the eye. Source: *Visual Impairment: An Overview.* New York: American Foundation for the Blind, 1990.

vice versa, is also impaired in elderly people. Overall, then, older people tend to need more intense light to see as well as they once did.

The vitreous body is normally transparent and semigelatinous, consisting mainly of water with some salt and albumin. In advanced years, this body loses hydration and sometimes detaches from its connections to the retina, a situation that can eventually lead to a more serious retinal detachment from the choroid. An additional complication can be hemorrhaging of retinal blood vessels into the vitreous. Another common occurrence with vitreal degeneration is the appearance of opacities in the vitreous that take on the shape of dots, lines, or cobwebs and are referred to as "floaters." Although annoying to the individual, the presence of floaters is normal and not a serious health concern. Problems with color vision, particularly difficulties in matching blues and greens, are sometimes a consequence of changes in the vitreous, lens, and aqueous humor that accompany aging.

The eyelids also undergo age-related changes that can impair vision. As a result of decreased elasticity, the loss of muscle tone, and less orbital fat, lids can droop or turn inward or outward. In addition to interfering with vision, these conditions can result in eyelashes' contact with the conjunctiva, the membrane over the surface of the eye, or too much of the conjunctiva's being exposed and becoming inflamed. Minor cosmetic surgery on the eyelids can usually correct these problems.

Dry eye is another age-related complication associated with the lacrimal apparatus. As the name implies, dry eye is a condition resulting from a decrease in the secretion of tears from the lacrimal glands and is seen more often in elderly women than in elderly men. The result can be discomfort and possible inflammation. The usual treatment, hourly administration of artificial tears, is not always a satisfactory solution to the condition.

Eye Diseases Associated with Aging

The four eye diseases or conditions that are the primary causes of visual impairment in elderly people are cataracts, diabetic retinopathy, glaucoma, and age-related macular degeneration. It is not unusual for older people to suffer from more than one of these conditions, either consecutively or simultaneously.

CATARACTS

Cataract is defined as a painless, progressive clouding of the lens of the eye. The condition usually develops in only one eye at a time, and the degree of impairment can vary greatly among individuals. Fortunately, most people are not affected to the point of significant visual disability.

It is not known how cataracts are formed. Basically, the opacity is caused by some change in the internal structure of the lens, as if lens fibers coagulate and lens protein becomes insoluble and opaque. Also, water may accumulate between the lens fibers. If the opacity progresses and the lens becomes opaque, it is referred to as a "mature" cataract. At this stage, vision is lost, and the individual cannot see much more than light and dark. In uncommon circumstances, the lens may swell in mature cataracts and result in increased intraocular pressure or may even begin to disintegrate and liquify.

The treatment for cataracts is removal of the lens. Today it is a safe surgical procedure that can be performed under local or general anesthesia. The usual procedure, performed by an ophthalmologist, includes removing the clouded lens and, in most cases, replacing it with an intraocular implant, or artificial lens. Better vision results in 98 percent of all patients, and the complication rate is low. For those who do not receive intraocular implants, corrective eyeglasses or contact lenses are required.

DIABETIC RETINOPATHY

Diabetic retinopathy is almost always a condition affecting both eyes and appearing, to some degree, in most people who have had diabetes mellitus for at least 15 years. Longstanding diabetes may cause vascular changes that affect the small blood vessels supplying the retina and other ocular structures. Because diabetes is better controlled today and patients live longer, there is an increased frequency of diabetic retinopathy among individuals with diabetes. However, following prescribed regimens carefully, particularly in regard to dieting and exercising, seems to lessen the severity of retinal damage.

In retinopathy, the actual retinal pathology is seen as micro-aneurysms, or small hemorrhages, and yellow-white exudates. Abnormal new vessels that are also formed leak fluid and distort vision. Although there is no cure for the retinopathy, drugs are used to remove exudates, and photocoagulation by means of laser surgery helps to close new and leaky blood vessels.

GLAUCOMA

Glaucoma, another serious eye ailment in elderly people, is a condition in which loss of the visual field and damage to the optic nerve result from elevated intraocular pressure. The watery fluid between the cornea and the lens of the eye, the aqueous humor, is formed in the posterior chamber behind the iris and then circulates through the pupil into the anterior chamber. Here it is drained through the canal of Schlemm at the angle between the rim of the iris and the back of the cornea. The balance between the secretion and the outflow of this fluid, which nourishes the cornea and the lens, determines intraocular pressure. An increase in pressure can compress the blood vessels within the eyeball and thereby deprive the retina of an adequate blood supply, resulting in impaired vision and even blindness.

The most common form of primary glaucoma, affecting about 1 percent of people over age 40, is referred to as chronic, simple (open-angle) glaucoma. The condition is generally symptomless to the individual until late in its course; however, infrequently, blurred vision, not correctable with lenses, or complaints of a halo effect around lights, may be the first sign of a problem. Therefore, the routine measurement of intraocular pressure every 1 to 2 years after age 35 is recommended for everyone, but especially for people with a family history of glaucoma. In this open-angle form of glaucoma, the anterior chamber angle, where fluid is absorbed and drained, is open, but the outflow of fluid through the trabecular meshwork is blocked.

Treatment for open-angle glaucoma usually involves medication to lower intraocular pressure. Pressure generally can be reduced by increasing aqueous outflow with miotics, causing the pupil of the eye to contract, or by decreasing aqueous formation with carbonic anhydrase inhibitors or beta blocking agents. If this treatment fails, a drainage pathway through the trabecular meshwork can be created with laser surgery or by conventional glaucoma surgical techniques.

The second, less common, form of primary glaucoma is closed-angle glaucoma. As the name implies, this condition is the result of intermittent contact of the iris and the inner surface of the trabecular meshwork that obstructs the outflow of aqueous fluid. The result is an acute crisis in which the pressure within the eyeball rises suddenly. The attack, usually occurring when the pupil is dilated in response to darkness, is accompanied by pain around the eye, headache, nausea, and vomiting. Immediate treatment with appropriate medication given within hours is necessary to relieve the pressure. Once the eye is stabilized, surgery is often performed to correct the reduced angle and to restore the free flow of aqueous fluid within the eye chamber.

MACULAR DEGENERATION

Age-related macular degeneration can occur at any age but is most common in elderly people. The symptoms are a progressive loss of reading vision and of sharp distance vision, usually in both eyes. The macula is at the center of the fovea centralis, the most sensitive spot for visual acuity within the retina. Because this area of the retina degenerates in this disease, central vision is eventually lost, even though peripheral, or side, vision is maintained. Although the cause of this degeneration is unknown, the process is believed to be associated with a sclerosis of the choroidal blood vessels that supply nutrients to the macula area. Treatment for the condition has not yet proved remarkably successful, although laser coagulation treatment in selected cases (approximately 13 percent of the cases) may slow or stabilize the progress of the disease if it is started soon enough. Low vision devices, such as magnifying glasses and telescopes, may be helpful.

Functional Aspects of Vision

The term "visual impairment" is often based on the definitions of legal blindness—20/200 vision in the better eye with the best possible correction or a visual field constricted to a diameter of no greater than 20 degrees—which has been used since 1935 to determine people's eligibility for a variety of governmental and private services for visually impaired persons. The recent literature has suggested that functional vision assessments, rather than isolated clinical measurements of distance vision, provide more relevant information about an individual's ability to use vision in daily life. Actually, no strong relationships have yet been found to exist between visual functioning and clinical measurements of ocular health (Faye, 1984). In the past decade, the term "low vision" has been used to describe persons who are neither totally blind nor fully sighted and who may or may not meet the clinical criteria for legal blindness but whose vision cannot be corrected to normal by regular eyeglasses or contact lenses.

According to the World Health Organization (WHO) (1981), "blindness" can be broadly defined as the absence of vision or significantly usable vision; "low vision," although imposing a visual impairment, involves at least some residual vision. This approach is superior to the traditional one, which relies only on measurements of visual acuity and restrictions in the visual field as quantitative determinants of the loss of vision. The various definitions of visual impairments are, of necessity, broad and nonspecific. What represents significantly usable vision depends not only on visual functions that might be measured clinically but also in large measure on the individual's abilities and circumstances.

Because reading is such a valued leisure activity for a great number of elderly persons, many older people are unwilling to accept visual impairment as a natural consequence of age. They are demanding more attention from their health care professionals to make the best use of their remaining vision for reading. It is important for those who are involved in planning services and caring for elderly persons to understand the implications of visual impairment for an individual's functioning. Four aspects of the problem are considered in the remainder of this discussion:

1. the incidence and consequences of visual impairment among elderly people,

2. changes in visual functioning in elderly people,
3. adaptation to visual impairment, and
4. implications for professionals working with elderly visually impaired persons.

Incidence and Consequences of Visual Impairment

Demographic aging is a phenomenon of the 20th century. In 1900, 3.1 million people in the United States were age 65 and over, making up about 4.1 percent of the population. By 1980, more than 23 million people were age 65 and over, representing 11 percent of the population. Today, 31 million are in the 65-and-over age group, and it is estimated that, by 2030, 66 million people will be in this age category (American Association of Retired Persons, 1990; U.S. Department of Health and Human Services, Office of Human Development Services, 1980).

Given the universality of aging and the increasing number of older persons in society, the causes and consequences of visual changes that accompany age assume greater significance. The decline and selected severe deterioration of vision occurs with age, and virtually all persons must adjust to some reduction in visual function as they age. The impact of visual impairment is often felt more keenly because of other problems associated with aging, such as physical and psychological changes, economic limitations, loss of social independence, and altered roles in the family, the workplace, and the community.

Research has documented the prevalence of multiply impaired persons and found increases in chronic health conditions, such as hearing loss, arthritis, high blood pressure, heart conditions, and orthopedic impairment, among elderly blind persons (Kirchner & Peterson, 1988; Kirchner & Phillips, 1988). These impairments are only part of the difficulties visually impaired elderly people cope with on psychological and physical levels. The difficulties handling problems commonly associated with the aging process include separation from family members, the loss of a spouse, withdrawal from earlier life roles, retirement, a decrease in overall income, and the loss of family and friends. The onset of vision loss exacerbates the other problems associated with attempts to maintain an independent life-style.

Many visually impaired elderly people become separated from the traditional social and financial support mechanisms of society. Data from a recent study conducted by the Michigan Commission for the Blind indicate that the majority who participated in an independent living program for elderly people were women (average age, 76 years), two-thirds of whom were widows who had additional chronic health conditions at rates higher than the general aging population (Crews, 1988).

Individual adaptations to changes in visual functioning are affected by the nature and extent of the vision loss, whether it is stable or progressive, and the presence of other problems influencing the person's ability to cope with the demands of daily living. Barraga (1976) distinguished between the reorganization of visual perceptual impressions and the learning process in visual perceptual development.

When a person has had "normal" visual abilities earlier in life and has lost visual function in later years, the adaptation involves a reorganization of cognition based on unclear, distorted, or limited visual input. Such a person must rely on earlier visual memories to attend to forms and outlines of objects that involve more limited visual cues. The more a person concentrates, associates with visual memory, and continues to move through and maintain contact with familiar objects and environments, the more efficient his or her perceptual reorganization will be.

The person who is motivated to continue functioning visually and who is encouraged to use residual vision maximally will accomplish the necessary perceptual reorganization more rapidly. Barraga (1976) noted that the person who continues to read, even with difficulty or quite slowly; continues to write for his or her own use and for others; and continues to watch television with the expectation of being able to interpret what he or she sees will continue to do these activities with greater efficiency. Low vision devices, combined with rehabilitation that involves adaptive training and related services within a multidisciplinary framework, obviously maximize a person's ability to utilize residual vision.

When a person has had a visual impairment from birth or from early years, his or her visual perceptual development is different. The extent to which visual memories are used to reinforce environmental cues determines the level of adaptation to the visual demands of daily life.

Each visually impaired person is unique. Therefore, few generalizations can be made about functional capabilities in traveling or other activities or about the quality of perceptual development or reorganization in elderly visually impaired people. The more important variables that determine the effective use of residual vision are (1) motivation to use vision as the primary source of learning, (2) intelligence and cognitive ability, (3) personality, attitudes, and self-concept, (4) age at onset of the visual impairment and the nature and effects of the ocular disease or defect, (5) past experiences, vocation, and avocation, and (6) family structure, needs, support, and attitudes (Barraga, 1976).

Changes in Visual Functioning

Age-related sensory and perceptual changes can greatly influence the older person's life and his or her ability to interact with the environment. Changes in vision may isolate the individual and lead to complex psychological reactions, such as depression, apathy, and social isolation. (See Chapter 5 for a more complete discussion of the psychological aspects of aging and visual impairment.)

As noted earlier in this chapter, with increased age come ocular changes, such as a decrease in the size of the pupil, refractive changes involving increases in hyperopia (farsightedness), changes in astigmatism, the loss of lens transparency, and increased thickening of the lens and its capsule. The consequence of these ocular changes is a reduction in the amount of light that reaches the retina, which reduces the person's apparent absolute sensitivity to light. Partial compensation for this elevated visual threshold may be achieved by increased illumination.

The evaluation of visual functioning in elderly persons depends, in part, on the design and instrumentation of tests. For example, the clinical assessment of a person's visual acuity usually involves the use of the Snellen eye chart. This test determines only a person's ability to discriminate fine detail (high spatial frequency) at a maximum level of contrast involving black letters on a white background. It is also important to measure such contrast sensitivity among older persons. This type of test is a subjective measure of the older persons's ability to discern objects and fine detail under reduced-contrast or low-contrast conditions.

OPTICAL VERSUS NEURAL FUNCTIONS

Many of the "normal" changes in vision that come with aging exacerbate the impairment created by ocular disease that affects vision (Rosenbloom, 1986). Therefore, a fuller understanding of the nature of visual impairment requires a differentiation between optical and neural functions. For example, a person with an optically induced vision loss caused by irregularities in the eye's refractive surfaces or ocular media, the transparent substance through which light passes prior to stimulation of the retina, can be expected to suffer reduced visual acuity and decreased contrast sensitivity caused by excessive intraocular scatter. Such a person experiences greater difficulty in seeing fine details and large objects of low contrast. In some patients with optically based losses of vision, visual acuity may remain virtually unaffected while contrast sensitivity is diminished. This situation can lead to impaired visually guided mobility. Cunningham and Johnson (1980) found that the detection of low-contrast objects, such as steps and pavements, is critical to the mobility of pedestrians. Marron and Bailey (1982) showed that the loss of contrast sensitivity and of visual field contributed almost equally to impaired mobility from decreased vision and that visual acuity is a relatively poor predictor of one's ability to be mobile.

Vision losses from disorders of the neural pathways typically produce defects in the visual field that may or may not be accompanied by a decrease in visual acuity. Central field losses affect a large number of visually impaired elderly people and are often associated with metamorphopsia (a condition in which objects appear distorted or misshapen), poor tolerance to variations in luminance, dependence on high levels of luminance, reduced contrast sensitivity, and poor mobility even though the peripheral visual field may be intact. The size and extent of scotomas (blind areas) limit retinal sensitivity because only objects of sufficient size, illumination, or contrast will be recognized within these areas. In cases in which scotomas are numerous, the correct localization and evaluation of visual information may become so difficult that some persons, despite relatively good visual acuity, are unable to read even with the use of magnification.

Although not as common as central field losses, peripheral field losses are important. Mobility skills and the ability to orient oneself are hindered by such defects. Furthermore, ocular changes reduce an elderly person's ability to adapt appropriately when going from bright to dark surroundings. Poor adaptation to the dark leads to problems in walking or driving at night that can be compounded by a defective sense of balance. Adaptation difficulties can be minimized in the domestic environment by ensuring that there is adequate artificial and natural lighting and that hazards, such as loose banisters, worn steps, torn linoleum, loose rugs, and highly polished floors, are avoided or eliminated.

Various physiological changes in the body also affect visual functioning. The wasting and weakness of skeletal muscles influence not only ocular mobility but also the general patterns of body movement and mobility. Concurrently, the reduced speed with which nerve impulses can influence the power of muscles and balance results in decreased neuromuscular performance. (See Chapter 2 for a more complete discussion of the physiological aspects of aging.)

DEPTH PERCEPTION

Another important aspect of human vision is depth perception. The localization of objects in the visual field can be made using cues of relative size, gradients in texture, the overlay of near or far objects, motion parallax, light, and shadows. Binocular information concerning the position of the observer depends on the binocular cues of convergence, retinal disparity, and cortical integration and interpretation. Age differences in stereopsis, or the ability to perceive depth or the relative position of objects in space, can be attributed to physical and functional changes in the eye, such as accommodation, convergence, transmissiveness of the lens, scatter of light, and sensitivity to glare. A loss of depth perception is probably a function of visual impairment, not of age. In general, it is difficult to determine whether age per se or visual impairment causes various decrements in visual performance.

LUMINANCE

Because of increased intraocular scatter, the absorption of light by the ocular media (the transparent substance of the eye through which light passes prior to stimulation of the retina), and a reduction in the size of the pupil with age, older people need higher than normal luminance levels to function efficiently. However, changes in the media may limit the degree to which increasing illumination can improve visual acuity. Light scatter in the eye also produces glare, a veil-like distribution of light superimposed on the retinal image that degrades and reduces the brightness of objects in the visual field. A typical 60-year-old person requires approximately twice as much illumination as does a 20-year-old to achieve the same level of visibility. By age 80, a person may need three or four times as much luminance as does a 20-year-old. However, the increased glare that results from such levels of light may, in turn, reduce both visual clarity and comfort.

These various changes in visual functioning have important implications for health professionals who provide counseling to newly visually impaired persons. If an older individual's environment includes poorly designed light fixtures and inappropriate distribution of light, glare and inadequate lighting may cause edges to become less distinct and boundaries of objects to blur. The depth of steps may also be difficult to judge. Moreover, glare from shiny surfaces, such as linoleum and glossy paint, will cause more trouble, as it does when originating from the light from oncoming cars at night. The need for higher levels of illumination that are properly controlled and directed has been well established but frequently overlooked. Lovie-Kitchin and Bowman (1985) and Merz (1982) described the role of the optometrist in the assessment of the response of older persons to levels of illuminance and the appropriate standards for domestic lighting requirements. Cullinin (1978) identified the effects of poor lighting control on elderly visually impaired people. He found that among those surveyed who had recently been seen at a specialist's clinic, over 60 percent apparently had poorer vision at home than they did at the time of examination. Thus, it is obvious that poor lighting in the home is a prevalent problem that can dramatically inhibit visual functioning.

Research has consistently reported a differential loss of discrimination for the colors of short wavelengths, such as green, blue, and violet, in elderly persons. For older persons, colors often appear faded. Warmer colors, such as reds and oranges, may seem less faded than do the cooler blues and greens. It seems likely that the age-related impairments in the discrimination of blue and green are associated, in part, with changes in the mechanisms of the eye and with a loss of the photoreceptors of the retina. Thus, increasing the saturation of colors may help elderly people distinguish colors (Ordy & Brizzee, 1979). The use of saturation of colors in the environment can be particularly helpful to an older visually impaired person. Rehabilitation teachers who go into the homes of elderly clients can be helpful in identifying the need for environmental modifications to minimize hazards caused by inappropriate lighting and glare and the use of inadequately contrasting colors.

THE COMPLEXITY OF THE VISUAL PROCESS

Various studies have shown that with advancing years, the visual perception of more complex patterns or configurations alters significantly (Ordy & Brizzee, 1979). Because the term "visual perception" refers not only to complex visual discriminatory tasks but also to specific visual recognition and visual learning and memory, the extent to which the reported age difference in visual perception is the result of vision, cognitive ability, personality, or even changes in psychosocial relations is not clear.

Although the role of the central nervous system in the decline of visual performance with age is not fully understood, decreased visual functioning cannot be adequately explained on the basis of morphological and physiological changes. The complexity of the visual process in its normal and impaired states has been graphically illustrated by Corn (1983). Her model organizes various interrelated factors into a pliable, three-dimensional structure composed of visual abilities, available resources, and past experiences and environmental cues (see Figure 2). Corn (1983) suggested that this model provides "a systematic approach to locating components that compensate for minimal or reduced visual abilities, allows choices for the use of environmental cues, and contributes to an understanding of how individuals with low vision function visually" (p. 376).

An elderly person's adaptations to the effects of visual impairment are highly individualized. Some decline in visual performance in later years is present in many functions. Figure 3 identifies many of the visual perceptual abilities that are affected in various degrees.

Although age-dependent changes in sensory processes play a critical role in an elderly person's adaptation to the physical and social environment, systematic epidemiological and clinical research on individual differences is still scarce and fragmentary (Ordy & Brizzee, 1979). Longitudinal studies with normal human subjects suggest that the decline in sensory capacity resulting from age may have been grossly

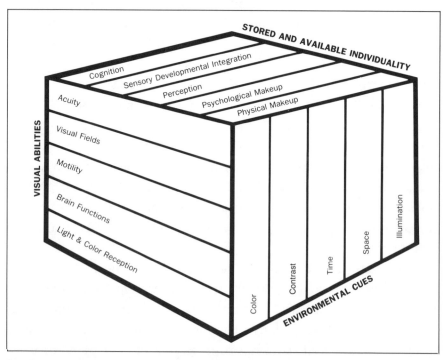

Figure 2: Corn's model of visual functioning. Source: *Foundations of Education for Blind and Visually Handicapped Children and Youth.* New York: American Foundation for the Blind, 1986.

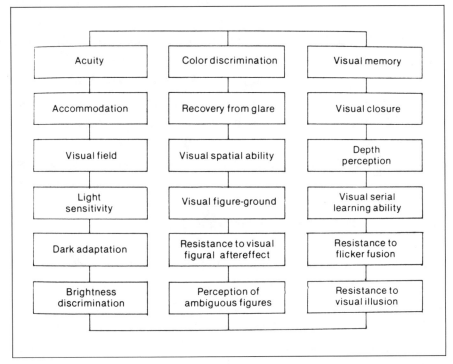

Acuity	Color discrimination	Visual memory
Accommodation	Recovery from glare	Visual closure
Visual field	Visual spatial ability	Depth perception
Light sensitivity	Visual figure-ground	Visual serial learning ability
Dark adaptation	Resistance to visual figural aftereffect	Resistance to flicker fusion
Brightness discrimination	Perception of ambiguous figures	Resistance to visual illusion

Figure 3: Visual functions affected by the aging process.

overestimated in earlier cross-sectional studies. Therefore, it is important to know not only the degree of visual impairment with age but the effect of these visual decrements on the adaptive behavior of the individual. From a behavioral standpoint, some reductions in visual acuity, color vision, and depth perception might not result in significant personal handicaps that have important social consequences. It is particularly true in situations in which the visual impairment is of gradual onset and some compensation is made by using low vision devices, by developing other skills, and by making changes in the environment (Botwinick, 1975).

Elderly persons vary widely in their adaptive capacity, social expectations, and occupational demands. Hence, eye care professionals must focus less on measurements of residual vision and more on the needs, life-styles, stated interests, and goals of elderly persons. They must ask what a particular patient can continue to do or do better in real-life situations at home, in vocational pursuits, or in social relationships. The emphasis should be on assessing the qualitative differences in the needs of individuals and not on assuming that individuals with similar reductions in visual abilities will have similar functional difficulties. Because older persons often suffer from multiple visual problems, it can be difficult to identify age differences regarding specific visual functions. Differentiating between changes caused by aging and ocular disease remains a formidable challenge. However, with the development of more sophisticated tests for the early detection of ocular disease, more effective intervention is now possible and will continue to develop.

Adaptation to Visual Impairment

Often, elderly persons with declining visual function can no longer rely on visual cues to compensate for other sensory and physiological losses. Mobility problems derived from visual loss may exacerbate an already unsteady gait and existing balance problems. Lip reading may no longer be possible to compensate for auditory deficits. The loss of visual stimulation may even bring about a decrease in the sense of taste and a loss of appetite. The cumulative stress, anxiety, and depression produced by these losses make it more difficult for elderly persons to utilize their remaining strengths and assets to cope with their visual impairments.

Visual impairment can affect a wide range of activities in the older person's life, including reading restaurant menus or theater programs in dim light, identifying grocery store labels and prices under fluorescent lights, and distinguishing gray curbs from gray sidewalks. Reading and writing letters, signing checks, and identifying labels on medicine containers can become increasingly difficult with age and associated visual dysfunction.

Although elderly persons may find it difficult to compensate for vision loss through increased reliance on their other senses, the augmentation of the quality and quantity of sensory stimuli enhances their information about the environment and should facilitate their adjustments to new roles in life. For example, auditory informational input, such as that provided by cassettes and Talking Books or computers with speech synthesizers, is used increasingly. Additional environmental information can be gained through the tactile senses; thus, the use of a cane or walker may provide a great deal of information through the sense of touch as well as adding stability.

Overall, there are several mechanisms for coping with vision loss. Other sensory modalities may be used more extensively; adaptations can be made to the environment; low vision rehabilitation involving the ophthalmologist, the optometrist, and allied health care providers can be obtained; and social support systems can be used. In recent years, an increasing number of optometrists have been helping persons with low vision maximize their use of residual vision. A comprehensive low vision examination is an essential service for the older visually impaired person. Low vision rehabilitation includes not only the prescription of appropriate low vision devices but also instruction and supportive services to enhance the person's performance in the tasks of daily living (Rosenbloom, 1984). Adaptive training involves relearning processes that may include altering eye movements with the use of low vision devices at various fixation distances, determining the appropriate illumination for a particular task, and developing a modified procedure for the recognition of letters and words.

Various studies have reported a greater than 80 percent success rate in rehabilitating low vision patients who previously were thought to be "hopeless" (Fried, 1980; Kirchner & Phillips, 1988). Both the team approach and a professional's positive attitudes toward low vision rehabilitation are essential contributing factors. (See Chapter 10 for a more complete discussion of low vision assessment and rehabilitation.)

Implications for Working with Elderly Visually Impaired Persons

If serious vision loss occurs without adequate support from friends, relatives, or professionals; the timely intervention of caregivers; and referral for rehabilitation or other services, elderly persons may adopt inappropriate coping behaviors that might be difficult to change. In addition, severe visual impairment may develop as the older individual is experiencing emotional reactions to old age that seem to be part of the developmental processes involved in late-life adjustment, and this fact also needs to be considered. One such process—the life review—appears to be universal. It takes place through reminiscence accompanied by feelings of nostalgia, regret, and pleasure. Although untoward complications can include extreme emotional pain, despair, guilt, obsessive rumination, panic, and, in extreme instances, suicide, a resolution through life review may bring atonement, serenity, constructive reorganization, and creativity.

The health care professional who works with the older visually impaired person has an important counseling role in ascertaining that the person has factual, concise, and clear information about the visual impairment and its causes and effects. Consideration and discussion of the person's feelings about his or her treatment by family and friends are also important. The elderly visually impaired person may need to realize that friends and family members will require time to understand and adjust to his or her vision loss and its functional implications as well.

As each visual impairment is unique, so is the individual's reaction to the impairment. Members of rehabilitation teams working with elderly visually impaired individuals should encourage them to become aware of the potential for living more independently and help them to learn alternative life-styles and understand the anxieties and uncertainties associated with adapting to their visual impairment. This process of adapting, constructing a new environment, and modifying one's self-image may be uneven and stressful. However, the ebb and flow of formulating and reformulating new priorities and goals are an inevitable part of healthy functioning and adaptation. Perhaps one important role the professional can play in assisting the person to adjust successfully to visual impairment is to be warm and empathic, have a positive attitude toward the person, and be pragmatic in counseling and planning efforts.

References

American Association of Retired Persons. (1990). *A profile of older Americans.* Washington, DC: Author.

Barraga, N. C. (1976). *Visual handicaps and learning.* Belmont, CA: Wadsworth.

Birren, J. E., & Williams, M. V. (1982). A perspective on aging and human function. In R. Sekuler, P. Kline, & K. Dismukes (Eds.), *Aging and human visual function.* New York: Alan R. Liss.

Botwinick, J. (1975). Behavioral processes. In S. Gershon & A. Raskin (Eds.), *Aging.* Vol. 2. New York: Raven.

Corn, A. L. (1983). Visual function: Theoretical model for individuals with low vision. *Journal of Visual Impairment & Blindness, 77*(8): 373-377.

Crews, J. E. (1988). No one left to push: The public policy of aging and blindness. *Journal of Educational Gerontology, 14*(3): 399-409.

Cullinin, T. (1978). *Low vision in elderly people: Light for low vision.* Proceedings of a symposium. London: University College.

Cunningham, P., & Johnson, A. (1980). *Edge detection: A new test of visual function.* Paper presented at the ANZAAS Jubilee Conference, Adelaide, Australia.

Faye, E. (1984). The effect of the eye condition on functional vision. In E. Faye (Ed.), *Clinical low vision* (2nd ed., pp. 172-189). Boston: Little, Brown.

Fried, A. N. (1980). Rehabilitation: An essential component of low vision care. In *Low vision ahead: Proceedings of the First Australian Pacific Conference on Low Vision.* Melbourne, Australia: Australian National Council of and for the Blind, Association for the Blind.

Kasper, R. L. (1983). Eye problems of the aged. In W. Reichel (Ed.), *Clinical aspects of aging* (2nd ed.). Baltimore: Williams and Wilkins.

Kirchner, C. (1988). *Data on blindness and visual impairment in the U.S.* (2nd ed.). New York: American Foundation for the Blind.

Kirchner, C., & Peterson, R. (1988). Data on visual disability from NCHS, 1977. In C. Kirchner (Ed.), *Data on blindness and visual impairment in the U.S.* (2nd ed., pp. 19-24). New York: American Foundation for the Blind.

Kirchner, C., & Phillips, B. (1988). Report of a survey of U.S. low vision services. In C. Kirchner (Ed.), *Data on blindness and visual impairment in the U.S.* (2nd ed., pp. 285-293). New York: American Foundation for the Blind.

Lovie-Kitchin, J., & Bowman, K. (1985). *Senile macular degeneration: Management and rehabilitation.* Woburn, MA: Butterworth.

Marron, A., & Bailey, I. (1982). Visual factors and orientation mobility performance. *Journal of Optometry and Physiological Optics, 59*(5): 413-426.

Merz, B. (1982). Lighting in homes: A study of quantity and quality. *Lighting in Australia, 2*: 26-28.

Ordy, J. M., & Brizzee, K. R. (1979). Functional and structural age difference in the visual system of man and nonhuman primate models. In J. M. Ordy & K. R. Brizzee (Eds.), *Sensory systems and communication in the elderly.* New York: Raven.

Rosenbloom, A. (1984). An overview of low vision care: Accomplishments and ongoing problems. *Journal of Visual Impairment & Blindness, 78*(10): 491-493.

Rosenbloom, A. (1986). Care of the visually impaired elderly patient. In A.

Rosenbloom & M. Morgan (Eds.), *Vision and aging: General and clinical perspectives* (pp. 337-348). New York: Professional Press.

World Health Organization. (1981). *The use of residual vision by visually disabled persons: Report of a WHO meeting.* Euro Reports and Studies No. 41. Geneva, Switzerland: Author.

U.S. Department of Health and Human Services, Office of Human Development Services. (1980). *Facts about older Americans, 1979.* Washington, DC: U.S. Government Printing Office.

CHAPTER 4

Social Aspects of Aging and Visual Impairment

Jon Hendricks

If we live long enough, nearly all of us will experience changes and problems with vision, some fairly serious. Most older people are not seriously impaired; most retain sufficient visual function to perform activities of daily living independently or with limited assistance. But eye problems increase as people grow older; indeed, age is the single best predictor of visual impairment and blindness (Lowman & Kirchner, 1988).

Seventy percent of the visually impaired people in this country are beyond retirement age, and well over 90 percent of newly visually impaired persons fall into this age category. Accordingly, as the number of elderly people increases, the number of visually impaired persons can be expected to climb at a corresponding rate (U.S. Department of Commerce, Bureau of the Census, 1983).

To appreciate the extent of visual impairments among elderly persons, one should have an idea of how many people are in that age category, what changes have occurred in life expectancy, and what the future may hold in this regard. This chapter begins with an overview of some demographic parameters affecting the lives of older persons, particularly those who are visually impaired. These factors include financial status, health, family and support network, and housing. It then summarizes what is known about rates of visual impairment by social categories and ends with suggestions for services and intervention to enhance well-being. The discussion also touches on some factors influencing the quality of life of elderly people, particularly those age 85 and over, who are referred to as the "old-old," or the frail elderly.

The Numbers and Their Significance

Older persons constitute one of the most rapidly growing segments of the population. By the year 2000, persons 65 and over are expected to represent 13 percent of the population. By the year 2030, 66 million older persons, or 21.5 percent of the population, will be age 65 and over—two and one-half times the number in 1980. In 1989, 31 million persons were 65 years or older. This represents 12.5 percent of the U.S. population, about one in every eight Americans. In 1989, there were 18.3 million older women and 12.6 million older men, a ratio of 145 women to every 100 men (American Association of Retired Persons, 1990).

Why is it insufficient to note that there are many older people and that life expectancy is increasing? First, longevity rates for the 31 million persons age 65 and over differ by sex, race, social characteristics, and economic position. These variations in longevity pose interesting questions. Why do women constitute 60 percent of the elderly population, and how do we account for the widening "longevity gap" between the sexes? Why do black persons have shorter life expectancies than do white persons, and why is this trend reversed at age 75? Why do people of higher socioeconomic status and those who have higher levels of education live longer than do those who are less advantaged?

If there is something about being wealthy, white, or female that promotes greater life expectancy, then identifying that something may improve everyone's chances of living longer. Aging is never merely a biological event; by taking sociocontextual factors into account, professionals enhance their understanding of the entire process. The psychologist and the sociologist have as much or more than the biologist to say about why people age the way they do.

THE OLD-OLD

The thorny question of the quality versus the quantity of life must be addressed. If advances in life expectancy could automatically be accompanied by continuing good health, financial security, and social fulfillment, most people probably would opt for a bonus decade or two. But if advances in life expectancy meant ever-diminishing vigor in return for the gift of longer life (as in the story of the mythical Tithonus), how many would take the option?

Persons age 85 and over are currently the fastest growing segment of the American population and the most vulnerable to health problems. Chronic conditions such as heart disease, arthritis, and diabetes are prevalent among the old-old, and the debilitating effects of these conditions tend to increase with age. The rate of hospital use as well as nursing home admissions increases steadily and will continue to do so.

Will advances in modern medicine enable the future old-old to enjoy reasonably good health, or must they inevitably face ill health? Although this question has not been resolved, evidence suggests a lengthening of the number of years in which poor health and disabilities are daily companions (Schneider & Brody, 1983). Advances in high and low technological assistive devices for independent living can, however, help the older disabled person achieve a higher level of independent functioning.

WOMEN

Gerontologists sometimes say that the problems of old age are women's issues. Women live longer than do men, and the differential has grown wider in recent years. By the end of the 20th century, the gap will amount to approximately 10 years.

Currently, at age 65 there are 3 women for every 2 men; by age 75, there are 66 percent more women than men. After age 85, there are 224 women for every 100 men still living. A white woman has a one in three chance of living to age 85; a nonwhite woman has a 28 percent chance of reaching 85. Unfortunately, their male counterparts will have died; regardless of race, men's chances of celebrating their 85th birthday are no better than one in six (White House Conference on Aging, 1981).

Some believe that the longevity gap will narrow now that women are a greater part of the workplace and may suffer the same stress and acute diseases, such as heart attack and stroke, as men. However, the data do not yet reflect such a narrowing. Most women who become widowed after age 65 will not remarry. Being single and female is a fact of life in old age. And, for many, old age can be accompanied by loneliness and financial hardship.

MINORITIES

It is important to consider the special situation of minority populations when discussing the aging of America. In 1989, 10 percent of elderly persons represented minority populations. Eight percent were blacks,
and the remaining 2 percent were American Indians, Eskimos, Aleuts,
Asians, and Pacific Islanders. Persons of Hispanic origin, regardless
of race, represented 3 percent of the older population. Hispanics and
Asians represent the fastest growing minority groups within the elderly
population. Given the tremendous growth of minorities in the U.S.
population, the figures concerning these groups are bound to increase
greatly (U.S. Department of Commerce, Bureau of the Census, 1989).
The numbers are important; many of these subpopulations are at particular risk. Not only do they have shorter life expectancies and higher
age-specific mortality and morbidity rates than does the majority
population, but many become old following a lifetime of difficulties.
Many experience the results of years of depressed earnings, fewer
educational opportunities, and a higher prevalence of serious illnesses,
such as hypertension, heart disease, stroke, and diabetes. The disadvantages become apparent when some of the particulars are examined.

First, life expectancy at birth has traditionally been far more favorable
for whites than for minorities. In the past 40 years, however, the differential has been reduced by over half. Today, only an average of five
years separates whites from blacks. By age 65, the differential has all
but disappeared. As mentioned, after age 75, blacks have a better chance
of survival. There is still a gap between the two groups, but blacks are
catching up, experiencing a one-third gain in the number of people
age 65 and over, compared to a 23 percent gain for whites during the
past four decades. In all likelihood, the differences would disappear
if the socioeconomic status (and all that it portends) of whites and blacks
were comparable throughout life (Kitagawa & Hauser, 1973; U.S.
Department of Commerce, Bureau of the Census, 1983).

VISUALLY IMPAIRED PERSONS

If the current prevalence rates of visual impairment continue, the extension in life expectancy suggests that the number of elderly persons with

severe visual impairments will increase dramatically. According to the National Center for Health Statistics (NCHS) Health Interview Survey (HIS), there were 2,038,000 older persons who were severely visually impaired in 1984 (Nelson, 1988). However, it can be estimated that there are currently well over 3 million severely visually impaired older persons in the country. This considerable undercount of older visually impaired persons exists largely because of difficulties in identifying and counting this population.

It is likely that there will be a 78 percent increase in the number of elderly people who will be forced to face visual disabilities in the year 2000. The greatest proportion of these people will be the old-old and women, who will outnumber visually impaired men by roughly two to one (Lowman & Kirchner, 1988). Logic also suggests these elderly people will be at the lower end of the socioeconomic scale, will be more disadvantaged in regard to most of the standard indicators, will suffer multiple health impairments, will have their activities limited for a month or more out of every 12 months, and disproportionately will be members of minority groups.

How can such a claim be made? Like so many other characteristics of elderly persons, visual impairment is probably influenced by a person's relative position in the social structure. For example, the prevalence rates for severe visual impairments among the total population of Americans age 65 and older are higher among women not only because there are more older women than older men, but because the rates are higher among women in general and increase with every successive age interval. As for income, elderly people in the lowest income groups are nearly three times as likely to report visual impairments as are those in the highest income group. The same holds true for educational levels—those with fewer than nine years of schooling report the highest rate, followed by college graduates, high school graduates (an inexplicable departure from the pattern), and those with an education beyond the college level. In terms of race, the rate of visual impairment among elderly minority group members is 90 percent higher than among whites (National Center for Health Statistics, 1981).

Quality of Life

What is life like after age 65? What hurdles or challenges do elderly people face? From national surveys, we know that older people are concerned about income, health, safety, the possibility of being dependent, and a variety of other frailties affecting everyday life (National Council on the Aging, 1981). In many ways, elderly persons are not much different from younger people in what captures their attention. A review follows of some of the topics that are especially relevant to professionals who work with blind and visually impaired elderly persons. Although the statistics cannot offer a truly sensitive portrait of daily life, they present an overall picture and a reference point for evaluating specifics. They also indicate some of the social and physical contexts of visual impairment among elderly people.

ECONOMIC CIRCUMSTANCES

The economic position of elderly people in general reflects the peripheral position older people occupy relative to American society. Although they were never intended to be more than a means to buttress financial well-being, social security payments have become a mainstay in the economic life of elderly persons in this country.

A large number of older persons depend primarily on social security, which constitutes over half their income. In fact, social security accounts for over 90 percent of the total income of 20 percent of white elderly persons and 40 percent of the total income of black elderly persons (Hendricks & Hendricks, 1986). Despite the indexing of benefits to cost-of-living indicators, a fifth of all elderly couples and nearly one-half of all single elderly persons who receive social security live below the poverty level. At best, only a scant minority of older persons are able to retain high or even stable incomes in their later years. Across the board, about 16 percent of all old people have incomes below federally established poverty levels, and another 25 percent are in the next higher income category.

Often, economic security varies by age, sex, race, education, and related socioeconomic status. The reasons for these fluctuations revolve around individual attributes and structural features of American society.

The further into old age one moves, the lower one's annual income is likely to be. For a great number of people, income starts to decline when they are approximately age 55, falls by nearly half during the decades of their sixties, and continues its decline thereafter. For people over age 72, poverty rates are double those of people in their sixties (U.S. Department of Commerce, Bureau of the Census, 1982). Furthermore, it is not surprising that most of those who are old, alone, and poor are women and members of minority groups. They have had lifetimes of interrupted work histories, lower incomes on which social security payments are based, low-paying jobs that have made saving difficult, and high medical costs.

Regardless of age, women generally have lower incomes. White men have the highest incomes, and black women the lowest. The income of older black people in general is about 44 percent that of older white people. Roughly one-third of elderly black people and one-quarter of elderly Hispanic people live below the poverty level (U.S. Department of Commerce, Bureau of the Census, 1982).

Generally, two trends hold true. First, since the mid-1970s, sources of income for elderly people have been shifting from earnings to private and public pensions and the conversion of assets. Second, because privately held assets are used up in the years immediately following retirement, there is an ever greater reliance on social security and related public benefit programs over time. Consequently, serious financial hardships are likely to have a major impact on those in their seventies and older (U.S. Department of Commerce, Bureau of the Census, 1982, 1983; White House Conference on Aging, 1981).

About 3.4 million older persons (approximately 12 percent of this group) were in the labor force working or actively seeking employment in 1989, including 2 million men (17 percent of older men) and 1.4 million women (8 percent of older women). Approximately half (52 percent) of older workers in 1989 were employed part time. Approximately 25 percent of older workers in 1989 were self-employed. Many older persons would like to continue working to support themselves and their families or to supplement retirement income. Others seek employment for psychosocial reasons—to remain active and productive in their later years. Unfortunately, their efforts to find jobs are often blocked, usually in subtle ways. Although legislation has been enacted that eliminates age discrimination, in practice, employers continue to favor younger workers. By age 55 or so, unemployment is a real and present threat. In the past decade, unemployment rates among men ages 55 to 64 increased by over 10 percent and grew faster than for any other segment of the population. So precipitous is the shift that the commissioner of labor for the New York federal region asserted that technological displacement accompanying structural changes in the nature of work has fallen disproportionately on male workers age 45 to 64 (Ehrenhalt, 1983). Whether it is due to their inability to be reemployed or to a true desire to retire, almost two-thirds of all new social security claimants are men age 62 to 65. Among women, roughly four-fifths request payment before they are 65 (U.S. Department of Commerce, Bureau of the Census, 1983).

HEALTH AND HEALTH CARE CONSIDERATIONS

Most older people are healthy; over two-thirds perceive themselves as having no serious health problems. There are differences by sex, race, and social class, but the stereotype of the sickly older person is not valid. In 1988, 29 percent of older persons assessed their health as fair or poor. Although there was little difference between the sexes, older blacks were much more likely to rate their health as good or excellent (48 percent) than older whites (28 percent). In general, one-sixth indicated having some difficulty doing routine tasks. Over 80 percent reported having chronic conditions, but these conditions generally did not impose restrictions on daily activities (NCHS, 1982).

Behind the overall statistics are interesting patterns. White people are healthier than nonwhites, and the wealthier are healthier than the poor. The diseases that affect aged men are most often seen as causes of death, but those of aged women predominate as causes of illness. Generally, the health conditions of elderly black people are appreciably less favorable; older black persons have higher incidence rates than do whites across a broad range of health measures and more often have multiple impairments.

Perceptions of physical well-being are directly related to income; 25 percent of those in the lower income levels say they feel excellent, compared to more than 40 percent of those with incomes over $25,000. As might be expected, people with greater financial resources also visit their physicians more frequently to ensure sound health. Finally, acute illnesses, relatively rare among older people, have been replaced by chronic ailments. The most frequently diagnosed chronic illnesses are arthritis and rheumatism; cardiovascular conditions; hypertension; impairment of the lower extremities, back, or hip; visual impairments; and diabetes (U.S. Department of Commerce, Bureau of the Census, 1983).

In spite of these limiting conditions, the majority of older people, even those age 85 and over, are not particularly constrained in carrying out daily tasks. If they can continue to dress, bathe, use the toilet, and eat without assistance, they are capable of maintaining an independent life-style. Undoubtedly, the need for assistance in one or another of these daily living activities increases as people move into their eighth decade and beyond, but the desire to retain a sense of autonomy does not decrease.

Accompanying increased life expectancy and its concomitant health and physical conditions are major health expenditures for physician visits, hospitalization, and other health care. Because the United States is the only remaining industrialized country in the world without national health insurance of some kind, all Americans face bankrupting out-of-pocket expenditures related to health care. Elderly persons are especially hard hit. Aggregate expenditures from all sources run twice as high among older persons as among the rest of the population, accounting for one-third of all money spent on health care in the United States. Among those 75 and over, curtailed resources and the likelihood of major health care costs impose real financial hardships (Social Security Administration, 1983; U.S. Department of Commerce, Bureau of the Census, 1983).

An interesting controversy has arisen about improvements in life expectancy and morbidity among the 75-and-over population. For years, gerontologists have contended that the period of diminished vigor thought to characterize old age would be compressed into the furthest reaches of life expectancy (Fries, 1980; Hendricks & Hendricks, 1986). For 150 years, improved housing, nutrition, sanitation, medical practices, and other factors have helped add years to lives. Today this country approaches a point at which the death rates for all ages will be low until old age is reached. As Strehler (1979) made clear, advances occurred because of the control of various causes of death, such as childhood diseases, epidemics, and tuberculosis, that in the past affected specific earlier parts of the life cycle.

But, as mentioned, it seems unlikely that longer life expectancy will be accompanied by extended years of good health. To improve the health status of elderly persons, advances must take place in such diverse domains as those relating to the physical causes of ill health; mental and emotional well-being; and the social, political, and economic contexts. If we assume that health care professionals do devote their full energies to the physical maladies of aging, based on the presumption that they are the primary detractors of total well-being, then the secondary factors affecting life expectancy would have to improve at a similar rate if maximum benefits were to accrue to the elderly population. To ward off or recover from illness involves more than a physical process; even under ideal conditions, medical care is not a panacea. As long as ancillary life-change events promote stress, both physical and psychosocial, people will not function optimally (Garrity & Marx, 1979). The compounding of the physical, social, economic, and emotional displacements that are too frequently associated with advancing old age is an outgrowth of the circumstances of a potentially dependent segment of the population that lacks the resources to attend to its needs.

STRUCTURE OF DAILY LIFE

Social scientists in all fields contend that an appreciation of the social context of elderly individuals is essential for an adequate understanding of what it means to be old. Changes in living arrangements, shifts in social roles and support networks, alterations in mobility and psychomotor processes, and many other dimensions of social interaction structure the daily lives of elderly people. The well-being of older Americans is colored by where they live, with whom they live, how often they see their friends and families, and how frequently they get out of their homes. An exhaustive enumeration of all these and other factors is not possible and may not even be necessary. But the consideration of a few select elements that shape life-style and the quality of life after age 65 will be useful.

Family and Social Interaction

One myth about the later years is that they are a time of loneliness and isolation. It is true that there are many more older women than older men because women in general outlive men by approximately seven years. About half of older women below age 75 are widowed; but regardless of gender, the death of a spouse is in all likelihood followed for the individual by at least a temporary decline in physical health and general well-being.

Nevertheless, widowhood does not deprive elderly people of family ties, because their bonds with adult children remain strong. The notion of the empty-nest years as a time of noncontact is not factual. Less than 10 percent of elderly people—largely women—actually live under the same roof as their adult children; yet they see each other frequently. Three-quarters of elderly persons who have children live within a half hour's travel of them and see them at least weekly (Hanson & Saver, 1985; White House Conference on Aging, 1981).

Although relatives are the primary source of support and contact for many older persons, friends also play an essential role. When family members are unavailable to help, friends and neighbors fill in. They are a source of strength for older people, protecting them from many of the negative definitions imposed by the larger society and from some of the protean liabilities that may stem from the attrition of social roles. Often, older people's reluctance to move to improved housing grows out of neighborhood ties based on long-term residence and bonds of friendship and community. After middle age, links to friends seem to grow in importance. Visiting back and forth, at least weekly, is one mechanism known to buttress morale (Hendricks & Hendricks, 1986).

Residence and Institutionalization

Where do elderly people live? Mostly they live where they have for the past 30 or 40 years. Find out where young families bought houses in the years after World War II, and you will find neighborhoods with many elderly residents. If you want to know where people who will be old in 2025 will be living, look where those with preschool children are buying houses today. In most cases, people settle down somewhere between ages 35 and 40 and stay. Of course, houses and neighborhoods age also. The locale and accessibility of people's homes determine a great deal about their behavior. Approximately two-thirds of elderly persons live in urban areas, but they are not particularly concentrated into inner-city ghettos. They live in older neighborhoods in core areas but not disproportionately so. The exception is elderly blacks; over 55 percent live in the heart of the central city, and another 12 percent live in other metropolitan areas (Hendricks & Hendricks, 1986). Because of recent trends concerning the movement of many people to suburban areas, we expect to find "gray belts" around the cities of tomorrow, a feature sure to affect the delivery of needed services (Hendricks & Hendricks, 1986).

Why does it matter where older people call home? For one thing, accessibility to essential services—such as shopping, medical care, and social services—is crucial. As older communities decay and lose population to suburbia and exurbia, many of the services that older people seek no longer exist. The homes older people occupy, often thought to be a hedge against inflation, are also older, require more maintenance, and are more costly to heat or cool. Fewer than one-sixth of all older people move out of homes they have lived in for years. Consequently, elderly people face fixed costs that may account for about 35 percent of their incomes. Until the recent inflationary surge the comparable rate for younger homeowners was about 25 percent. When more recent statistics are compiled, both estimates may have jumped dramatically (U.S. Department of Commerce, Bureau of the Census, 1983).

Those older persons who move to a new location often find the relocation process traumatic and likely to induce additional stress. A move to a new home involves far more than new physical surroundings; it reshapes one's entire life. The experience need not always be negative. If handled well and planned over time, the move can prove beneficial, as evidenced by the continuing influx of older people to retirement communities and the Sunbelt states. Another kind of move, usually with negative connotations, is the move to a nursing home. With the group 85 and over growing at the fastest rate, thoughts and questions about institutionalization and its alternatives become increasingly common.

Women and those who must face life on their own are most likely to find themselves in nursing homes. On any given day slightly more than 5 percent of the nation's elderly population reside in institutions of some sort. Many move in, some move out, and others die; the population of nursing homes turns over regularly. With advancing age, the prospect of institutionalization increases. In the 10 years after retirement, the rate of institutionalization is only 1.3 percent; by age 85, it is 23 percent (Eustis, Greenberg, & Patten, 1984; U.S. Department of Commerce, Bureau of the Census, 1983).

Among the more critical factors leading to nursing home admission are poor health or disability that limits independent functioning, the absence of a spouse or other family ties, and the lack of sources of financial support. The trajectory that culminates in institutionalization is not easily understood. Elderly persons prefer to remain in their own homes as long as possible, and gerontologists and health care professionals continually attempt to ameliorate the trend toward institutionalization by developing alternative systems, such as home health care, adult day care, respite care, and other supportive community-based care models, as well as support for family caregivers. Despite these alternatives, it seems certain that the utilization of nursing homes, at least by the old-old, will be the fastest growing component of the health care system between now and the year 2000. The number of residents will increase by one-half the current levels (Eustis, Greenberg, & Patten, 1984; U.S. Department of Commerce, Bureau of the Census, 1983). Rehabilitation coordinated by agencies for blind and visually impaired persons has tremendous potential for keeping older visually impaired persons from being placed in nursing homes prematurely and unnecessarily.

Patterns of Living

If most elderly people remain independent, what do they do with their days? Among elderly sighted persons, 80 percent or more spend time watching television. On a daily basis, television, visiting, and reading account for the greatest share of leisure time; together they add up to over six hours every day (White House Conference on Aging, 1981). Older people are also the most frequent subscribers to daily newspapers and seem to keep themselves informed about current affairs. Their leisure pursuits reflect efforts to remain involved in society and life and are extensions of lifelong patterns. Many occupy themselves with crafts and hobbies regularly.

Intellectual growth and development continue throughout the life span. Many older persons are involved in adult education and attend some kind of classes. Wellness and health promotion are important to elderly people, and their participation in exercise and physical fitness programs is growing along with that of the rest of the population. The need to be productive and to contribute to the community and to society continues into old age; many elderly persons, free from the constraints of a job or raising a family, have time to do volunteer work.

When asked what they routinely think about, older people say they think about their families, death, current events, crime, and the meaning of their lives—what people of all ages think about. Ties with children and grandchildren are a great source of comfort for those who have them, but the absence of these ties is not particularly troublesome to those without such links. When elderly people spend time thinking about death, they do so without a heightened sense of fear. In most instances, their views focus on realistic details, not apprehension. Also, contrary to popular opinion, those who live in nursing homes or in retirement communities, where death is an obvious fact of life, are not more disconsolate over their impending demise than are their peers who live in the community (Kalish, 1976).

However, some elderly people do worry. Many are concerned about the cost of living and plan carefully how they spend their money. They also worry about crime and being victimized. Fears about crime affect the way in which a great number of elderly people structure their lives. Many older persons restrict activities outside the home, including shopping, banking, visiting friends and neighbors, and participating in community events, to the daylight hours. The threat of crime may prevent some older persons, like their younger counterparts, from taking advantage of cultural and social programs in the evening. Thus, like everyone else in the country, the issues older people think about are those closest to their daily lives; age does not bring many changes in that respect.

Visually Impaired Elderly Persons

There is infinite variety among individual older persons, whether visually impaired or sighted. Neither chronological age nor functional disability determines behavior. One overriding stereotype of visually impaired people in general, and elderly persons in particular, is that they disengage from active involvement in the world around them. This belief is generally incorrect (Josephson, 1968; Scott, 1969). Although evidence is scattered and disparate, the social life of elderly blind and visually impaired people is probably not so disadvantaged when compared with that of sighted members of their social class. Many older persons with severe impairment who do not receive training in adaptive techniques to carry out daily activities frequently do withdraw from the community and begin to describe themselves as homebound. As noted earlier, the demographic pattern of blindness is skewed toward categories of less advantaged persons. Whether it is cause or consequence is unclear. Nevertheless, the activities, involvements, and concerns of blind and visually impaired people and of individuals without impairments in comparable socioeconomic circumstances are similar (Josephson, 1968).

Changes in vision that accompany the aging process do have an impact on the quality of life. Bader (1986) cogently noted that adequate vision and socioeconomic stability are among the most treasured resources of elderly people because they help individuals retain independent life-styles. Yet loss of vision does not automatically result in reduced life satisfaction or greater dependence. Much depends on the individual and how he or she copes with life's problems. Individual differences are not diminished with age; if anything, they are heightened (Greenblatt, 1979; Sekuler, Kline, Dismukes, & Adams, 1983). Those older persons who successfully handled life crises in the past and who maintain ego strength and inner security are likely to meet the challenges of vision loss and remain independent. Those who were actively involved in social and community affairs while they were sighted will probably continue this pattern even after they have lost their vision. Participation in available rehabilitation services from an agency for blind and visually impaired persons can enhance the possibility for continued involvement.

The agenda for future research on vision and aging needs to address a number of issues. Although we know that early treatment is essential to help detect and prevent eye disease, it has been reported that 40 percent of elderly people did not visit an eye care specialist in the year prior to having been surveyed, and nearly one-sixth had not done so in three years. We do not know which barriers stand in the way or how to surmount them (Eger, 1976). But outreach to older persons, to tell them annual eye examinations are essential, is critical as people live longer and have a greater chance of having eye problems as they age.

There may be several reasons why older persons do not seek assistance as their eyesight fails. Some believe that the loss of vision is a natural outgrowth of the aging process and suspect nothing can be done. Others may be reluctant to admit to themselves and friends that they have a vision problem. Some do not know where to go to find help and have no information about rehabilitation or other services. Bader (1986) suggested that barriers to obtaining service represent a combination of practical constraints, such as transportation difficulties; inaccessibility of services; insufficient knowledge about services; and negative attitudes, stereotypic thinking, and myths about blindness, both by and about elderly individuals.

SOCIAL LIFE SPACE AND VISUAL IMPAIRMENT

When an older person is diagnosed as having a severe visual impairment, great attention is given to the physical losses involved. But the emotional and psychological impact of the loss of vision is often overlooked. Many older persons have at least one other chronic health condition or disability. With vision loss added, there may be a compounding effect not readily identifiable on the basis of physical health alone.

Age-related deficits in visual capability are among the impairments that are potentially more disruptive to elderly persons. These changes have a significant impact on cognitive functioning, including learning, memory, information processing, and spatial representation. Without a cognitive map of one's environment and its elements, mobility, inter-action, and a sense of competence often suffer (Fozard, Ernst, Bell, McFarland, & Podolsky, 1977; Poon, 1980; Sekuler et al., 1983; Walsh, Krauss, & Reneger, 1981).

For elderly individuals, the loss of vision may occur when other losses—diminished hearing, unsteadiness of gait, and lessened physical strength—are becoming apparent. These losses result in more acute difficulties in conducting daily activities. Home presents new hazards. Once-simple tasks—cooking, taking a bath, and paying bills—are difficult. Many who lose their sight are afraid to leave home to visit friends, shop, go to a senior citizens center, or take advantage of services, particularly if their vision loss is combined with other sensory impairments. These problems are often compounded by other losses that are a natural part of aging—the death of a spouse, diminished family life, and retirement from a valued job. As a result, it is reasonable to hypothesize that the social "life space" of elderly visually impaired persons tends to contract. To this factor add the social reactions to the lack of sight. The attitudes of persons who interact with visually impaired persons—family, friends, professionals, and society as a whole—have a profound effect. Increasing isolation and inactivity are two formidable problems faced by people who are visually impaired, especially elderly persons. Much of the shift from independence to dependence relates to how others react to them and their new life situation.

Family members and friends are well intentioned but often tend to overprotect. They may assume dependence is an inevitable outgrowth of the loss of sight, particularly among elderly persons. Consequently, they do not encourage (or actively discourage) the older person in maintaining independence. A family member, for example, may fear leaving a relative at home alone and also fear the consequences of the person's venturing outside alone. These attitudes reinforce dependence. Sooner or later the visually impaired person believes he or she can no longer function without assistance. Many older visually impaired persons are prematurely admitted to nursing homes. Through encouragement and support of desires for independence and the learning of independent living skills, involvement of family members, and the receipt of available rehabilitation services, there is great potential for feelings of independence and interdependence.

Behavior among many visually impaired people and those who interact with them often reflects a learned "blind attitude" rather than the actual inability of visually impaired persons to relate to the environment (Monbeck, 1973; Scott, 1969). Such attitudes prompt an expectation of homogeneity among those with limited vision. These social definitions of what it means to be blind, in addition to being elderly, result in rigid stereotypes about individuals as well as their needs, including what services need to be provided.

In relation to the perceptions of others, being old or being both old and blind constitutes jeopardy. Stereotypically, people expect elderly people and blind people to behave in certain ways. But neither case has a factual basis. In setting out some of the stereotypic beliefs people have about blindness, Scott (1969) noted that these beliefs revolve around helplessness, docility, dependence, melancholia, aestheticism, and serious-mindedness. Stereotypic beliefs about aging might add loneliness and fearfulness, but the list would otherwise be similar (Levin & Levin, 1980; National Council on the Aging, 1981; Salmon, 1981). Unfortunately, stereotypes may become reality when the young interact with the old and sighted people have opportunities to interact with visually impaired persons.

COUNTERVAILING MEASURES

A variety of mechanisms counteract the isolation and dependence of visually impaired elderly persons. For instance, telephone contacts are in themselves enough to redress some of the affective disorders that appear to result from restricted and isolated social involvements (Evans,

Werkhoven, & Fox, 1982). Other forms of assistance, such as self-help groups, that place a strong emphasis on avenues for independence and self-esteem have been effective (Oehler & Fitzgerald, 1980). The establishment of peer support groups is increasing at agencies for blind people and is a way of assisting older visually impaired persons, particularly in the rehabilitation process.

Two themes underline nearly all attempts to expand the shrinking boundaries of social life space. One is the integration of visually impaired elderly persons into ongoing service programs rather than relegating them to well-intentioned but insulating situations designed to accommodate impairment. Many programs for seniors have inadvertently excluded visually impaired persons, believing that they are unable to participate in such activities as art classes, bingo, and exercise. By socializing with other elderly people, however, visually impaired older persons develop a valuable reference point for affirming competence.

A second, related theme of expanding social life space is the use of new or renewed skills as a means of enhancing self-esteem in visually impaired people and those with whom they interact (Freedman, 1975; Stern, 1969). For example, older visually impaired people can make important contributions as volunteers. Serving on a telephone reassurance team to call homebound elderly persons might be a logical volunteer activity. Often, in our rush to assist visually impaired persons, we forget that they, too, have needs to make contributions. As they work with local agencies for blind people, senior citizens centers are growing responsive to older visually impaired persons.

Too frequently, service agencies designed to aid blind and visually impaired people have concentrated on the young and on vocational training. Consequently, elderly people have had less access to rehabilitation than have their younger counterparts. Recognition of the need for rehabilitation among older persons grew in the late 1980s, but increased funds are necessary to meet the rehabilitation needs of the growing numbers of older visually impaired persons.

Regardless of the person's disability, rehabilitation services are most successful when they promote self-care; help eliminate environmental barriers; and ensure economic support, social interaction, and a meaningful sense of purpose and productivity. The person who is both old and visually impaired faces multiple disadvantages and thus can profit immeasurably from efforts that incorporate elements identified as optimal services among aging and blindness agencies (Benedict & Ganikos, 1981).

In the ideal world, neither disabilities nor age would be stigmatized as a form of deviance. But now those who are old or visually impaired are considered distinct from the mainstream and must prove they are not different. Friedson (1965) noted the dilemma confronting service programs and, by extension, confronting all entitlement legislation aimed at alleviating problems of disabled persons. To receive appropriations for governmental programs and to create public awareness of the needs of disabled persons, policymakers and service providers find that they must call attention to the people's disabilities, dependencies, and differences. Although this process helps meet many of the needs of disabled persons, it reinforces social stereotypes. Those who receive services are labeled "different," and with this label come all the connotations leading to symbolic redefinition. Through our definitions, we construct our world. One outcome is that aged and visually impaired people are set apart and given a separate (probably unequal) status (Grove, 1976). What starts as a physiological fact acquires social character (Krause, 1976).

As both Josephson (1968) and Scott (1969) noted, blindness and visual impairment are social phenomena. As such, society's attitudes toward them are subject to change, and perceptions of what elderly visually impaired or blind people are like, want, or can do are riddled with misconceptions. Yesterday's reality may be today's misconception (Freedman, 1973).

But outdated stereotypes need not determine quality of life for elderly people, especially those who are visually impaired. Older persons in our society value their independence and do not wish to be a financial or psychological burden on their families. They want to live in their own homes and be a part of their communities as long as possible. Visually impaired older persons are probably no different from their sighted peers, but many of them need access to services and physical and emotional support to remain independent. If family members and service networks can break away from stereotypic thinking and intervene at an early stage, the chances for greater numbers of visually impaired older people to adjust to independent living will be far greater.

Services for blind and visually impaired older people have been slow to develop. But as elderly people and their families, aging and blindness networks, and health care institutions all become more aware of the prevalence of visual impairment among older persons, the value of early treatment of eye disease, and the possibility of independent living, new services may emerge to meet the changing needs of older visually impaired persons. Older persons have become a major political and social force, and "gray power" has done much to counteract the stereotypes of old age. Older visually impaired persons can play a key role in changing negative images about aging and visual impairment by showing that they can, with a minimum of assistance, lead lives of independence, productivity, and dignity.

References

American Association of Retired Persons. (1990). *A profile of older Americans.* Washington, DC: Author.

Bader, J. E. (1986). Socioeconomic aspects of aging. In A. Rosenbloom & M. Morgan (Eds.), *Vision and aging: General and clinical perspectives.* New York: Professional Press.

Benedict, R. C., & Ganikos, M. L. (1981). Coming to terms with ageism in rehabilitation. *Journal of Rehabilitation, 47:* 10-18.

Eger, M. J. (1976). Vision and care and our senior citizens. *Journal of the American Optometric Association, 47:* 711-712.

Ehrenhalt, S. M. (November 28, 1983). Older men left in job squeeze. *USA Today,* p. 1A.

Eustis, N., Greenberg, J., & Patten, S. (1984). *Long-term care for older persons: A policy perspective.* Monterey, CA: Brooks/Cole.

Evans, R. L., Werkhoven, W., & Fox, R. H. (1982). Treatment of social isolation and loneliness in a sample of visually impaired elderly persons. *Psychological Reports, 51:* 103-108.

Fozard, J. L., Ernst, W., Bell, B., McFarland, R. A., & Podolsky, S. (1977). Visual perception and communication. In J. E. Birren & K. W. Schaie (Eds.), *Handbook of the psychology of aging* (pp. 497-534). New York: Van Nostrand Reinhold.

Freedman, S. (1973). *Realities and misconceptions.* Paper presented at the meeting of the American Foundation for the Blind, New Orleans.

Freedman, S. (1975). The assessment of older visually impaired adults by a psychologist. *The New Outlook for the Blind, 69*(8): 361-364.

Friedson, E. (1965). Disability as social deviance. In M. Sussman (Ed.), *Sociology and rehabilitation*. Washington, DC: American Sociological Association.

Fries, J. F. (1980). Aging, natural death, and the compression of morbidity. *New England Journal of Medicine, 303*: 130.

Garrity, T. F., & Marx, M. B. (1979). The relationship of recent life events to health in the elderly. In J. Hendricks & C. D. Hendricks (Eds.), *Dimensions of aging* (pp. 98-113). Cambridge, MA: Winthrop.

Greenblatt, S. T. (1979). The person who happens to be old and blind. *Journal of Visual Impairment & Blindness, 73*(3): 113-114.

Grove, W. R. (1976). Societal reaction theory and disability. In G. L. Albrecht (Ed.), *The sociology of physical disability and rehabilitation* (pp. 57-71). Pittsburgh: University of Pittsburgh Press.

Hanson, S. M., & Saver, W. J. (1985). Children and their elderly parents. In W. J. Saver & R. T. Coward (Eds.), *Social support networks and the care of the elderly* (pp. 41-66). New York: Springer.

Hendricks, J., & Hendricks, C. D. (1986). *Aging in mass society: Myths and realities*. Boston: Little, Brown.

Josephson, E. (1968). *The social life of blind people*. New York: American Foundation for the Blind.

Kalish, R. (1976). Death and dying in a social context. In R. H. Binstock & E. Shanas (Eds.), *Handbook of aging and the social sciences* (pp. 483-507). New York: Van Nostrand Reinhold.

Kitagawa, E. M., & Hauser, P. M. (1973). *Differential mortality in the United States: A study of socioeconomic epidemiology*. Cambridge, MA: Harvard University Press.

Krause, E. A. (1976). The political sociology of rehabilitation. In G. L. Albrecht (Ed.), *The sociology of physical disability and rehabilitation* (pp. 202-221). Pittsburgh: University of Pittsburgh Press.

Levin, J., & Levin, W. C. (1980). *Ageism and prejudice and discrimination against the elderly*. Belmont, CA: Wadsworth.

Lowman, C., & Kirchner, C. (1988). Elderly blind and visually impaired persons: Projected numbers in the year 2000. In C. Kirchner (Ed.), *Data on blindness and visual impairment in the U.S.* (2nd ed., pp. 45-52). New York: American Foundation for the Blind.

Monbeck, M. E. (1973). *The meaning of blindness: Attitudes towards blindness and blind people*. Bloomington, IN: Indiana University Press.

National Center for Health Statistics. (1981). Prevalence of selected impairments. *Vital and health statistics*, Series 10, No. 134. Hyattsville, MD: Author.

National Center for Health Statistics. (1982). Current estimates from the National Health Interview Survey, United States, 1981. *Vital and health statistics*, Series 10, No. 141. Hyattsville, MD: Author.

National Council on the Aging. (1981). *Aging in the eighties: America in transition.* Washington, DC: Author.

Nelson, K.A. (1988). Visual impairment among elderly Americans: Statistics in transition. In C. Kirchner (Ed.), *Data on blindness and visual impairment in the U.S.* (2nd ed.). New York: American Foundation for the Blind.

Oehler, J., & Fitzgerald, R. G. (1980). Group therapy with blind diabetics. *Archives of General Psychiatry, 37*: 463-467.

Poon, L. W. (1980). *Aging in the 1980s: Psychological issues.* Washington, DC: American Psychological Association.

Salmon, H. E. (1981). Theories of aging, disability, and loss. *Journal of Rehabilitation, 47*: 44-50.

Schneider, E. L., & Brody, J. A. (1983). Aging, natural death, and the compression of morbidity: Another view. *New England Journal of Medicine, 309*: 854-856.

Scott, R. A. (1969). *The making of blind men. A study of adult socialization.* New York: Russell Sage Foundation.

Sekuler, R., Kline, D., Dismukes, K., & Adams, A. J. (1983). Some research needs in aging and visual perception. *Vision Research, 23*(3): 213-216.

Social Security Administration. (1983). Relative importance of the aged, 1980. *Social Security Bulletin,* p. 46.

Stern, M. F. (1969). Activity or idleness: Restoration of social contacts among elderly blind. *The New Outlook for the Blind, 3*(6): 185-189.

Strehler, B. L. (1979). Implications of aging research for society. In J. Hendricks & C. D. Hendricks (Eds.), *Dimensions of aging* (pp. 84-90). Cambridge, MA: Winthrop.

U.S. Department of Commerce, Bureau of the Census. (1982). Current population reports, Series P-60, No. 134. *Money, income and poverty status of families and persons in the United States: 1981.* Washington, DC: Author.

U.S. Department of Commerce, Bureau of the Census. (1983). Current population reports, Series P-23, No. 128. *America in transition: An aging society.* Washington, DC: Author.

U.S. Department of Commerce, Bureau of the Census. (1989). *Projections of the population of the United States by age, sex, and race, 1988-2080,* Series P-25, No. 1018. Washington, DC: Author.

Walsh, D. A., Krauss, I. K., & Reneger, V. A. (1981). Spatial ability, environmental knowledge, and environmental use: The elderly. In L. S. Lisbon, A. H. Patterson, & N. Newcombe (Eds.), *Spatial representation and behavior across the lifespan* (pp. 321-357). New York: Academic Press.

White House Conference on Aging. (1981). *Chartbook on aging in America.* Washington, DC: Author.

CHAPTER 5

Psychological Aspects of Aging and Visual Impairment

Steven H. Zarit

Many people believe that the aging process results in irreversible and catastrophic declines in psychological abilities. Fortunately, this negative perception does not apply to the majority of individuals who are over age 65. Although some persons suffer serious psychological declines reflected in such feelings as despair and extreme depression as they age, the majority of older people remain competent and able to respond to the various challenges in their lives, including the physical, environmental, social, and psychological challenges related to the aging process.

Expectations of decline with aging have been widely exaggerated for several reasons. First, many people confuse senile dementia with the effects of aging and believe that all older persons have major psychological impairments. Second, a significant proportion of the differences in the abilities of older persons compared to younger persons is the result of generational factors, not age-related declines. Third, the effects of aging are highly variable. Some people experience decremental changes, but others show little change or improve in some abilities even into the eighth decade of life.

This chapter reviews findings on psychological changes taking place during aging. It addresses why aging is so frequently associated in the popular mind with decline and then draws on research to present a balanced perspective on aging that includes the possibilities both of decline and of continued development throughout the life span. In addition, it reviews findings on the psychological aspects of aging, discussing cognitive abilities such as intelligence and memory, as well as personality and social behavior. Finally, it examines common problems in the assessment and treatment of older persons with visual impairment.

Dementia

To understand the effects of aging on psychological functioning and behavior, it is critical to distinguish between the normal aging process and senile dementia. Senile dementia is a syndrome involving the progressive impairment of memory and other cognitive functions. Personality changes and the loss of the ability to carry out even the most basic activities of daily living, such as dressing and feeding oneself, also result. Individuals with dementia will be recognizable by their extreme forgetfulness. Unlike the average older person, who like anyone else forgets occasionally but with little consequence for everyday functioning, the person with dementia may be unable to remember from one minute to the next.

Although senile dementia was once considered the outcome of the aging process, it is now known to be caused by a group of diseases that produce degenerative changes in the brain and the permanent, persistent loss of memory (Cummings & Benson, 1983; Zarit, 1980). These diseases affect only a minority of older persons; most epidemiological surveys place the prevalence of dementia at 4 to 7 percent of the older population (Mortimer, Schuman, & French, 1981).

The most prevalent type of dementia is Alzheimer's disease, or senile dementia of the Alzheimer type, as it is sometimes called. Alzheimer's disease accounts for approximately 50 to 60 percent of all cases of dementia. It is the fourth leading cause of death in this country. The disorder is characterized by peculiar pathologies in the brain that are absent or found only to a minimal degree in normal aging (Roth, 1980). These changes include senile plaques, neurofibrillary tangles, granulovascular structures, and the substantial loss of brain neurons. The disease is progressive, leading to widespread pathology in the brain and concomitant decrements in cognition and behavior.

When first described around the turn of the century, Alzheimer's disease was called presenile dementia—a speeding up of the aging process—and was believed to affect people ages 40 to 55 years. Recent advances have revealed that the changes in the brain found in presenile dementia are similar or identical to those in the majority of persons over age 65 with symptoms of dementia. Patients with Alzheimer's disease have been as young as 30, but the prevalence is greatest past age 70.

The cause of Alzheimer's disease is not known and is currently under intensive scientific investigation. Possible causes being studied include genetic predisposition, a slow virus or other infectious agent, immunological changes, or environmental toxic agents. Scientists are conducting research in molecular genetics, virology, neurology, pharmacology, epidemiology, biochemistry, and psychiatry to find the cause, treatment, and cure for the disease. Until a cure is discovered, good medical and social management can lessen the burden on family caregivers. A calm, well-structured environment can help the Alzheimer's patient along with social activity and physical exercise.

The other common kind of dementia is multi-infarct dementia, which accounts for approximately 10 to 20 percent of the cases. Multi-infarct dementia is produced when the person suffers a series of small strokes, or transient ischemic attacks, that damage brain tissue. As with Alzheimer's disease, multi-infarct dementia is progressive. Although the cause is not known, it is assumed that the same risk factors in stroke and heart disease are involved, including hypertension, elevated cholesterol level, excessive weight, lack of exercise, and smoking. Although there are currently no cures, early treatment of concomitant factors such as hypertension might retard the progression of the condition (Roth, 1980).

Several rarer diseases, including Pick's disease and Jacob Kreutzfeldt disease, can result in dementia. Diseases that affect the subcortical regions of the brain, including Huntington's chorea and Parkinson's disease, also lead to symptoms of dementia in some cases. (For more complete descriptions of such dementing illnesses, see Cummings & Benson, 1983.)

The diagnosis of dementia must be made carefully. There are no definitive tests for Alzheimer's disease or multi-infarct dementia, and confirmation of the diagnosis can be made only at autopsy. A number of treatable problems can also cause symptoms of dementia, or delirium, which is a syndrome of fluctuating consciousness and impairments in intellectual functions, and is sometimes misidentified as senile dementia in older patients. Among the treatable causes of dementia and delirium are drug toxicities, metabolic and endocrine disorders, infections, metallic poisoning, malnutrition, fractures, and alcohol intoxication (NIA Task Force, 1980). Sensory deprivation caused by the sudden loss of hearing or vision can also lead to transitory symptoms of dementia or delirium. Depressed older persons are sometimes mistakenly labeled as having dementia because they are lethargic and often complain about failing memory. Their complaints, however, are the result of distractibility, rather than a permanent impairment of memory. A diagnosis of dementia should be made only after a careful medical and psychological evaluation rules out these treatable conditions.

Such reversible problems can also make symptoms worse in someone with an irreversible dementia. All too often, treatable problems, such as drug toxicities, are overlooked, and increased symptoms are ascribed to the dementia. Although primary treatments are not yet available, prompt treatment of other health problems in someone with dementia minimizes cognitive disturbances.

The distinction between senility and normal aging has practical implications. When older persons forget or act in ways that are unusual or that other people find upsetting, there is a tendency to ascribe the cause to age or senility and not to look for other reasons for their behavior, including environmental and interpersonal factors. In clinical settings, for example, older patients are often described as "a little bit senile" when they do not respond readily to the clinician. But the term "senile dementia" needs to be reserved for the minority of older persons with brain diseases that impair the memory and intellect.

Ascribing an older person's behavior to "senility" in a casual way will lead to overlooking the many possible causes for someone's troubling behavior. These causes include anxiety, depression, loneliness, distractibility, poor hearing, limited education, and inadequate social skills. Behaviors that are the result of the loss of vision, such as not finding one's way around or not recognizing familiar faces, may even be mistaken for signs of senility. By identifying possible causes of problem behavior, professionals can implement appropriate interventions. If the older person does have dementia, interventions can be designed that take into account the individual's cognitive deficits. Treatment plans can be simplified, and it may be necessary to teach family members to prompt the patient to follow through with the regimen. Another consideration is to maintain patients in familiar, predictable environments where the cognitive demands do not become overwhelming or frustrating (Zarit, Orr, & Zarit, 1985).

In contrast to dementia, the changes in normal aging are not as extensive or rapid. As will be discussed in this chapter, memory and other cognitive abilities may decline with age, but these changes do not impair the older person's overall competence.

Generational Differences

Many of the effects ascribed to the aging process are actually the result of differences between generations or cohorts. When people compare old and young individuals, they typically ascribe any difference to aging, but it may be that older persons have not changed as they have aged. Rather, the difference may be the result of earlier learning, environmental or life-style influences, or other factors that shape the abilities and character of the older generation.

Most research on aging uses a cross-sectional research design—a comparison of younger and older persons at one point in time. According to Schaie (1976), cross-sectional comparisons confound age and cohort. Although differences may be the result of aging, the possibility of differences in cohorts cannot be ruled out. Another strategy for studying the aging process is to conduct a longitudinal study in which the same persons are followed over time. The changes that are identified may be the result of the aging process, although it is not possible to rule out other factors, such as intervening historical events and the uniqueness of the observed changes to the cohort. To overcome these limitations in cross-sectional and longitudinal studies, Schaie suggested following several cohorts over time, using what he called a cohort-sequential research design. By observing how several cohorts change over time, it is possible to separate the effects of aging, cohort, and historical events.

Using a cross-sequential design, Schaie and his associates (Baltes & Schaie, 1976; Schaie, 1990; Schaie, Labouvie, & Buech, 1973; Schaie & Labouvie-Vief, 1974; Schaie & Stone, 1982) demonstrated the importance of generational differences in several dimensions of intelligence. A sample of persons, ages 20 to 70 years at the time of the initial testing, has been followed for 35 years and was retested at 7-year intervals. The measure of intelligence was the Primary Mental Abilities (PMA) test (Thurstone & Thurstone, 1949). This test consists of five subtests that measure different factors of intelligence: verbal meaning, spatial abilities, reasoning, arithmetic abilities, and word fluency. Although there has been attrition in the sample through death (especially in the older groups) and failure to locate some subjects at retesting, the results are striking. If one considered only cross-sectional findings, a comparison across age groups for one time of testing, the older subjects had lower scores on all five subtests. But looking at scores over time, there was an age-related decline on only one subtest, word fluency. The other subtests of the PMA were stable at least up to age 60 or 67. Even at more advanced ages, many subjects had stable or improved scores between test intervals. The differences between cohorts observed at the first-time testing remained stable over time. In other words, cohorts had different levels of these mental abilities at the outset, and the differences between younger and older persons were not the result of age-related decline.

These findings have caused a major revision of thinking about the relation of intelligence to age. Before these studies, findings of cross-sectional studies had been interpreted to indicate that mental abilities peaked during the third decade (Wechsler, 1958). Schaie and Labouvie-Vief (1974) place the period of decline much later in the life span for many components of intelligence (see also Schaie, 1990). Even then, some individuals continue to show stability of scores.

Cohort differences in personality have also been found. Schaie and Labouvie-Vief (1974) reported cohort differences in two dimensions of rigidity, motor-cognitive and perceptual-personality rigidity. A third measure, psychomotor speed, showed an age change. It is interesting to note that the older cohort had better overall psychological adjustment when they were 19 and 44 years of age than did the younger cohort at age 19.

These studies point out how important it is to consider that differences between old and young individuals may have causes other than age-related decline. If older persons are more conservative, for instance, at least some of the difference may be the result of their adopting these values when they were young, rather than because they have grown older. One way to improve intergenerational communication is to understand some of these generational differences and to learn about the cultural, societal, and historical events that shaped the lives of today's older persons when they were young.

Individual Differences

In evaluating how much decline occurs in aging, it is important to take into account the considerable individual differences among older persons. On virtually any psychological test, and many physiological indicators as well, there is a greater variance among older persons than among younger persons (Schonfield, 1974; Tobin, 1977).

One possible implication of these observations is that age-related declines occur at different ages for different people. The extent of change may also vary from person to person. The findings from Schaie's cohort-sequential study suggest that people do not decline at the same age. A related hypothesis is that some portion of decline is related to changes in health, rather than solely to aging. The significant changes caused by dementing illness have already been noted. In addition to dementia, studies have found that persons with cardiovascular disease perform more poorly on a variety of measures, including intelligence (Birren, Butler, Greenhouse, Sokoloff, & Yarrow, 1963; Wilkie & Eisdorfer, 1973). In contrast, healthy older persons differ little from younger persons. These findings suggest that health status and the level of physical functioning may be more important for determining psychological functioning than chronological age. Also, older people may differ more from one another than from the young because their experiences have made them different. Although children move through an age-graded school system in which they have experiences similar to others in their cohort, the adult years are marked by fewer age-graded events that are shared by most people. People have widely different careers and marital, familial, and leisure-time experiences. The result of these variations in experience is that people become more different from one another as they age.

Because older people differ considerably from one another, it is not easy to generalize that all older people are a certain way. Their psychological functioning may be good, poor, or anything in between, and age will be a relatively weak predictor compared to other factors, such as health and past experience. Therefore, each individual needs to be viewed as unique. In regard to the following discussion, it is important to keep in mind how changes vary from person to person.

Age-Related Differences in Cognitive Abilities

INTELLIGENCE

The most studied question in the psychology of aging is whether changes in intelligence take place as we age. As was noted, there seems to be little change on some dimensions of intelligence, especially those involving verbal abilities, until late in life. On dimensions involving nonverbal or novel tasks, substantial age-related differences have usually been reported.

Some theorists, particularly Horn and Cattell (1967), have proposed that tests using verbal, familiar material represent a different type of intelligence than do tests of nonverbal and novel tasks (see also Horn & Donaldson, 1976). The verbal tasks are considered to represent stored or acquired knowledge and are called "crystallized intelligence." The novel tasks represent the ability to apply a generalized intellectual ability to new problems or situations. This type of intelligence is called "fluid intelligence."

From this perspective, it is assumed that the decline in fluid abilities is the result of age-related changes in the brain. There is some loss of brain neurons with aging, although the amount of loss is minor compared to what occurs in dementing illnesses. An alternative hypothesis is that the results may be an artifact of testing. Speed is typically a factor in tests of fluid intelligence. Older persons may be at a disadvantage when they must respond quickly and within brief time limits, although the allowance of more time has not resulted in significantly improved performance (Storandt, 1977).

It is also argued that older persons are less familiar with and have less practice in fluid tasks than do the college students with whom they are usually compared. One study that investigated this proposition by training older persons in a task of fluid intelligence (Willis, Blieszner, & Baltes, 1981) found that the performance of older persons improved as the result of training and on a related test of fluid intelligence for which they had no training. The researchers interpreted these findings to suggest that intellectual performance is modifiable throughout the life cycle and that some of the age differences in fluid intelligence may be the result of a lack of experience or practice.

The overall picture is that selective abilities decline with age. Although this decline might be related to age changes in the brain that accompany aging, it is also possible that many older persons are able to improve their abilities when given the proper training.

MEMORY

Perhaps the most widely held belief about aging is that memory declines. As with other abilities, the change is not as extensive as previously thought. In part, the expectation of memory loss is the result of viewing dementia as the outcome of aging, rather than as a disease. Although there is substantial memory loss with dementia, changes in the memory of a healthy older person are more benign.

The most significant age-related differences in memory involve the ability to take in new information. Once material is learned, the older person's subsequent recall is the same or almost the same as that of younger persons (Botwinick, 1978; Craik, 1977). These age differences are greater or smaller, depending on the testing conditions and the type of material to be remembered. In divided-attention experiments in which subjects are distracted by competing stimuli, learning and memory are more disrupted for older persons than for younger persons. The pacing of exposure to material is also important. When older persons are given more time to study verbal stimuli and to give their responses during the test period, age-related differences are reduced (Canestrari, 1963). Another factor that affects age differences in memory is whether the information to be learned and remembered is meaningful. The performance of older persons is substantially poorer than that of younger persons when less meaningful material, such as nonsense syllables, is used. But it is the same or nearly the same when more familiar material is used (Hulicka, 1967). In everyday situations, hearing and vision loss are likely to make learning and remembering information more difficult.

A common observation made by and about older persons is that they remember the past but cannot recall what happened recently. When older persons say they remember the past as if it were yesterday, they may be thinking about major life events, such as marriage or the birth of a child, that have important personal significance. What happened in the past week usually pales in comparison. Another factor is that all people reminisce, which enhances old memory. People may remember best those memories that are periodically rehearsed.

Some recent studies have highlighted problems that older persons have in recalling old information. For instance, the recall of the names of persons in one's high school class decreases over time (Bahrick, Bahrick, & Wittlinger, 1975). Older persons also experience more "tip of the tongue" responses for names of well-known persons—they feel they know the name but cannot recall it. It is interesting to note that when presented with a multiple-choice question on items for which they had a tip-of-the-tongue response, older persons can usually pick the correct name; they also will pick wrong answers for the items they initially stated they did not know (Lachman, Lachman, & Thronesberry, 1979). Overall, they appear to have a large fund of information from which to draw.

In another experiment, Botwinick and Storandt (1974) asked historical questions that were organized by decades, for example, the 1930s and

1940s. Their subjects tended to recall best the events that occurred when they were 15 to 25 years old. It has been speculated that the problems observed in regard to memory of newly learned items are related to the changes in the brain that occur in normal aging, especially alterations in the hippocampus, which is involved in memory. At a psychological level, one hypothesis is that older people cannot encode new information as "deeply" as can younger persons. They are unable to make as many associations to stimuli and therefore do not learn or remember as efficiently as do young people (Hartley, Harker, & Welsh, 1980). An alternative hypothesis is that older people simply do not use efficient learning strategies. For instance, they are less likely than are younger people to try to remember by organizing the stimuli or by using mnemonics, and their performance improves if they use some strategy (Denny, 1974; Hultsch, 1969, 1975; Whitbourne, & Slevin, 1978).

These findings suggest a number of practical steps that may be helpful for improving memory. First, recall is improved if the material to be remembered is presented slowly and the older person has sufficient time to study it. Second, older persons also do better if there are fewer distractions. Third, when there is vision or hearing loss, stimuli can be presented in ways that overcome these deficits to whatever extent is possible. Fourth, the use of mental strategies improves performance. Finally, basic strategies, such as making notes and keeping an appointment book, should not be overlooked for dealing with specific memory problems.

One clinically relevant dimension of memory is that older people's evaluations of their abilities can be misleading. Persons with dementia, for instance, are less likely to complain about failing memory than are older persons with no evidence of dementia, even though persons with dementia have significantly more memory problems (Kahn, Zarit, Hilbert, & Niederehe, 1975). Furthermore, persons who complain more of failing memory are not more likely to develop dementia than are those who report fewer problems. Older persons who are depressed also complain more about failing memory, even though their performance on tests differs little or not at all from nondepressed persons (Kahn, Zarit, Hilbert, & Niederehe, 1975; Popkin, Gallagher, Thompson, & Moore, 1982; Zarit, 1982).

There are several reasons for the discrepancies between complaint and performance. Persons with dementia may complain less than do normal older persons because their memory is so poor that they cannot remember. Their refusal to acknowledge their problem may also be part of a protective denial. Trying to make dementia patients aware of their deficits is often upsetting to them, and they typically will not acknowledge any problem. In contrast, normal older people notice everyday instances of forgetting. If they are concerned about the loss of memory or with becoming senile, they may be more upset when they forget ordinary things. They may not be forgetting much more than they ever did, but they worry that they are suffering from a major decline. This tendency to magnify the significance of complaints is especially pronounced in those who are depressed. The reassurance that a certain amount of forgetting is normal is often sufficient to lessen the older person's concerns about failing memory (Zarit, Cole, & Guider, 1981; Zarit, Gallagher, & Kramer, 1980).

REACTION TIME

Perhaps the most consistent finding in research on aging is the slowing of reaction time. Although there is considerable individual difference in the amount of slowing down, most persons have slower reactions as they age. Slowing is apparent even in the simplest experiments, such as those involving the pressing of a lever when a light comes on. When more complex decisions are required, older persons may be disproportionately slower than younger persons.

The significance of reaction time is that it reflects the speed at which the nervous system processes information. Reaction-time experiments can be divided into premotor and motor components. The premotor component is the time it takes to decide to act; the motor component is the time of the action itself, such as the moving of one's arm to press a lever. With aging, slowing occurs primarily in the premotor or decision-making time (Botwinick, 1978; Botwinick & Thompson, 1966). Decreased reaction time appears to be the result primarily of a slowing in the central nervous system, rather than in the peripheral neural pathways (Birren & Botwinick, 1955).

As stated earlier in this chapter, speed is a factor in age-related differences in intelligence and memory. It is also likely that many older persons have increased difficulties with tasks that have to be completed at a fast pace or decisions that must be made quickly.

Personality and Aging

Personality refers to the characteristic ways that people view themselves and adapt to different situations. In our culture, there are both positive and negative expectations for personality changes in aging. On the positive side is the expectation that one may overcome the problems of early life and approach events with confidence and the wisdom that comes from experience. Belief in the role of the wise elder who can see beyond immediate events to universal principles or truths is found in many cultures. At the other extreme, there are also the beliefs that people's faults become more pronounced as they age and that the problems they had when they were young will be magnified in old age.

ERIKSONIAN THEORY

For a long time, the dominant view was that personality development is completed before adulthood and little change occurs after that time until there is generalized decline in late life. Most theorists now agree with the position articulated by Erikson (1963) that personality development continues through the adult years. Erikson views a life cycle of eight distinct stages, each involving a different psychological conflict. The conflict grows out of the interaction between the social and cultural demands placed on the individual at that period of life and his or her biological and psychological capacities. The conflict in each stage is resolved either in a positive or negative way. For instance, Erikson suggested that early adulthood presents the conflicts of intimacy versus isolation. One can develop a close, caring relationship with another individual or retreat into oneself, feeling lonely and disappointed in relationships. Moreover, the effects of the stages are cumulative. In each stage, one builds on the strengths and weaknesses that one carries from the past. Erikson's eight stages of life and the psychosocial conflict in each are as follows:

- *Infancy:* basic trust versus mistrust
- *Toddlerhood:* autonomy versus shame and doubt
- *Early childhood:* initiative versus guilt
- *School-age years:* industry versus inferiority
- *Adolescence:* identity versus identity confusion
- *Young adulthood:* intimacy versus isolation
- *Middle age:* generativity versus stagnation
- *Old age:* integrity versus despair.

The psychological task that Erikson considers paramount in old age is integrity versus despair. Integrity is the belief that one has lived one's life as well as one could. Because older people do not have time to start over if they have not achieved their goals or are dissatisfied with parts of their lives, their psychological well-being depends on accepting these limitations without undue regret or guilt. The alternative is a sense of despair.

DISENGAGEMENT THEORY VERSUS ACTIVITY THEORY

Although Erikson focused on subjective psychological conflict, other theories have been concerned with the role of activities and social involvements in old age. The theory that has provoked the most controversy is the disengagement theory of aging proposed by Cumming and Henry (1961). As is implicit in Erikson's ideas, the disengagement theory proposes that the major psychological issue in later life is the possibility of physical decline and death. According to this theory, it is best for aging individuals and for society if older persons gradually give up or disengage from activities and involvements, rather than be forced to give them up because of physical or mental impairments. Cumming and Henry, on a sample of healthy middle-aged and older persons, suggested that disengagement might begin as early as the fifties and occur before the person has suffered any major losses in health. Moreover, Cumming and Henry believed that disengaged persons were better adapted in later life.

The disengagement theory has been the subject of considerable criticism. Most studies have not replicated the findings of Cumming and Henry. In contrast to the theory, disengagement has sometimes been found to be associated with poor health, the loss of income or of a spouse, or other negative changes. One major study, however, partially supported the theory. Lowenthal, Thurnher, and Chiriboga (1975) reported that among older persons approaching retirement, those with the least responsibilities and demands had the highest morale. In contrast, individuals who sought out challenges and were viewed by the raters as the most creative and psychologically healthy had lower morale.

The antithesis of the disengagement theory is the activity theory. The activity theory posits that successful aging is associated with maintaining as many involvements as one had when younger, if possible, or replacing those that are lost through retirement or other changes with new activities. Many older people endorse this position and suggest that activity contributes to their health and morale. Increasingly, older people seem to lead more active and productive lives. One reason for this change is that older people are healthier and have more lifestyle options than older people in previous generations. According to Neugarten (1972), the young-old, those 65 to 74, are less likely to have the physical and mental frailties associated with aging. These persons often maintain high levels of activities and social involvement.

Activity level, however, is not sufficient by itself to account for one's overall adaptation to later life. Neugarten, Havighurst, and Tobin (1968) proposed that personality style is more important than activity level; for example, persons who are rigid or defensive will adapt poorly, whatever their level of activity. Other factors include the availability of an intimate relationship, good health, opportunities for creativity, and a social network. Poor health, of course, can limit one's activities and satisfaction with life.

ADAPTABILITY AND OTHER TRAITS

Research on personality and age has also considered how specific traits or characteristics might change with age. Despite the contradictory or inconclusive results that have been found for many of the characteristics studied, investigations on four traits—rigidity, cautiousness, extroversion, and neuroticism—are worth noting. As was stated earlier in this chapter, older people may appear more rigid than younger persons, but these results are attributable primarily to cohort differences rather than to the aging process. Cautiousness has been studied in test-taking behavior, as has risk taking in games or simulated life situations. In their response to tests of memory and other cognitive abilities, older persons are more reluctant to guess than are younger persons and will make more errors of omission (Botwinick, 1978). Errors of omission account for at least part of the difference in cognitive performance between younger and older persons. Similarly, older people have been observed to take fewer risks in games (Okun & DiVesta, 1976) and to be more cautious about making life changes in hypothetical situations (Botwinick, 1966; Wallach & Kogan, 1961). When risk taking is encouraged or rewarded, however, older persons respond appropriately and take more risks (Birkhill & Schaie, 1975).

An important indicator of the adaptability of older persons is rate of psychopathology. With the exception of brain disorders, the prevalence of major psychiatric disorders does not significantly increase with age. The rates of such disorders as serious depression are high, with estimates ranging from 5 to 15 percent (Blazer, 1982), though some recent studies (Blazer, Hughes, & George, 1987) place the prevalence much lower. Rates among elderly people are comparable to or lower than those found in middle age (Weissman & Myers, 1978). If only those patients whose symptoms have occurred for the first time in old age are considered, then the rates are even lower. Overall, older people generally report higher morale and more satisfaction with their lives than do persons in other age groups.

The adaptability of older persons is borne out by studies of their response to major life changes, such as widowhood and retirement. Neither of these events is associated with significant rates of mental illness. The major problems reported by widows are lowered income and loneliness (Lopata, 1973). Studies of retired persons suggest that many people are happy with retirement. Dissatisfaction is related to having retired involuntarily, having an inadequate income, or being in poor health (George, 1980; Kimmel, Price, & Walker, 1978; Palmore, 1972; Shanas, 1970; Streib & Schneider, 1971).

Social Relationships

Social relationships are an important mediator of stressful life events in old age. The family plays the largest role. Rather than withering away, as some social scientists predicted, the family remains a viable support for most older persons. The majority of older people live within driving distance of one or more children and have regular contact with them (Shanas, 1979). Furthermore, families provide considerable assistance to older persons who are in poor health. Assistance will be provided first by a spouse or, if there is no spouse, by adult children. If there are no children, siblings or other relatives help out (Shanas, 1979). Even when there is a devastating illness, such as Alzheimer's disease, family members, particularly adult daughters or daughters-in-law, often serve as caregivers (Zarit & Zarit, 1983). In addition, it should not be overlooked that the relationship between aged parents and adult children is reciprocal, and older parents continue to give assistance to their children in a variety of ways (Bengtson, 1982). This reciprocal relationship allows the healthy state of interdependence between parent and adult child.

A critical type of support is provided by a confidant, either a relative or a friend. Older men tend to name their wives as confidants, whereas women are more likely to name friends (Lowenthal & Robinson, 1976). Having a confidant has been found to be associated with better adaptation to retirement and widowhood. It does not, however, buffer the effects of illness (Lowenthal & Haven, 1968).

Although many families are a source of support to older persons, some are in conflict. Increased dependence because of an illness, for instance, can exacerbate long-standing marital or family problems. In some cases, the family's positive strengths can be brought out by providing information about the relative's health problems and by keeping discussions focused on the immediate problems, rather than letting family members bring up long-standing conflicts (Zarit & Zarit, 1983; Zarit, Orr, & Zarit, 1985). In other instances, marital or family therapy can lessen tensions that are aggravated by stressful events (Gilewski, Kuppinger, & Zarit, 1985).

Overall, many older people are able to respond and adapt to the changes in their lives. In the absence of serious debilitating illness, psychological changes tend to be mild and benign. Some persons, however, lose their capacity to adapt because of illness or other adverse circumstances. Others will carry into old age the problems and conflicts that restricted their earlier lives. It is important to avoid stereotyping older persons as a group. People are not good and wise or mean and rigid just because they are old. They are, rather, the products of their own generational and life experiences, and they respond in unique ways to the changes and limitations placed on them as they age at their own individual rates.

Vision Loss and Adjustment in Old Age

In the preceding sections, many of the positive findings about psychological changes with aging were highlighted. Probably the most serious obstacle to successful adaptation is poor health. Eye disorders in later life present special challenges. The loss of vision at any age requires considerable changes in how one manages everyday life. Given the psychological changes that occur with aging, there are reasons to believe that older persons are disadvantaged in adjusting to the loss of vision. For instance, such qualities as increased caution and slower learning do not have any adverse effects on the healthy older person, but they may make adaptation to the loss of vision or readiness to participate in a rehabilitation program more difficult. It is also likely that the older person with a vision loss may have other health problems that make adaptation harder. The effects of impairments are cumulative; someone with arthritis and poor vision will have more problems with mobility than will someone with only poor vision. Older people with both hearing and vision loss present special challenges to service providers.

VARIABILITY OF REACTIONS

Older persons who experience vision loss in late life have various reactions, depending on other life circumstances. Some find it difficult to consider contacting an agency for blind or visually impaired persons or to receive services, such as rehabilitation teaching, orientation and mobility instruction, and the use of low vision devices. Many others make an excellent adjustment to their vision loss and are able to lead fulfilling lives. The case of Mrs. B is an example:

> Mrs. B, a 70-year-old woman, suffered a vision loss related to glaucoma and cataracts. Surgery to correct her condition was not successful. Although her visual acuity was fairly good when measured under ideal conditions (about 20/80), she had restricted fields and was photophobic, and both limited her mobility outdoors. She also had severe back problems and could not walk long distances. Because of these limitations, she virtually had not left her apartment for the year since her eye surgery, except for weekly shopping trips in a van provided by a senior center. She also had a limited income, receiving only social security and Supplemental Security Income.
>
> After she was examined at a low vision center, Mrs. B began to receive rehabilitation services that began with mobility training so she could use buses to travel to appointments. She also was prescribed low vision devices for near tasks and for use in sunlight. But her life was still restricted to her apartment and the occasional visits to the clinic. She longed for more stimulation and especially for companionship. She expressed a desire to paint, something she had not done previously but that had always interested her.
>
> With the help of the staff at the clinic, Mrs. B located a painting class at a senior center and worked out bus routes so she could get there. The instructor, however, was upset by her visual impairment and told her she could not take the class because she could not see well enough. She was dismayed by this response but soon found another class, which proved to be a success. She developed quickly as an artist, working as much as four hours a day at home, and subsequently won prizes for her work. She also now participates in other activities, such as taking courses at a community college.

This example is noteworthy because Mrs. B overcame multiple disabilities to make a satisfactory adjustment. It also illustrates the potential that many older visually impaired people have for responding to interventive efforts. In addition, it provides support for the activity theory of aging. The implication is that activities are the best antidote to the sadness caused by the irreversible losses associated with aging and illness. Helping older persons overcome their limitations and increase their activity level is often the goal of rehabilitation efforts. There are times, however, when more activity may not be appropriate. Some individuals have genuinely accepted their losses and do not seem to need or want more activity. They may be satisfied with their current levels of activity, but it is still important to convey to them the benefits of available rehabilitation and related services so that they are aware of this option.

Rehabilitation interventions are complex, and positive results are not always apparent at the onset. Usually out of fear, some older patients with vision problems are unwilling to learn new ways of carrying out routine tasks or to try new activities, often out of fear. As already mentioned, multiple health problems and impairments may be complicating factors. But it is important that older visually impaired persons know what services are available to them and the kinds of skills that can be learned so they have the option of taking advantage of these services when and if they are ready.

ASPECTS OF ADAPTATION

Lack of knowledge of one's condition or denial of visual impairment is a frequent obstacle to successful adaptation. Many older patients believe that what they need is a new pair of eyeglasses, and they may reject other approaches to help them. A thorough explanation of their condition and information about the alternatives available to them are often useful in breaking down barriers to accepting help. Many older patients must first exhaust all possibilities for a "cure" of their condition before beginning a rehabilitation or intervention program.

Another reason why an older person may experience difficulty adjusting relates to his or her learning skills. Important skills and traits involve being able to break down tasks into small steps, not giving up too quickly on something new, and not being self-conscious. These abilities can be illustrated in relation to the task of learning to read with magnification. Initially, some persons experience considerable frustration using magnification because they are unable to read fast or accurately enough. If they practice with simple material first, such as pairs of words or sentences, they will be better able to master more complex reading matter. Sometimes, older persons complain that magnification does not allow them to see as before, and they will give it up, even when they might benefit considerably. Their only goal is complete recovery, and they reject anything that falls short. By helping them formulate more limited and realistic goals, such as being able to read slowly, professionals can help them overcome their initial frustration. Sometimes patients give up because they find low vision devices awkward to use. Encouraging them to be patient, to give themselves time to become comfortable with a device, and to measure their progress in small steps can make a difference. Finally, some feel self-conscious using devices in public. But often they overcome their reluctance when they meet others who are using devices successfully.

The last reason for poor adaptation to the loss of vision is demoralization or depression. Although some patients become markedly depressed, a more common pattern is to become passive and withdrawn. Demoralization is likely to be part of the various problems just described. Demoralized older patients can be particularly frustrating to other people. They complain a lot but do little to help themselves. The reason for their complaints and passivity is that they do not believe anything they do makes a difference. It is important to help them verbalize these beliefs and identify ways in which their lives can continue to have meaning. For more severely depressed older persons, psychiatric treatment, including the use of antidepressant medications and psychotherapy, is beneficial (Gallagher & Thompson, 1983; Zarit, 1980).

As with other aspects of aging, response to vision loss is highly variable. And as with patients of any age, the time and effort spent with older patients is often rewarded. Neither the effects of aging nor the impact of vision loss is too insurmountable to overcome.

References

Bahrick, H. P., Bahrick, P. O., & Wittlinger, R. P. (1975). Fifty years of memory for names and faces: A cross-sectional approach. *Journal of Experimental Psychology: General, 104*: 54-57.

Baltes, P. B., & Schaie, K. W. (1976). On the plasticity of intelligence in adulthood and old age: Where Horn and Donaldson fail. *American Psychologist, 31*: 720-725.

Bengtson, V. L. (1982). Bridging the generation gap. In S. H. Zarit (Ed.), *Readings in aging and death: Contemporary perspectives* (2nd ed., pp. 129-138). New York: Harper & Row.

Birkhill, W. R., & Schaie, K. W. (1975). The effect of differential reinforcement of cautiousness in intellectual performance among the elderly. *Journal of Gerontology, 30:* 578-583.

Birren, J. E., & Botwinick, J. (1955). Age differences in finger, jaw, and foot reaction time to auditory stimuli. *Journal of Gerontology, 10:* 429-432.

Birren, J. E., Butler, R. N., Greenhouse, S. W., Sokoloff, L., & Yarrow, M. (1963). *Human aging: A biological and behavioral study.* Washington, DC: U.S. Department of Health, Education, and Welfare.

Blazer, D. G. (1982). *Depression in late life.* St. Louis: C. V. Mosby.

Blazer, D. G., Hughes, D. C., & George, L. K. (1987). The epidemiology of depression in an elderly community population. *The Gerontologist, 27:* 281-287.

Botwinick, J. (1966). Cautiousness in advanced age. *Journal of Gerontology, 21:* 347-353.

Botwinick, J. (1978). *Aging and behavior* (2nd ed.). New York: Springer.

Botwinick, J., & Storandt, M. (1974). *Memory, related functions, and age.* Springfield, IL: Charles C Thomas.

Botwinick, J., & Thompson, L. W. (1966). Components of reaction time in relation to age and sex. *Journal of Genetic Psychology, 108:* 175-183.

Canestrari, R. E., Jr. (1963). Paced and self-paced learning in young and elderly adults. *Journal of Gerontology, 18:* 165-168.

Craik, F. I. M. (1977). Age differences in human memory. In J. E. Birren & K. W. Schaie (Eds.), *Handbook of the psychology of aging* (pp. 384-420). New York: Van Nostrand Reinhold.

Cumming, E., & Henry W. (1961). *Growing old: A process of disengagement.* New York: Basic Books.

Cummings, J. L., & Benson, D. F. (1983). *Dementia: A clinical approach.* Boston: Butterworth.

Denny, N. W. (1974). Evidence for development change in categorization criteria for children and adults. *Human Development, 17:* 41-53.

Erikson, E. H. (1963). Childhood and society (2nd ed.). New York: W. W. Norton.

Gallagher, D., & Thompson, L. W. (1983). Depression. In P. M. Lewinsohn & L. Teri (Eds.), *Clinical geropsychology* (pp. 7-37). New York: Pergamon.

George, L. K. (1980). *Role transitions in later life.* Monterey, CA: Brooks/Cole.

Gilewski, M. J., Kuppinger, J., & Zarit, S. H. (1985). The aging marital system: A case study in life changes and paradoxical intervention. *Clinical Gerontologist, 3*(3), 3-15.

Hartley, J. T., Harker, J. O., & Welsh, D. A. (1980). Contemporary issues and new directions in adult development of learning and memory. In L. W. Poon (Ed.), *Aging in the 1980s: Psychological issues.* Washington, DC: American Psychological Association.

Horn, J. L., & Cattell, R. B. (1967). Age differences in fluid and crystallized intelligence. *Acta Psychologist, 26:* 107-129.

Horn, J. L., & Donaldson, G. (1976). On the myth of intellectual decline in adulthood. *American Psychologist, 31*(10): 701-719.

Hulicka, I. M. (1967). Age differences in retention as a function of interference. *Journal of Gerontology, 22:* 46-51.

Hultsch, D. F. (1969). Adult age differences in the organization of free recall. *Developmental Psychology, 1:* 673-678.

Hultsch, D. F. (1975). Adult age differences in retrieval: Trace-dependent and cue-dependent forgetting. *Developmental Psychology, 11:* 197-201.

Kahn, R. L., Zarit, S. H., Hilbert, N. M., & Niederehe, G. (1975). Memory complaint and impairment in the aged. *Archives of General Psychiatry, 32:* 1569-1573.

Kimmel, D. C., Price, K. F., & Walker, J. W. (1978). Retirement choice and retirement satisfaction. *Journal of Gerontology, 33:* 575-585.

Lachman, J. L., Lachman, R., & Thronesberry, C. (1979). Metamemory through the adult life-span. *Developmental Psychology, 15:* 543-551.

Lopata, H. Z. (1973). *Widowhood in an American city.* Cambridge, MA: Schenkman.

Lowenthal, M. F., & Haven, C. (1968). Interaction and adaptation: Intimacy as a critical variable. *American Sociological Review, 33:* 20-30.

Lowenthal, M. F., & Robinson, B. (1976). Social networks and isolation. In R. H. Bionstock & E. Shanas (Eds.), *Handbook of aging and the social sciences* (pp. 432-456). New York: Van Nostrand Reinhold.

Lowenthal, M. F., Thurnher, M., & Chiriboga, D. (1975). *Four stages of life.* San Francisco: Jossey-Bass.

Mortimer, J. A., Schuman, L. M., & French, L. R. (1981). Epidemiology of dementing illness. In J. A. Mortimer & L. M. Schuman (Eds.), *The epidemiology of dementia* (pp. 3-23). New York: Oxford University Press.

Neugarten, B. L. (1972). Personality and the aging process. *The Gerontologist, 12:* 9-15.

Neugarten, B. L., Havighurst, R. J., & Tobin, S. S. (1968). Personality and patterns of aging. In B. L. Neugarten (Ed.), *Middle age and aging* (pp. 173-177). Chicago: University of Chicago Press.

NIA Task Force. (1980). Senility reconsidered. *Journal of the American Medical Association, 244*(3): 259-263.

Okun, M. A., & DiVesta, F. J. (1976). Cautiousness in adulthood as a function of age and instructions. *Journal of Gerontology, 32:* 451-455.

Palmore, E. B. (1972). Compulsory vs. flexible retirement: Issues and facts. *The Gerontologist, 12:* 343-348.

Popkin, S. J., Gallagher, D., Thompson, L. W., & Moore, M. (1982). Memory complaint and performance in normal and depressed older adults. *Experimental Aging Research, 8:* 141-145.

Roth, M. (1980). Senile dementia and its borderlands. In J. O. Cole & J. E. Barrett (Eds.), *Psychopathology in the aged* (pp. 205-232). New York: Raven.

Schaie, K. W. (1976). Age changes and age differences. *The Gerontologist, 7:* 128-132.

Schaie, K. W. (1990). Intellectual development in adulthood. In J. E. Birren & K. W. Schaie (Eds.), *Handbook of the psychology of aging* (3rd ed., pp. 291-310). New York: Academic Press.

Schaie, K. W., & Labouvie-Vief, G. (1974). Generational versus ontogenetic components of changes in adult cognitive behavior: A fourteen year cross-sequential study. *Developmental Psychology, 10:* 305-320.

Schaie, K. W., Labouvie, G., & Buech, V. U. (1973). Generation and cohort-specific differences in adult cognitive functioning: A fourteen year study of independent samples. *Developmental Psychology, 9:* 151-166.

Schaie, K. W., & Stone, V. (1982). Psychological assessment. *Annual Review of Gerontology & Geriatrics, 3:* 329-360.

Schonfield, D. (1974). Translations in gerontology—From lab to life: Utilizing information. *American Psychologist, 29:* 796-801.

Shanas, E. (1970). Health and adjustment in retirement. *The Gerontologist, 10:* 19-21.

Shanas, E. (1979). The family as a social support system in old age. *The Gerontologist, 19:* 169-174.

Storandt, M. (1977). Age, ability, level, and method of administering and scoring the WAIS. *Journal of Gerontology, 32:* 175-178.

Streib, G. F., & Schneider, C. J. (1971). *Retirement in American society.* Ithaca, NY: Cornell University Press.

Thurstone, L., & Thurstone, T. (1949). *SRA Primary Mental Abilities.* Chicago: Research Associates.

Tobin, J. B. (1977). Normal aging: The inevitability syndrome. In S. H. Zarit (Ed.), *Readings in aging and death: Contemporary perspectives* (pp. 39-48). New York: Harper & Row.

Wallach, M. A., & Kogan, N. (1961). Aspects of judgment and decision making: Interrelationships and changes with age. *Behavioral Science, 6:* 23-36.

Wechsler, D. (1958). *The measurement and appraisal of adult intelligence.* New York: Psychological Corp.

Weissman, M. N., & Myers, J. K. (1978). Affective disorders in a U.S. urban community. *Archives of General Psychiatry, 35:* 1304-1307.

Whitbourne, S. K., & Slevin, A. E. (1978). Imagery and sentence retention in elderly and young adults. *Journal of Genetic Psychology, 133:* 287-298.

Wilkie, F., & Eisdorfer, C. (1973). Systemic disease and behavioral correlates. In L. F. Jarvik, C. Eisdorfer, & J. E. Blum (Eds.), *Intellectual functioning in adults: Psychological and biological influences* (pp. 21-30). New York: Springer.

Willis, S. L., Blieszner, R., & Baltes, P. B. (1981). Intellectual training research imaging: Modification of performance on the fluid ability of figural relations. *Journal of Educational Psychology, 73:* 41-50.

Zarit, S. H. (1980). *Aging and mental disorders: Psychological approaches to assessment and treatment.* New York: Free Press.

Zarit, S. H. (1982). Affective correlates of self-reports about memory of older persons. *International Journal of Behavioral Geriatrics, 1:* 25-34.

Zarit, S. H., Cole, K. D., & Guider, R. L. (1981). Memory training strategies and subjective complaints of memory in the aged. *The Gerontologist, 21:* 158-164.

Zarit, S. H., Gallagher, D., & Kramer, N. (1980). Memory training in the community aged: Effects on depression, memory complaint and memory performance. *Educational Gerontology, 6:* 11-27.

Zarit, S. H., Orr, N. K., & Zarit, J. M. (1985). *Families under stress: Interventions for Alzheimer's disease and related dementias.* New York: New York University Press.

Zarit, S. H., & Zarit, J. M. (1983). Families under stress: Interventions for caregivers of dementia patients. *Psychotherapy, 19:* 461-471.

CHAPTER 6

Hearing Impairment among Older Persons: A Factor in Communication

Harold L. Bate

Although the focus of this book is on aging and visual impairment, it is important that service providers in the fields of aging and blindness have an understanding of hearing impairment and its impact on the older individual. Many older persons encounter both hearing and vision loss. As a consequence of various age-related changes in the auditory system, older persons encounter certain kinds of auditory disturbances that are less characteristic of younger people. Even when the auditory problems that develop are the same as those experienced by younger persons with hearing impairments, the degree of difficulty experienced by older persons is greater. These auditory problems include the following:

- difficulty in hearing speech and other sounds of daily living because they are not loud enough,
- difficulty in understanding speech, even in quiet situations, because of a lack of clarity attributable to the loss of the ability to hear high frequencies,
- difficulty in understanding speech in the midst of background noise because of the particular pattern of hearing loss (e.g., good hearing in low frequencies, poorer hearing in high frequencies),
- greater difficulty in understanding speech (lack of clarity) than would be expected on the basis of the hearing sensitivity per se,
- difficulty in understanding speech amid any kind of distracting or competing background noise, irrespective of any loss of hearing sensitivity,

- greater difficulty in understanding speech through one ear than through two ears,
- difficulty in understanding speech in poor acoustical environments, such as reverberant rooms, especially when there is some background noise,
- difficulty in understanding speech emanating from the radio, television, telephone, and other reproductive sources unless fidelity is exceptionally good and there is little background noise, such as music,
- difficulty in understanding any form of "distorted speech," such as a foreign dialect, the inarticulate speech of a child, rapid speech, speech through a window or other medium (such as in box offices), or speech from another room or from a distance.

Many of the foregoing difficulties may not be recognized as hearing-related problems. Family members and friends may misinterpret the hearing-impaired person's signs of confusion and inappropriate responses as early signs of senility. It is equally important to recognize that various communication disturbances resemble hearing impairment associated with aging. Bollinger's (1982) behavioral indexes of communication disorders among elderly individuals list approximately 40 indexes for seven areas of disorders. Because of the wide variety of possible disturbances and conditions, a differential diagnosis made by a speech/language pathologist and an audiologist may be needed. To understand the impact on older persons of the range of auditory difficulties they may experience, one needs to understand the impact of acquired hearing loss on any individual and then consider the aspects that are unique to older persons and that combine to create special problems for that population.

Psychological and Practical Aspects of Hearing Impairment

Few aspects of daily living are unaffected by a hearing difficulty. On the one hand, the impact of the hearing problem is often so subtle that it escapes not only the realization of those closest to the hearing-impaired person but the affected individual as well. But the hearing loss may be blamed for a variety of problems, experiences, and feelings that may not really be attributable to the loss per se or that may be compounded or exacerbated by the loss.

The most disabling effect of hearing impairment has been noted, repeatedly, to be its interference with easy communication. A breakdown in communicating easily with other people can result in isolation from social interaction and loss of opportunities for love, work, and recreation that are more readily available to those with normal hearing. Some persons begin to withdraw and eventually become isolated from the mainstream of life. In some cases the result can be stagnation and despair, which affect both mental and physical health.

The list of auditory problems presented earlier helps one appreciate the potential impact of a hearing impairment on activities of daily living and on many aspects of life. When one realizes the kinds of hearing loss that are possible, one can recognize how often persons who are hearing impaired may miss something because of the inability to hear or sort out messages from a public address or paging system in an airport, bus station, or train station or when at a physician's office, the movies, the theater, lectures, or religious services. One can also better understand the fear, apprehension, and confusion that hearing-impaired hospital patients must feel when they cannot hear or can only half hear the quiet, concerned discussions at their bedside; when they are startled repeatedly because they did not hear an approaching nurse or attendant; or when they do not understand the conversation of nurses and physicians whose lips are hidden and whose speech is muffled by surgical masks.

Until hearing loss affects them personally or is experienced by a family member, many people are oblivious to the many little ways that hearing serves them in their daily lives. For example, when cooking, hearing enables one to monitor the boiling water, the sizzling bacon, the bubbling dish in the oven, the bell of the microwave oven, the buzz of another timer, or the bottle or can falling off the shelf. One of the great values of hearing is that it bestows on the individual the ability to listen to something or someone while attending to something else visually. If you have a hearing loss, you may not be able to do two things at once. For instance, you cannot easily run the water for a bath while attending to something in another room, because the bathtub may overflow, and you cannot freely talk to a friend while preparing a meal.

Also associated with hearing impairment may be apprehensions and problems arising from the inability to hear alarm clocks, timers on ovens and clothing dryers, doorbells, telephones, knocks on the door, crackling sounds of fire, pets wanting to go in or out, prowlers, smoke alarms, weather conditions, children crying, and the multitude of other sounds that constantly bombard those who can hear. In addition, hearing loss can present certain problems for those who drive. Hearing-impaired persons may have difficulty knowing whether the car has been started and is running, whether it is running properly, and whether they have actually turned the motor off. Because they must visually attend to the road, they cannot communicate with their passengers because they can neither lip-read nor use sign language. The inability to hear the sirens of emergency vehicles while driving is another source of concern.

Entertaining others at home and attending family gatherings, receptions, parties, and other events involving small talk with a rapid exchange of comments, often against a general background of noise, are all situations that the hearing-impaired person approaches with mixed feelings and considerable anxiety. The demanding task of tracking conversations while attempting to avoid embarrassment and the appearance of being dull can be fatiguing and anxiety provoking. It is not uncommon for the older hearing-impaired person to avoid these situations, thus limiting opportunities for socialization.

These experiences would be difficult enough in encounters with people who readily understood the problem and who employed various courtesies to help one cope and compensate. However, because hearing loss is an invisible impairment, people do not readily recognize the nature of the difficulty. If they do, they often do not know how to respond. Complicating the situation is the tendency of hearing-impaired persons to hide the problem. As a consequence, people frequently are annoyed when they are asked to repeat what they have said, irritated by misunderstandings, and unwilling to be patient and apply good speaking behavior when talking to a person with a hearing loss.

The extent to which a hearing loss affects a given individual is dependent on several factors, including the support and understanding of friends and family; the person's age, personality, basic intellectual skills, social and economic status, education, and general knowledge; the occupational and social demands placed on the individual; and the presence of other sensory impairments. For older individuals, the combination of hearing and visual impairment can have a dramatic impact on the ability to function independently and on the perception of independent functioning.

Impact on Older People

The effects of hearing loss on older persons are similar to those experienced by hearing-impaired persons of any age group, but the effects may be complicated by additional factors. One important factor is physical and social isolation. Isolation attributable to the various psychosocial aspects of aging is commonly noted. The extent to which that isolation is attributable to or intensified by hearing impairment is unclear, but studies indicate that there seems to be a correlation between isolation and impaired hearing (Ventry & Weinstein, 1982). It is reasonable to assume that the two types of isolation may combine and intensify in certain individuals to such an extent that these persons become severely depressed. The isolation experienced by the hearing-impaired older person in a nursing home, for example, can be quite severe unless special efforts are made to educate the staff members on the need to counteract it. The sense of aloneness and abandonment felt by some nursing home residents can be significantly increased by impaired hearing.

A second factor is the sense of disappointment and frustration that many older hearing-impaired persons feel. As Hull (1982) noted, the frustration that hearing-impaired older people experience because of the difficulty of understanding what their children and grandchildren are saying at a family gathering is often acute. The older person may feel a great sense of disappointment when he or she finds that the long-awaited opportunity to interact with a grandchild is not very enjoyable because of the high-pitched, soft, inarticulate speech of the child, which may not be heard well, if at all. This experience may prompt still another sense of loss among many that may occur with increasing age.

Another factor is the association of certain behaviors caused by the hearing loss with behaviors that are characteristic of senility. Older people may worry that their families believe they have lost the ability to function independently and to handle their own affairs. They may also be concerned that certain responsibilities may be taken away from them (Hull, 1982). Someone's difficulty in communicating is often seen as an inability to function predictably and rationally. Other feedback and reactions may cause elderly people to begin to doubt their own abilities.

Compared to younger persons, many older persons seem to accept hearing loss as another of the many inevitable consequences of growing old, and they do not want to be a bother to others. As a consequence, they may give up various struggles in life more easily and lose the motivation and determination to cope.

Another notable aspect of hearing impairment in older persons is related to the reactions of others. As mentioned previously, people's reactions to requests by any hearing-impaired person to repeat what they have just said and their response to what seems to be confusion and rude behavior (such as talking aloud at church or a play or interrupting when someone else is talking) are generally negative. When the same behaviors are manifested by older persons, listeners appear to be even less understanding, patient, and compassionate. The older person is more likely than is someone younger to be regarded as rude, stubborn, or even senile, rather than hearing impaired (Hull, 1982).

In addition, older persons with a hearing impairment may have more difficulty than do younger persons because of other sensory deficits. For elderly people with a hearing loss, vision plays a significant supplementary, and sometimes compensatory, role. If vision is impaired, the impact of the hearing loss is even greater.

Other physical and mental changes that may be more common among older people can also make hearing loss more significant. Decreased manual dexterity and tactile sensitivity can cause problems in manipulating and inserting hearing aids. Likewise, older persons may have greater difficulty forming the letters and signs for effective communication via the manual alphabet. Changes in perception, memory, psychomotor performance, and learning may intensify the impact of the hearing impairment and affect various compensatory and rehabilitation efforts.

Implications of Visual Impairment

Vision changes associated with normal aging and the high prevalence of visual impairment among older persons cause added problems for the older person who also has a hearing impairment. The primary effect of impaired vision is on the use of speech reading (lipreading) to supplement impaired hearing. The more dependent the individual is on speech reading, the more significant the impact of the vision problem. Depending on the nature of visual impairment, the older person with a hearing loss may have more difficulty understanding speech under certain lighting conditions and at certain distances or angles. Likewise, those who have a reduced ability to adapt to light and dark may need a longer time than do others before they can communicate easily when going into or leaving a dark restaurant on a bright, sunny day.

Vision problems among older hearing-impaired persons may make it difficult for them to see hearing aid batteries and to determine the positive and negative sides, as well as to see the various controls that need to be manipulated on the hearing aid. As a consequence, a vision problem can interfere with the successful use of a hearing aid, especially when combined with reduced tactile sensitivity and manual dexterity.

Vision loss and decreased mobility may also add to the sense of isolation arising from a hearing loss and from other factors associated with aging. It should be recognized that many of the same diseases and conditions, such as diabetes and hypertension, that cause visual impairment can also cause hearing impairment.

Tinnitus and Vestibular Functioning

Another problem related to hearing ability among elderly persons is tinnitus. "Tinnitus" refers to any of the types of "head noise" that may occur even when a hearing impairment is not obvious. It ranges from ringing and whistling noises to roaring and buzzing sounds. The noises may be minimal and infrequent or loud and disruptive of attention and sleep. Such noises can occur whether a person is totally deaf or has normal hearing.

The source of the problem may be within or outside the ear. There are many possible causes for tinnitus, including the side effects of medications (not uncommon among older persons, especially regular users of aspirin) and vascular or neural problems. The specific cause in a given case is difficult to ascertain and is usually not identified. As a consequence, treatment is likely to be by trial and error.

Another area of concern is disequilibrium, or balance problems, among older persons. About 50 to 75 percent of older people may experience symptoms of dizziness (Traynor, 1982). This loss of equilibrium is often referred to as "presbystasis." Ocular difficulties may well play a primary etiological role. Episodic dizziness can be disturbing to the person who experiences it. Like tinnitus, it may result in a worried concern about health and even the fear of an impending stroke or death. As a consequence, vestibular rehabilitation services are sometimes offered. Such rehabilitation may involve counseling regarding the problems associated with the condition and certain labyrinthine exercises (Traynor, 1982).

Prevalence of Hearing Impairments

Most people associate the loss of hearing with aging. The popular portrayal of elderly people includes some obvious manifestation of hearing difficulties. Similarly, a person age 25 to 55 who misunderstands or fails to hear something is often teased about "getting older." A valid basis exists for this common association between hearing impairment and increasing age. The prevalence of hearing impairment among the older population is markedly greater than it is among younger persons. What surprises most people, however, is the prevalence of hearing impairments in the general population.

GENERAL PREVALENCE

In most countries, hearing loss affects more people than does any other chronic health condition. Because it is an invisible impairment, most people simply do not recognize the extent of its occurrence or the nature and extent of its impact. A recent "best estimate" is that 8 percent of the civilian, noninstitutionalized population in the United States experiences some difficulty in hearing or understanding speech (Punch, 1983). Included in this estimate is the approximately 1 percent of the population who are deaf. The prevalence estimate of 8 percent is consistent with the often cited estimate that 15 to 20 million people in the United States have a hearing impairment. Indeed, the 1980 National Health Interview Survey estimated 17.4 million hearing-impaired people (Punch, 1983). With the growth in population reflected in the 1990 census, estimates of 20 to 24 million hearing-impaired people are becoming increasingly common.

PREVALENCE IN THE AGING POPULATION

Estimates of the prevalence of hearing impairment, regardless of the population, can vary considerably as a function of how the data were obtained and what definition of hearing impairment was used. Such variability in data collection is especially evident in the estimates of the prevalence of hearing impairment in older populations. Estimates of those affected range from 20 to 65 percent of those 65 and over. The findings of the National Center for Health Statistics, reported by Punch (1983), showed prevalence rates of hearing impairment in the civilian, noninstitutionalized population of this country that range from less than 2 percent of the population under age 14 to 10 percent of those ages 45 to 54 to nearly 39 percent of those 75 and over. Personal experience, as well as various published studies, suggest that these estimates are conservative, especially for older groups. Practicing audiologists estimate that 50 percent of those 65 and over have some degree of hearing impairment (Hull, 1977); the estimates are even higher for each subsequent decade of life.

The prevalence of hearing impairments varies among particular subgroups of older people. For example, a greater percentage of men than of women are hearing impaired. Hearing impairment is more prevalent among white persons than it is among black persons (Punch, 1983) and more prevalent among persons with low incomes. In addition, Chafee (1967) estimated that 90 percent of the residents of long-term care facilities have some degree of hearing impairment.

PROJECTIONS

It is important for health care professionals and others who provide services to older people to recognize the likelihood of hearing impairments among that population and the increase in the proportion of the total population with impaired hearing. It is estimated that the number of persons with hearing impairments will increase at a faster rate (102 percent between 1980 and 2050) than will the total U.S. population (36 percent) as a direct result of the aging of the population (Fein, 1983). Given the statistics on the high percentage of blindness and visual impairment among elderly people, it is obvious that a large proportion of persons will have at least some degree of deficiency in regard to both major senses.

Type of Hearing Loss or Impairment

The ear or, more accurately, the auditory system is incredibly complex. Its intricacies of function and dysfunction are still not fully understood. In many instances of permanent hearing loss the cause of the loss is unknown. Even when the cause is known, the exact nature of the damage to the auditory system is not always able to be determined. Yet, as a result of various investigations during the past 30 years, professionals do have helpful information regarding the nature of hearing impairment among older persons.

Impairments of hearing may be caused by problems in various parts of the auditory system, from the ear to the brain. If the hearing loss is the result of a problem in the outer ear, the ear canal, the tympanic membrane (eardrum), or the middle ear, it is referred to as a "conductive" hearing loss. If there is a disorder in the inner ear or the auditory nerve up to the lower portion of the brainstem, the resultant hearing impairment is referred to as a "sensorineural" hearing loss. In some instances, an ear may have disorders in both the conductive and the sensorineural portions. In such instances, the term "mixed hearing loss" is used. Hearing impairments caused by problems higher in the brainstem or within the brain itself are generally referred to as "central disorders." (See Goodhill [1979] or Newby [1979] for details on the anatomy and physiology of the auditory system and the various disorders that may occur.) Most conductive hearing losses can be treated medically or surgically, but some cannot. Most sensorineural hearing losses and central auditory disorders cannot be treated medically or surgically, but some can. It is important for any individual who has a hearing impairment to have a medical examination, preferably by an otolaryngologist, an ear, nose, and throat specialist.

The type of hearing loss a person has will determine to a great extent the kinds of auditory problems experienced. Generally, the main hearing difficulty associated with conductive hearing loss is a reduction in the overall loudness of sounds. Persons with sensorineural hearing losses have a problem not only with reduced overall loudness of sounds. Some sounds, depending on the frequency or pitch, may be of normal loudness; others may be considerably softer or not heard at all. Such unevenness in the relative reduction of the loudness of various sounds can result in a lack of clarity of sounds, especially of speech, as well as distortions. Individuals with this problem are likely to have extreme difficulty understanding speech against a noisy background.

The impact of central auditory disorders may be subtler. Individuals with such disorders may function successfully in many situations and have little or no problem with a reduction in the overall loudness of sounds. However, under adverse listening conditions of one kind or another, such as when competing speech or background noises, rapid rate of speech, distorted speech over a telephone, or other difficult listening environments are factors, the individual may not be able to understand what is said. He or she may be able to hear the speech but simply cannot make sense of it.

In addition to the type of hearing loss, other parameters of hearing impairment are the degree of hearing loss and the pattern of hearing loss. As in vision loss, there are normal changes in the auditory system associated with the aging process. Different parts of the system, such as the auditory nerves and the structures of the inner ear, may be affected. The term typically used to refer to the hearing impairment associated with aging is "presbycusis." But not all hearing losses in older persons are due to or complicated by aging. Older persons are subject to the same conditions, diseases, and accidents that give rise to the kinds of hearing losses also incurred by younger persons. There are, however, changes in the auditory system and resultant hearing problems that are more common, if not unique, in the older population.

Identification and Measurement of Impairments

It is beyond the scope and purpose of this chapter to elaborate on the methods and procedures for identifying and measuring hearing in older people. A variety of audiology texts deal with such information in great detail. It is important, however, for health care practitioners to be aware of some of the methods and resources that are available and the problems that may be encountered.

Older persons who have a hearing impairment can be identified in a number of ways. One way is for the persons to identify themselves on the basis of the difficulties they experience. Another way is through the recognition, by friends and family members, health care professionals, or others, of certain behaviors that are symptomatic of hearing difficulty. Other methods of identification are interviews and a variety of assessment questionnaires or surveys. Such surveys attempt to identify not only the presence of a hearing impairment but also the extent to which the individual perceives that the impairment is creating a problem or disability. Some questionnaires are, however, designed to be completed by family members, nursing home staff, or other individuals. (For a discussion of most of the questionnaires, see Alpiner [1987].)

More traditional forms of identification of a hearing impairment in older people are audiometric screening programs and audiologic evaluations. Screening programs using pure-tone audiometry are conducted in nursing homes, retirement centers and residences, shopping centers, senior citizens centers, and mobile hearing-test vans that go to a variety of screening sites, including rural areas. Sometimes, identification is accomplished in a pass-fail hearing screening test; in such instances, individuals who fail need further hearing tests to provide more helpful information. Other forms of audiometric identification go beyond the usual pass-fail screening tests of hearing and quickly determine approximate hearing threshold levels.

The most complete assessment of hearing impairment in older persons can be provided by audiologists, who are generally found in community speech and hearing clinics, university speech and hearing clinics, hospitals, rehabilitation centers, and private practice. Such evaluations are typically nonmedical. However, many audiologists work in medical settings, including the offices of otolaryngologists, and may conduct hearing evaluations as part of complete medical assessments. The location of audiologists and the identification of services they provide usually can be determined from listings in the yellow pages of a telephone directory. Information regarding certified audiologists and agencies providing their services also may be obtained from the American Speech-Language-Hearing Association, which is located in Rockville, Maryland. This association also is the certifying body for speech/language pathologists and audiologists. Referrals to audiologic facilities may originate from any source, including self-referral, personal physicians, and university-affiliated medical centers. In addition to hearing tests, audiologists also may provide various rehabilitation services, including the selection and fitting of hearing aids.

Modifications of the Auditory Environment

Older persons experience special difficulty under adverse listening conditions, such as in reverberant rooms and noisy environments. Much can be done to help them hear better by improving the acoustics of the environment in which they live and are expected to function. For example, it is frequently difficult to persuade hearing-impaired persons to go to social halls for various activities because such rooms are acoustical "nightmares." Any effort to reduce noise in the room and from outside the room will do much to improve the listening conditions. If the special acoustical treatment of rooms and ventilation systems is not feasible or affordable, there are many inexpensive and helpful measures that can be used. For instance, if the room is reverberant, the addition of various sound-absorbing items, such as wall hangings, area rugs, upholstered furniture, and draperies, will help.

Architects and interior design specialists who plan and build facilities for older persons, such as nursing homes, retirement complexes, and senior citizens centers, are becoming increasingly aware of the need to create accessible environments for older persons in general and for those with vision, hearing, and physical disabilities. Advances in technology are making accommodations increasingly possible.

Guidelines for Effective Communication

An effective and helpful way of reducing the impact of a hearing impairment on an older person is through informational counseling for those individuals who play primary roles in the life of the person, including family members and friends. The information provided can cover the following guidelines for conversing with and assisting hearing-impaired older persons, which will help reduce the usual concomitant problems of hearing impairments. These guidelines are particularly helpful to professionals working with elderly persons:

- Be patient and understanding. People with a hearing loss do not want sympathy. They simply want to be able to talk intelligently with you.
- Determine which mode of communication the person prefers— lipreading, paper and pencils, or sign language. Speaking loudly is not always the answer.
- Open your mouth sufficiently when speaking, but do not exaggerate your lip movements.
- Speak slowly and clearly, taking care to round off words without exaggerating. Be careful in the pronunciation of proper names because they are especially difficult to pick up. You may have to raise your voice a little, but shouting only distorts your words and could cause severe discomfort to the listener.
- Do not speak with anything in your mouth, such as a pipe or cigarette. Make sure your hands are away from your mouth.
- Move away from background noise or competing speech. Turn down the radio, television, or record player before speaking. Select seating in restaurants and other places in areas that have the least background

noise and distraction. Always face the person, and make sure your face is illuminated by adequate light.

- Do not attempt to talk to hearing-impaired persons from another room. Not only are the distance and intervening obstacles too great for them to hear you adequately, they cannot see your face and, therefore, cannot lip-read if they are able to do so.
- When someone with a hearing loss joins a group already in conversation, make sure that person understands what is being discussed, even if you have to write it down.
- Some people have difficulty hearing certain speech sounds. When you suspect that this is the case, try rephrasing what you have said. Do not endlessly repeat the same words.
- Never ridicule an attempt to hear. It could do untold damage to confidence.
- Do not hesitate to ask what you might do to make yourself better understood.
- Modifications of the auditory environment often help hearing-impaired persons. If a room is reverberant, add carpeting or area rugs, wall hangings, draperies, and upholstered furniture, which will help minimize the echo.
- Encourage the hearing-impaired person to take advantage of the various services that are available in the community.
- The use of a hearing aid does not mean that the individual hears normally when the device is worn. The person may still have difficulty hearing, especially in noisy situations and rooms with poor acoustics.
- Take care that you do not "talk down" to the person. There is sometimes a tendency to speak in a humiliating, patronizing, and degrading way, especially to older persons with hearing impairments.
- Whenever possible, be sure a microphone and public address system are used for meetings, lectures, and other large, public gatherings.
- Allow the older hearing-impaired person more processing time than is typical in normal conversations. The use of a slower-than-normal rate of speech and of more pauses will help greatly.
- Review the lists and descriptions of auditory difficulties experienced by hearing-impaired older persons. Try to understand what it must be

like to have such difficulties, and then be ready to help those who need assistance. Seek their suggestions without being patronizing.
• Remember that the loss of hearing is the sensory impairment you are most likely to experience during your lifetime. Think about how you hope others will relate to you when the time comes.

Conclusion

Given the prevalence of hearing impairment in the older population, it is important for all health care professionals and other service providers working with older persons to be aware of the nature and impact of hearing impairments and of the hearing aids and services that are available. Members of the speech and hearing profession need to exert effort to inform allied professionals of the availability of these services. Individuals who work with older persons, however, can seek information on the availability of devices and services from various sources, such as those listed in the Resources section of this book, as well as from local speech and hearing professionals, speech and hearing clients, otolaryngologists, self-help groups, clubs and organizations, and hearing aid dispensers. Despite increased public education, many older persons still are reluctant to seek help or do not know that help is available. Each person or professional who relates in some way to older people can serve as a resource or referral agent to help an older person with hearing impairment to find the appropriate services.

References

Alpiner, J. G. (1987). Evaluation of adult communication function. In J. G. Alpiner & P. A. McCarthy, (Eds.), *Rehabilitative audiology: Children and adults.* Baltimore, MD: Williams and Wilkins.

Bollinger, R. L. (1982). Nonauditory communication disturbances resembling presbycusis. In R. H. Hull (Ed.), *Rehabilitative audiology* (pp. 293-313). New York: Grune & Stratton.

Chafee, C. (1967). Rehabilitation needs of nursing home patients: A report of a survey. *Rehabilitation Literature, 18*: 377-389.

Fein, D. J. (1983). Projections of speech and hearing impairments to 2050. *ASHA, 25*(11): 31.

Goodhill, V. (Ed.). (1979). *Ear: Diseases; deafness, dizziness.* New York: Harper & Row.

Hull, R. H. (1977). *Hearing impairment among aging persons.* Lincoln, NE: Cliffs Notes.

Hull, R. H. (Ed.). (1982). *Rehabilitative audiology.* New York: Grune & Stratton.

Newby, H. A. (1979). *Audiology* (4th ed.). Englewood Cliffs, NJ: Prentice-Hall.

Punch, J. (1983). Sociodemographic and health characteristics of the hearing-impaired population. *ASHA, 25*(8): 15.

Traynor, R. J. (1982). Vestibular rehabilitation: The role of the audiologist. In R. H. Hull (Ed.), *Rehabilitative audiology* (pp. 479-489). New York: Grune & Stratton.

Ventry, I. M., & Weinstein, B. E. (1982). The hearing handicap inventory for the elderly. *Journal of Speech & Hearing Research, 25:* 593-599.

SECTION II

Service Delivery

CHAPTER 7

An Overview of the National Network on Aging

Raymond C. Mastalish

Early in the 1940s, demographers started recognizing a trend in our society. Changes in the birthrate began to reflect our fascination with mobility and its impact on the extended family structure and the emphasis on smaller families. Tremendous advances were occurring in the health field with the discovery of antibiotics and other wonder drugs, increased knowledge about the relationship between nutrition and health, and emphasis on preventive health practices, including sanitation.

All these factors have contributed both to the tremendous growth in the population of older people, particularly those age 75 and over, and a decrease in the availability of care provided by family members. But only during the last two decades have the private and public sectors recognized the implications of this demographic change—new buying patterns, shifts in population centers from the cold-weather industrial states to warmer retirement states, the growing political presence of the elderly population, and technological advances that create new approaches and devices to assist elderly people with debilitating physical conditions and sensory impairments.

The Private Sector and the Elderly

Typically, institutional changes follow demographic changes in our society. In the United States, the private sector was first to respond and to experience institutional change in the form of the creation of organizations by uniting elderly persons and those working with them or on their behalf. As early as 1927, the special interests of a group of retired employees of federal government agencies resulted in the formation of the National Association of Retired Federal Employees (NARFE). Today NARFE, located in Washington, DC, conducts legislative activities on behalf of approximately 467,000 members. Next, in 1945, came the formation of the Gerontological Society of America (GSA), which conducts scientific studies of the aging process and the social aspects of demographic change. GSA, also in Washington, DC, represents approximately 6,700 researchers, academicians, and service providers. It promotes research, policy development, and the education of those who work in the field of aging.

The National Retired Teachers Association, organized in 1947, preceded by 10 years the American Association of Retired Persons (AARP). Today AARP is the largest individual membership organization in the world, with more than 32 million members, age 50 and over. AARP works actively to promote programs supporting an enhanced and independent life-style for all older Americans. It sponsors educational and service programs, as well as legislative committees that work with government representatives to further the interests of older persons.

The National Council on the Aging (NCOA), instituted in 1950, represents professionals who provide direct services to elderly persons in a wide range of health, social work, and community action agencies. It also sponsors 10 constituent units, including the National Institute of Senior Centers (NISC), the National Institute on Senior Housing (NISH), the National Institute on Adult Day Care (NIAD), the National Institute on Community-Based Long-Term Care (NICLC), the National Center on Rural Aging (NCRA), the National Association of Older Worker Employment Services (NAOWES), the Health Promotion Institute (HPI), and National Voluntary Organizations for Independent Living for the Aging (NVOILA). These organizations provide networks for service providers in the field of aging who are committed to improving services for older persons.

Labor organizations demonstrated their interest in the growing elderly population when they established the National Council of Senior Citizens (NCSC) in 1961 as a membership organization of elderly union members. The National Association of State Units on Aging (NASUA), founded in 1964, was the first of a new kind of national organization representing public officials employed in state offices and agencies that interact with the elderly population. Members of this association include administrators of the state units on aging that were created by the Older Americans Act (OAA) and that will be discussed later in this chapter.

The most dramatic organizational response to the graying of our country came in the 1970s, when 13 new national organizations representing the interests of elderly people and those who work in the field of aging were formed. These organizations represent not only special segments of the elderly population, such as minorities via groups like the National Caucus and Center on the Black Aged, the National Hispanic Council on Aging, the National Pacific/Asian Resource Center on Aging, and the National Indian Council on Aging, but also specialized groups serving programmatic interests and geographic areas. The latter include the National Association of Nutrition and Aging Service Programs, the National Association of Meal Programs, and the National Senior Citizens Law Center. The National Association of Meal Programs represents private, nonprofit nutrition groups that provide home-delivered meals. The National Senior Citizens Law Center is an advocate for providers of legal services who help elderly persons.

Regional organizations of professionals in the field include the Southwest Society on Aging, the Southeast Society on Aging, the Northeastern Society on Aging, and the Mid-America Congress on Aging. They are individual membership organizations that bring together elderly persons, researchers, academicians, service providers, planners, advocates, and elected officials in their respective geographic areas. The former Western Gerontological Association is now the American Society on Aging, a national organization.

The Association for Gerontology in Higher Education consists of colleges and universities that offer training and conduct research in gerontology. As components of the network on aging increase and expand in response to the growing number of elderly people, the members of this association will play a critical role in preparing personnel to work in agencies and organizations.

The growing need for nursing homes and other residential facilities led to the development of national organizations in this area of service, including the American Association of Homes for the Aged, the National Association of Nursing Home Administrators, and the National Citizens' Coalition for Nursing Home Reform. Organizations concerned with home care, such as the National Home Caring Council and the National Association for Home Care, work for quality care for older persons at home.

Perhaps the most significant stimulus for institutional change was the involvement of local public officials and community organizers and planners who formed the National Association of Area Agencies on Aging (NAAAA) and aging affiliates of public interest groups like the National Association of Counties and the U.S. Conference of Mayors. Another national group, the Leadership Council of Aging, is a coalition of 32 organizations involved in aging issues. The council is a forum for expression of views related to service delivery to elderly persons and a clearinghouse of information.

Despite what might appear to be a fracturing of interests or duplications of efforts, a national network on aging has formed, with identifiable focal points and specific responsibilities at the national, state, and local levels. This national network, outlined in the discussion that follows, can be viewed as a federally mandated administrative network linked to a broader network of special interests, agencies of service providers, and elderly persons represented by the organizations just described.

The Public Sector

With the formation of organizations representing the interests of the elderly population, the public sector began to respond to the changing demographics of our society. As early as the 1920s, elected officials, demographers, academicians, and researchers advocated at the federal level for special commissions, agencies, and programs to address the concerns of the aging population. The Civil Service Retirement Act of

1920 led the way for other legislation to provide services and programs for elderly people.

Perhaps the most significant early action was the passage of the Social Security Act in 1935. Its primary goal was to provide economic security beyond retirement as a matter of right for American workers. The Social Security Act guarantees income to older persons in retirement as long as they have worked a certain length of time, usually 10 years, and have reached age 62. With the passage of amendments to the act beginning in the 1960s, additional benefits accrued.

The costs of health care escalated in the 1960s and impoverished many elderly persons, the population group most at risk of developing ill health. Medicare, the health insurance program for elderly people, was enacted in 1965 in response to this health care crisis. Designed to cover expenditures for health care of persons 65 and over, regardless of income level, it covers hospitalization, some other kinds of skilled nursing care, and payments to physicians. The Medical Assistance Act, known as Medicaid, is based on means testing and pays all health costs, including long-term care expenses, for persons below certain income levels. These two health care insurance programs are continually modified.

As inflation soared through the 1970s, many elderly people were unable to survive on social security alone. To assist them, as well as blind and disabled people, the Supplementary Security Income (SSI) program went into effect in 1974. It provides financial assistance, regardless of work history, to eligible elderly people with low income. In addition to providing supplements for poor people, policymakers decided to provide recipients of social security payments with automatic cost-of-living adjustments tied to rates of inflation.

The concept of social security has changed over the years and has been frequently misinterpreted. Critics continually question the financial structure of the system and its long-term fiscal status. Advocates for older persons continue to point to the need for a secure retirement income in old age and fight to preserve or increase payments to elderly persons. This debate is not ignored by the public. A "wrong" position on social security issues can mean the demise of an elected official's career or the defeat of someone seeking to be elected. Reactions from national aging organizations and from elderly individuals when legislators assume controversial positions on aging-related issues can have an overwhelming impact on elected officials at the federal, state, and local levels.

Congress has recognized the political force that the elderly population represents, as well as the needs and concerns of elderly persons, by creating two oversight nonlegislative committees, the Select Committee on Aging in the House of Representatives and the Special Committee on Aging in the Senate. The committees hold hearings on a range of topics, such as elder abuse, Alzheimer's disease, community-based long-term care, the impact of technology on the elderly population, and eroding retirement income. In 1985, a hearing before the House Select Committee addressed the issues of elderly visually impaired persons. The committee also publishes studies and working papers. The committees' influential role in calling attention to the plight of elderly people cannot be discounted.

The perceived or real political power of the elderly population—"senior power"—is also revealed in national conferences, which have become institutionalized events, that address issues of aging. In addition, most of the organizations representing the interests of elderly people have held national meetings and conferences around the country. Some draw thousands of elderly persons; others draw thousands of professionals in the field of aging. Perhaps some of the most significant events are the national meetings that bring together elderly people and professionals.

One of the first such national events was the federally sponsored National Conference on Aging held in 1950 in Washington, DC. This conference spurred Congress to create the Federal Committee on Aging and Geriatrics. Since then, Congress has provided for the White House Conference on Aging every 10 years—1961, 1971, and 1981. However, no such conference was held in 1991. Each conference can be credited with significant institutional change, but the recommendations of the 1961 White House Conference on Aging were perhaps the most far reaching. They resulted in the passage of the OAA of 1965 and the subsequent evolution of a national network on aging.

The Older Americans Act: Blueprint for a Network

After the 1961 White House Conference on Aging, several attempts to establish a federal agency as a focal point for aging were made in Congress. But no action was taken. In 1965, Senator Patrick McNamara (D-Michigan) and Congressman John Fogarty (D-Rhode Island) both introduced legislation that became the OAA. Many believe the OAA began the process for the most significant institutional change regarding elderly persons in this country. Through subsequent amendments, the OAA has spurred the evolution of the national network on aging.

The OAA provided for the creation of the federal Administration on Aging (AOA), located in what was then the U.S. Department of Health, Education, and Welfare to address the development and coordination of federal programs that directly affect the elderly population. Title III of the OAA provided for the creation of focal points for services for aging persons at the state level, the state units on aging. For a state to participate in OAA programs and receive federal funds for such activities, its governor was required to designate a state unit on aging. This unit, referred to by different names, such as the State Department on Aging, Division for Aging Services, Executive Office on Aging, and Commission on Aging, was to be an identifiable office within the state government. Each state unit was to develop a statewide plan to identify the elderly population within the state, their needs, resources to meet those needs, and proposals for OAA funding. Once the state plan was approved by the AOA, the state unit could directly fund service activities at the local level.

1973 AMENDMENTS

Even though the OAA was amended in 1969 and again in 1972, the next major set of amendments supporting the evolution of a national network on aging came in 1973. The 1973 amendments reflected a concern of several senators and members of Congress regarding the proliferation of federal and state programs that provided services for elderly people. The multiplicity of programs sometimes resulted in the duplication of efforts at the local level. Appropriations under the OAA alone had grown from $6.5 million in 1966 to $195.6 million in 1973. Appropriations in 1990 were $792.3 million.

The 1973 amendments were significant in that they also reflected the growing trend toward local decision making. The involvement and representation of recipients of service, in this case the elderly population, in decision making was now the order of the day. Therefore, Congress decided that funding decisions for programs under the OAA made at the state level were too far removed from those who received services. To enable the government to be more responsive to local needs, the 1973 OAA amendments required each state unit on aging to divide the state into planning and service areas and to designate an Area Agency on Aging (AAA) as the focal point for services within each area. Each area agency was to develop an area-wide plan on aging and to create an advisory council, at least half of whose members would be elderly persons. Again, the motive was to ensure input into the decision-making process from elderly persons at the local level.

Today, there are 670 AAAs across the nation. Their names vary. They may be called the County Office on Aging, Mayor's Commission on Aging, Council on Aging, Regional Development District Office on Aging, and so on. The size of the staff may vary from three to hundreds, but the average is eight. Each designated agency has the same roles and responsibilities and serves as a focal point for programs for elderly people. Thus, as a result of the 1973 OAA amendments, another administrative component of a national network on aging was created—AOA at the federal level, state units on aging at the state level, and AAAs at the local level.

ADDITIONAL AMENDMENTS

Other amendments to the OAA as well as other events have broadened the scope of the national network on aging to include the service-provider community and other entities representing specialized interests. In 1973, Congress appropriated money for the National Nutrition Program for the Elderly, enabling older persons to come together at nutrition sites for a nutritious hot meal each day. The program also offers older persons fellowship as well as opportunities to receive other services at the meal sites. Today there are over 12,000 congregate nutrition sites across the nation, located in housing projects, senior centers, church and synagogue facilities, and restaurants. In addition, the Meals-on-Wheels program delivers food to homebound elderly persons.

The AAAs are the planners, coordinators, and advocates for elderly people and the monitors of service agencies at the local level. They do not deliver services directly, except in special cases. To clarify this role, the OAA, as amended in 1978, required AAAs to designate community focal points for service delivery. The community focal points generally are multipurpose senior centers or service agencies where various types of nutrition services, counseling, information and referral, health screening, and recreation and socialization activities are available. AAAs also contract with over 15,000 service agencies in local communities to provide specific services, such as transportation, Meals-on-Wheels, counseling, information and referral, outreach, legal assistance, housing, case management, and homemaker, chore, and visiting nurse services.

Other Network Components

Although the OAA and its amendments have evolved into a broad-based national network on aging with an identifiable and distinctive administrative network, the act also generated the creation of other components that are directly or indirectly related to the network. For example, an advisory-level body, the Federal Council on Aging, was established to advise Congress, the president, and AOA on aging issues. The council is composed of 15 persons who are appointed by the president and Congress and represent older Americans, health care professionals, the service-provider community, and the research and academic communities.

As the field of gerontology expanded, the need for trained researchers and professionals to work in organizations on aging became increasingly apparent. Title IV of the OAA provides funds for gerontology training programs, research projects, and demonstration projects. They include university degree programs, a minority intern program, the development of training and technical assistance guidelines for the staffs of state agencies and AAAs, and senior centers and service agencies. Research on Alzheimer's disease and other chronic illnesses and projects to improve the management skills of administrators of programs for the elderly population are also included. There were approximately 150 grants under Title IV in 1987.

More and more low-income elderly persons need and want jobs to supplement limited retirement income. The Senior Community Service Employment Program for Older Americans, Title V of the OAA, which is administered through eight national contractors and designated state offices, supports 62,502 part-time employment slots for low-income elderly persons. These employment slots, often accompanied by training opportunities, provide for a broad range of jobs in aging organizations, service agencies, and private businesses.

Through Title VI of the OAA, funds are provided for approximately 125 Indian tribes. These funds support programs in such areas as nutrition, transportation, health screening, and in-home chore services for elderly Indians both on and off the reservation.

Other volunteer programs for older persons are under the auspices of the federal government agency ACTION, which funds the Retired Senior Volunteer Program (RSVP), the Foster Grandparents Program (FGP), and the Senior Companion Program (SCP). The ACTION programs, separate from OAA-funded programs, provide volunteer opportunities for elderly persons. The RSVP programs involve older persons in various volunteer activities, which include tutoring children in reading and math and working for drug abuse, crime prevention, health, and nutrition centers, with an emphasis on helping at-risk persons and refugees. The FGP and the SCP provide volunteer opportunities with a stipend for low-income older persons. The FGP pays older volunteers a stipend to provide personal, individual care to children. Approximately 27,100 FGP volunteers serve 73,100 children, with an emphasis on at-risk children. The SCP pays older persons a stipend to help adults with special needs in the home. Approximately 12,600 SCP volunteers provide long-term care services to 33,900 disabled and frail elderly persons.

The agencies, organizations, institutions, and tribal governments that receive OAA funds are part of the broadly based national network on aging. This fact is significant. The network comprises the multitude of planning and service agencies, related educational and research institutions, national aging organizations, and Indian tribes plus over 14,500 individuals who voluntarily serve on area agency advisory councils (see Figure 1). These individuals provide direction on how the responsibilities of the various components of the national network on aging work at the local level.

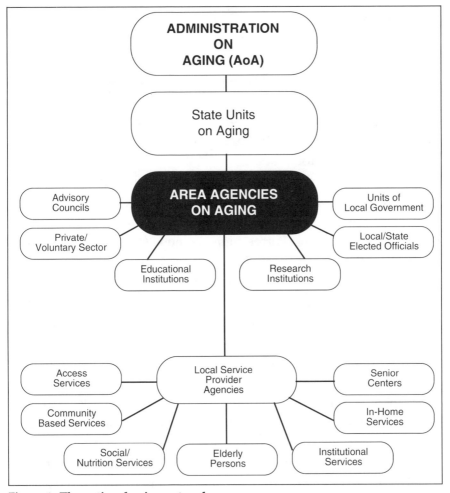

Figure 1: The national aging network.

National Network

An overall goal of the OAA is that the network on aging help elderly persons remain independent in their communities and homes and avoid inappropriate and premature institutionalization. To achieve this goal, the network develops comprehensive, coordinated service delivery systems on the federal, state, and local levels. The responsibilities of AOA, state units on aging, and AAAs are parallel and fall within four basic categories—planning, coordination, advocacy, and monitoring (Armor, Estes, & Noble, 1981).

PLANNING

Because AOA must relate horizontally on the federal level to Congress, other federal agencies, and national organizations, the carrying out of its responsibilities is a complicated process. For example, little happens in the area of nationwide planning simply because of the constraints within the federal bureaucracy and within the administration that is in office at the time. There has been no national plan on aging under any administration for years.

The lack of a national plan may not be an oversight by AOA but may reflect the reality of the OAA administrative structure. It is elderly persons at the local level who establish program priorities for their service delivery systems. Furthermore, because AOA is administratively several levels down in the U.S. Department of Health and Human Services (HHS) rather than at the top of the department, it has limited clout to ensure the responsiveness of other federal agencies to the needs of the nation's elderly population. This placement also limits its ability to carry out advocacy responsibilities, particularly with Congress. The need for advocacy from AOA is critical in the 1990s. Such advocacy must take place both within AOA and for programs outside its jurisdiction, such as SSI, whose administrative program lacks sufficient outreach and resources to reach all eligible older persons. Arthur Flemming, former U.S. commissioner on aging as head of AOA, has even proposed that a separate title be inserted within the OAA to pull together all advocacy functions, including ombudsman and legal services ("Flemming supports," 1991).

However, AOA also has vertical monitoring responsibilities in relation to the states, generally to the state units on aging. Monitoring is accomplished through the 10 AOA regional offices located in HHS regional offices, which review and approve state plans.

The responsibilities of a state unit on aging are also primarily horizontal; that is, the unit relates to other state-level agencies, the state legislature, and the governor's office. State units on aging develop statewide plans based on plans from the AAAs. The state plan addresses the overall needs of elderly people throughout the state and sets forth steps that the state unit must take to help fill the gaps in the service delivery system. The state unit may coordinate its efforts with those of another state agency that is administering other federal funds, such as the Medicaid and Medicare programs, or with those of agencies that administer state-financed programs. Each of those programs offers a focal point for delivering needed in-home supportive services and usually includes a case-management component and a tracking mechanism to ensure that appropriate services were indeed provided. If an area agency on aging has problems working with a local program administered through another state agency, the state unit may work with the appropriate state agency to encourage cooperative efforts at the local level.

The state unit may also have some difficulty carrying out its advocacy role with the state legislature because it is part of the state government and its director is appointed by the governor. Therefore, it may not always be able to advocate openly for elderly people on programs that the governor does not support. Yet its effectiveness in advocacy may be enhanced because of the personal relationship between its director and the governor, which may enable the director to garner the governor's support. The state unit also performs advocacy by working through the state advisory council or through AAAs that may be able to advocate measures that the state unit may not be in a position to support. In addition, the state unit on aging monitors the activities of the AAAs within the state.

The role of the area agency on aging is unique; it must implement directives emanating from the federal and state levels while responding to local needs and directives as it develops a comprehensive, coordinated community-based service delivery system for elderly constituents. One primary responsibility is the development of the area plan. The area agency first conducts a needs assessment of the entire population of elderly persons within the planning and service area to determine who they are, where they are, and what their needs are. The needs assessment process is done in various ways—through door-to-door surveys; scientific sampling of households in the area; and surveys conducted in senior centers, senior citizens clubs, or other places where elderly people congregate.

As a result, the AAA is usually in a position to provide the most comprehensive information about the elderly population in its planning and service area. Through the needs assessment process, AAAs can identify the growing number of older persons in their service areas who are experiencing vision loss. It is therefore important that survey methods include targeted questions to help identify special-needs groups, for example, questions about vision and vision loss and their impact on daily functioning for the older person. A few AAAs in the country have begun to enlist the assistance of a local agency for blind and visually impaired persons in conducting a needs assessment related to visually impaired elderly people. It is to be hoped that increasing numbers of AAAs will collaborate in needs assessment with agencies for blind persons as the number of older people experiencing vision loss continues to grow.

After needs assessment, the AAA conducts a resource assessment of the area's service delivery systems to identify existing resources, potential resources, and gaps in the delivery of needed services. All potential resources in the area are part of the assessment—public and private; federal, state, and local; and community- and family-support systems. The area agency then prepares a plan of action to fill those gaps through a comprehensive, coordinated community-based service delivery system. The area agency gives this area plan to the state unit for approval before getting OAA funding.

COORDINATION AND ADVOCACY

In implementing the area plan, AAAs coordinate with other planning agencies and networks of service providers at the local level, even with those who do not receive funds through the area agency. For example, an area agency may coordinate with a community mental health center on a transportation project to improve elderly people's access to counseling services by rerouting vans so they stop at the center. If that is impossible, the area agency may coordinate with the community mental health center and a multipurpose senior center to have a mental health counselor stationed at a nearby senior center. Coordination may be an area agency's most difficult responsibility. Even though coordination is one of the least visible activities, it may be the most productive in improving and expanding the delivery of services to elderly people.

The AAA's coordination role is complimented by another responsibility, advocacy. In its advocacy role, the area agency may operate under some of the same political and administrative constraints as do AOA and the state units. However, because of the independence of many AAAs, whose base of support is the broad representation of elderly persons and community leaders serving on the advisory council, AAAs may be influential advocates at the local, state, and national levels. Well-informed elderly persons can be their own best advocates; therefore, another role of the area agency is to ensure that its elderly constituents are knowledgeable about issues that affect them.

The effectiveness of an area agency's advocacy on an issue is directly linked to its other roles. Thus, the more information an agency has collected during the planning process about a particular issue, the more it may be able to advocate for it. Or, by coordinating efforts with other agencies in the community, the area agency can show unity and thereby advocate from a position of strength. For example, through the planning process, an area agency may have identified the need for housing for elderly people. The director may present the findings and plans on how to meet that need for housing to local elected officials. A well-prepared plan of action, however, may not convince the officials to take the necessary steps. Therefore, the agency may then work through its well-informed advisory council, together with supportive housing officials, to influence community leaders to support the housing program. Indirectly, the elderly constituents may have more influence in local decision making than does the staff of the area agency working alone. This is important for service providers in the blindness field to know when they want increased comprehensive services for older blind and visually impaired persons in cooperation with the local aging network.

MONITORING

When the AAA has identified gaps in services and worked to coordinate and advocate for community response to those gaps, it may decide to provide OAA resources or other resources it administers to fill those gaps. Other resources frequently are Medicare and Medicaid funds, Title XX social service funds, housing funds from the U.S. Department of Housing and Urban Development, and transportation funds from the U.S. Department of Transportation. Resources may also include state and local funds, such as those from state-legislated programs—state lottery funds, local levies, and special county or city allocations. In addition, many AAAs have generated funds from private sources, such as foundations, corporations, and individuals. Overall, the OAA portion of an AAA's budget is frequently only about 50 percent of the total service funds the agency administers. In monitoring the funded projects, AAAs may use a formal checks-and-balances procedure and on-site visits by staff and advisory council members.

Linkages: The Aging and Blindness Service Delivery System

Although links between the national network on aging and agencies serving the visually impaired community have slowly developed, there is much potential for collaboration at the federal, state, and local levels. Local projects seem to offer the most promise, because they are directly responsive to a community's needs.

In carrying out planning responsibilities, the AAA has numerous opportunities to link up with the blindness network. For example, when an area agency develops its needs assessment process and survey, it can work with officials from the blindness network to ensure the inclusion of questions regarding the needs of visually impaired elderly people, including their need for preventive eye examinations, eyeglasses, or other prosthetic devices; for assistance in planning how to manage with limited vision and maneuver in the community; and for information about blindness. If the two networks work together, the AAA can obtain valuable information to address the needs of elderly people with impaired vision.

In a recent review of the blindness field (Orr, 1990), 23 agencies providing services for blind persons around the country reported they had a cooperative and collaborative working relationship with the AAA. Some of the joint efforts involve educational programs about aging and vision loss, in-service training sessions, and needs assessment. These local collaborative efforts are major steps to ensure that older visually impaired persons receive the comprehensive services they need from both the aging and blindness service delivery systems. In the next step of the AAA's planning process, the AAA and the blindness network can work together to identify services in the community, both existing and potential, that can respond to the identified needs. Furthermore, the two networks can then move to the next step of determining how they would support each other in identifying or generating needed resources. Such coordinated efforts have the potential for far greater results than efforts conducted in a parallel process. They are particularly important in times of scarce financial resources.

During collaboration, the two networks can join together to address identified needs, making sure they are not working at odds or duplicating efforts. For example, the AAA might encourage a multipurpose senior center to provide vision screening for elderly people to detect impaired vision or urge a transportation project to extend its services to visually impaired elderly riders. The agency itself might use larger type in its newsletters, monthly calendar, posted fliers, or other publications for easier reading for all older people.

Likewise, the two networks can work together to ensure that local leaders and policymakers are aware of the needs of the visually impaired elderly population and how the two networks propose to fill gaps in services. Often the most effective advocacy occurs when two separate networks link together and policymakers realize that their responses will be met by a united community rather than by opposing networks. For example, library officials can be convinced to offer special programs for elderly people with visual impairments and to make those services available at senior centers and nursing homes and for homebound persons.

As the network on aging places more emphasis on community-based and in-home services as alternatives to institutional care, community leaders must recognize the need for such services and the savings they incur by supporting increased funds for these services. Increased funds for community-based services would help elderly blind persons continue to live independently in their homes and to avoid premature and unnecessary nursing home placement.

Finally, the AAA and the blindness network can link together to monitor funded service projects, to ensure that they provide appropriate outreach to elderly people with impaired vision and meet the requirements of Section 504 of the Rehabilitation Act of 1973 by ensuring physical access to service facilities. The AAA's monitoring of projects of particular interest to visually impaired elderly persons is enhanced when it has input from the blindness network.

Linkages can occur at all levels. AOA must work toward coordinating and advocating at the national level on behalf of the blindness network and support joint research and service projects for older visually impaired persons. It should also be working with national organizations representing the blindness network to encourage coordination at the state and local levels.

State units on aging must work with state agencies for the blind on behalf of visually impaired elderly people. For example, they can cooperate with representatives of the blindness network to ensure that the state legislature and the governor's office are responsive to the needs of this population and can work with state and local organizations to establish close working relationships concerning issues related to aging and blindness and visual impairment.

By working together, the networks enhance each other's understanding of the issues at hand and ensure that the community-based service delivery system includes accessible services needed by visually impaired elderly people. The aging and the blindness networks can establish a united front in advocating for their mutual constituents.

Each network complements the other's efforts; together the two can make great strides in addressing the needs of the visually impaired elderly community.

References

Armor, P. K., Estes, C. L., & Noble, M. (1981). Implementing the Older Americans Act. In R. Hudson (Ed.), *The aging in politics: Process and policy.* Springfield, IL: Charles C Thomas.

Flemming supports special OAA title on advocacy. (1991). *Older Americans Report,* p. 43.

Orr, A. L. (1990). *Innovative models of service delivery to older blind and visually impaired persons.* Unpublished paper.

CHAPTER 8

An Overview of the Blindness System

Alberta L. Orr

The blindness system today represents an array of services under public and private auspices. The number of agencies and services for blind persons varies tremendously from state to state. In some communities, there are both public and private providers of service; in others, only the state agency provides rehabilitation services. Every state has a state agency either in the form of a specific rehabilitation agency for blind persons or a special unit for blind rehabilitation as part of a generic vocational rehabilitation agency for disabled persons. The *Directory of Services for Blind and Visually Impaired Persons in the United States,* published by the American Foundation for the Blind (AFB) (1988), lists over 1,000 separate agencies and organizations providing services to blind people in the following categories—education, rehabilitation, library services, radio reading services, university programs, and low vision clinics. The list is a combination of autonomous freestanding voluntary agencies and others that are linked through fiscal, structural, and programmatic means.

Because a majority of these agencies did not exist before the twentieth century, a review of the development of the blindness system is in order. In addition to providing a historical perspective of the blindness field, this chapter describes the leadership organizations of and for blind persons in the field, resources for blind persons, services specifically targeted for the elderly visually impaired population, personnel preparation programs, and the current issues facing service providers and consumers in the blindness field today.

The Development of Services

Because this book is about the older visually impaired population, it is important to look at this country's response to the rehabilitation needs of older blind persons. In preindustrial agrarian American society, most older blind persons were cared for within the extended family structure; others were placed in almshouses. Boarding homes, typically associated with schools for blind children or with sheltered workshops, were another option. These homes were designed to provide housing for blind men while they were learning or working at a trade, most typically making brooms. Many boarding homes continued to provide shelter to former employees who were no longer able to work, particularly those who had no family resources or support. Today a few homes specifically for older blind persons exist throughout the country where the costs are covered by the older person's social security benefit or pension.

Mainstreaming, originally an educational concept, has also had an impact on aged blind persons, most of whom live independently in the community, either alone or with family members. The field of blindness, however, has its roots in educational services, and a review of the development of educational services will shed light on the development of the field in general.

EDUCATIONAL SERVICES

The development of organized services for blind persons began in education. In 1832, the first school for the blind, the New England Asylum for the Blind, opened in Boston, Massachusetts, and later became the well-known Perkins Institute in Watertown, Massachusetts. Dr. Samuel Gridley Howe, director, believed that he could prepare blind people to "participate in the economic and social life of their home communities" (Lenihan, 1977, p. 23). Dedicated to providing blind people with the necessary vocational skills for living in their own communities, Howe set up the first workshop in the United States at Perkins in 1837.

Two other prominent residential schools were also founded in 1832—the New York Institution for the Blind in New York City and the

Overbrook School for the Blind in Philadelphia. They were each financed privately through philanthropic efforts. In 1837, the first state school for the blind was opened in Ohio. These institutions established the trends and the pace for the 37 state-operated residential schools for blind children that existed at the close of the nineteenth century.

In 1879, the importance of educating blind children was recognized at the federal level when a federal statute established funds for the publication of free textbooks for blind children through the American Printing House for the Blind (APH) in Louisville, Kentucky. APH's initial appropriation was $10,000; today, APH's appropriation has grown to $5 million to serve over 4,300 primarily multiply disabled children in 50 residential schools and 41,600 visually impaired children in public schools.

By 1910, a small number of visually impaired children attended special classes referred to as "sight-saving classes" in public schools, rather than residential schools. This arrangement continued into the 1950s, when mainstreaming into the regular classroom with sighted peers became the primary educational trend. This major shift in educational method was the result of pressure from parents of visually impaired children to have their children be part of the mainstream of education. The epidemic of retinopathy of prematurity in the 1940s and 1950s resulted in visual impairment in 12,000 infants who were born prematurely to middle- and upper-class families. The excess of oxygen in incubators of premature infants resulted in blindness or visual impairment, as well as other disabilities that included varying degrees of retardation. The parents of these children advocated for their children to continue to live at home, attend public schools, and receive the necessary ancillary services by teachers trained in the special education of visually impaired students. In 1965, the Elementary and Secondary Education Act (P.L. 89-10) paved the way for the Education for All Handicapped Children Act of 1975 (P.L. 94-142), the landmark legislation that called for the right to equal educational opportunities for all handicapped children within their own communities.

The U.S. Department of Education's regulations governing P.L. 94-142 resulted in a series of lawsuits initiated by parents who were dissatisfied with the provisions made by their school districts on behalf of their blind children. Two famous cases—*Rowley v. Hendrick Hudson School Board* (1982) and *Irving Independent School District v. Tatro* (1984)—had a tremendous impact on the individualized nature of education for disabled students. The Supreme Court decision on *Rowley v. Hendrick Hudson School Board* resulted in a restrictive interpretation of P.L. 94-142. It was ruled that Congress had not intended to maximize the potential of each handicapped child. It took two years before the second case, *Irving Independent School District v. Tatro,* reversed the policy implications of the first decision by ruling that the meaningful access to education that Congress envisioned in P.L. 94-142 included whatever services were needed by each handicapped child to remain in school during the school day in order for each child to have the fullest potential for learning. P.L. 94-142 was amended in 1990 and renamed the Individuals with Disabilities Education Act (IDEA). IDEA also mandates coverage of all or part of low vision clinical evaluations, training in the use of low vision devices, and other related services, such as orientation and mobility (O&M) training for visually impaired children.

In the 1990s, blind and visually impaired children attend public school classes along with their sighted peers, facilitated by itinerant teachers, where needed, who provide additional assistance related to visual impairment. Each student proceeds through the educational process through an individualized education program (IEP). As visually impaired students reach high school, a focus on transition from school to the world of work becomes a regular part of the educational process to prepare them for postsecondary school, independent living, and employment. Transition is now a mandated service within the public education system, and efforts are under way to include transition services as part of rehabilitation services through the Rehabilitation Act of 1973, which is discussed later in this chapter.

VOCATIONAL REHABILITATION SERVICES

Prior to the early part of the twentieth century, blind persons who were employed worked in sheltered workshops. Extending vocational education to disabled persons gained considerable impetus during World War I. At that time many believed that vocational training would help individuals with a disability develop residual capacities needed for vocational effectiveness. Vocational rehabilitation was first viewed as a critical need for veterans when they returned from World War I.

The Soldier's Rehabilitation Act of 1918 was landmark legislation that authorized vocational rehabilitation services for all veterans disabled during the war, with employment as a real possibility after vocational rehabilitation training (Obermann, 1965). It was during the early history of organized labor that the need for vocational education programs was realized. Large numbers of unskilled laborers needed vocational training and retraining when skills they had for a particular task became obsolete.

In 1917, the Smith-Hughes Act made federal monies available on a matching basis to each state for vocational education programs and created the Federal Board for Vocational Education, which administered both the veteran and civilian vocational rehabilitation programs. Under the act, all participating states had to "designate or create a state board for vocational education which would have the necessary power to cooperate with the Federal Board for Vocational Education in the administration of the Act" (MacDonald, 1944).

Between 1918 and 1920, eight states passed laws establishing civilian vocational rehabilitation programs. In 1920, the first significant federal action for vocational rehabilitation was the Smith-Fess Act (P.L. 66-236), which authorized a joint federal-state vocational rehabilitation program for handicapped civilians. The implementation of the act was delegated to the Federal Board for Vocational Education. Only a few states passed legislation under P.L. 66-236, and the state services that were established were of minimal assistance to blind people because at that time blind persons were typically designated as unemployable and were therefore rejected.

In spite of the passage of rehabilitation legislation prior to the 1920s and 1930s, the belief and attitude prevailed that visually impaired persons had little potential for competitive employment, and they therefore received very little benefit from early legislative developments in rehabilitation. Blind individuals continued to be maintained in stereotypic occupations and were expected to work in sheltered workshops or home-industry settings (Risley & Hoehne, 1970).

Legislation in the 1930s had a significantly more powerful impact on assisting blind and visually impaired persons in this country than did legislation of the previous decades. Four significant pieces of legislation are noteworthy—the Pratt-Smoot Act of 1931 (P.L. 71-787), Title X of the Social Security Act of 1935 (P.L. 74-271), the Randolph-Sheppard Act of 1936 (P.L. 74-732), and the Wagner-O'Day Act of 1938 (P.L. 75-739). Since its inception, each of the programs provided for by these acts has developed significantly to benefit blind and visually impaired persons.

The Pratt-Smoot Act

The Pratt-Smoot Act of 1931 (P.L. 71-787) was significant in the development of services to blind persons in that it authorized the Library of Congress to finance the production of braille books to be distributed to blind persons through regional libraries. In 1933, the act was amended (P.L. 72-439) to include the recording of Talking Books for blind persons. Additional amendments in 1962 (P.L. 87-7650) have provided for children's books and musical scores.

During the first year of funding in 1932, the Library of Congress's appropriation for Books for the Blind was $10,000. In fiscal year 1990, the National Library Service (NLS) for the Blind and Physically Handicapped had a budget of 37.112 million. NLS is the department of the Library of Congress that oversees the production and distribution of books and magazines in braille and on recorded disks and cassettes, as well as special Talking Book machines and special cassette players used for the recorded materials. In 1990, more than 20 million recorded and braille books and magazines were circulated to a readership of 695,350.

In 1966, physically disabled and other print-handicapped persons were declared eligible for Talking Books. This action resulted in a major expansion of special library services. Today, Talking Books are widely used, and this service is highly valued among older visually impaired persons, whether living independently at home or in congregate settings.

The Social Security Act

The Social Security Act (P.L. 74-271) of 1935 recognized the special needs of blind persons in Title X, Aid to the Blind. The inclusion of Title X was the result of intervention and pressure on Congress on the part of leaders in the blindness field to recognize the financial needs of this special population. Because many blind persons had extremely limited earnings, spokespersons for blind people argued for the exemption of modest earnings from benefit calculation between 1935 and 1950. It was not until 1950 that blind people were permitted to earn up to $50 a month without reduction of their social security benefits. At the same time, welfare authorities attempted to abolish the separate Title X program administered by state agencies for blind persons and include it in a single category with other types of adult assistance. Advocates of blind and visually impaired persons fought against this change, more on the grounds that civil service welfare workers were not aware of the special needs of blind persons.

The 1965 amendments to the Social Security Act established Social Security Disability Insurance (SSDI). The SSDI program expanded social security coverage to those persons who are so disabled that they are not capable of engaging in "substantial gainful activity." Although the eligibility requirements for disability insurance were originally extremely narrow, they have gradually been broadened over the years to be more responsive to the conditions of disabled persons. By 1979, blind persons could earn up to $500 a month without losing insurance benefits.

In 1972, Supplemental Security Income (SSI) (P.L. 92-603) of the Social Security Act abolished Title X and established a national income security program for three groups of financially needy Americans—blind persons, older persons, and disabled individuals who meet the limited income and resources eligibility criteria. The 1972 amendment is also significant in that it extended Medicare coverage to SSDI recipients.

The Randolph-Sheppard Act

In 1936, the Randolph-Sheppard Act (P.L. 74-732), which came to be known as the legislation that created a showcase of productive blind people, was passed. The law enabled blind people to become small business entrepreneurs by licensing them to set up vending stands in federal buildings under the auspices of the U.S. Office of Education. The act also mandated that a survey be conducted to identify other types of employment for visually impaired persons (Risley & Hoehne, 1970). By 1941, there were 316 vending stands in federal buildings and over 600 stands operating in state and municipal buildings as a result of comparable state legislation. Today over 3,000 vending facilities are in operation. The increased emphasis on the rehabilitation of blind persons brought about by the Randolph-Sheppard Act represents the only significant program expansion for rehabilitation between 1920 and the start of World War II.

The Wagner-O'Day Act

When the Social Security Act of 1935 was passed, it committed the federal government to support efforts to create and expand a stable market for products made by blind persons in sheltered workshops. This foundation laid the groundwork for the subsequent Wagner-O'Day Act of 1938 (P.L. 75-739). This act combined training and employment opportunities for blind persons and established that workshops for blind persons would be given priority as vendors to federal departments for brooms, mops, and other products that the shops manufactured. During World War II, for example, these workshops produced and sold to federal departments $32 million worth of commodities. As a result of this legislation, more blind persons could find employment in these workshops. Both the Randolph-Sheppard Act and the Wagner-O'Day Act helped to dispel misperceptions regarding the abilities of people who were blind or visually impaired. Both expanded the opportunities for blind people to demonstrate their abilities in remunerative employment. The kinds of job opportunities that were created also increased the level of awareness in the civil service system of the potential of blind employees.

Because of expanded federal purchases from the workshops, an increasing need arose for an organization that would coordinate efforts in this area. The National Industries for the Blind (NIB), a private, nonprofit organization, was formed in 1938. NIB was established under the sponsorship of the American Foundation for the Blind to fill this need. In addition, President Franklin Roosevelt appointed a special committee, the Committee on Purchase of Blind-Made Products, to establish the appropriate quantities and fair-market prices for government purchases from these workshops.

The Wagner-O'Day Act was further modified in 1971, when Senator Jacob Javits spearheaded a movement to include people with other disabilities in the workshops. Priority for government purchase was still reserved for products made by blind persons. During the same year, the Javits-Wagner-O'Day Act (P.L. 92-28) broadened the original legislation by including the provision of services in addition to products by the workshops and by requiring military commissaries and post exchanges of all other government agencies to deal with the workshops on the same "fair price" basis.

World War II resulted in considerable growth in the development of rehabilitation services in general and the rehabilitation of blind persons most specifically. The war was significant in creating increased demand for industrial products necessary to maintain the war effort and in drawing 12 million people into military service who might otherwise have been working in the civilian labor force (Levitan, Magnum, & Marshall, 1976). The wartime labor shortage gave disabled persons an enormous opportunity to demonstrate to thousands of employers that a disability did not mean that an employee could not be successful at an appropriate job. In fact, the labor shortage made the increased presence of disabled persons in the labor force a national necessity.

In 1943, the Barden-LaFollette Act (P.L. 79-113) was passed. The act amended P.L. 66-236 and stands out as a major piece of legislation for providing the first federal-state vocational rehabilitation program support for the rehabilitation of blind persons. It created the impetus for services that would provide blind and visually impaired adults with education, training, job placement, and support for entrepreneurial opportunities. Federal support went either to the vocational rehabilitation agency or to separate agencies serving blind persons that had previously been set up under a state commission for the blind or a similar agency structure. A rapid growth in vocational rehabilitation services for blind persons followed, as well as a vast increase in the number of blind clients who were rehabilitated for gainful employment. P.L. 79-113 also extended federal-state rehabilitation services to mentally retarded and mentally ill individuals and expanded the types of physical restoration services that could be provided to disabled people.

The 1943 amendments were changed with the passage of the Vocational Rehabilitation Act Amendments of 1954 (P.L. 83-565). This legislation resulted in an increase in the federal share of the funding of federal-state vocational rehabilitation programs from 50-50 to three federal dollars for every two state dollars. It also authorized the provision of $30 million in 1955 to each state for rehabilitation and appropriation as well as expansion in the annual funding to $45 million in 1956, $55 million in 1957, and $65 million in 1958 (Obermann, 1967). A 1965 amendment raised the appropriation ceilings to finance the construction of new rehabilitation centers, the renovation and expansion of existing facilities, and the addition of new features such as reader services for blind students and professionals.

For blind and visually impaired persons who would not be employable after receiving rehabilitation services, rehabilitation for the purpose of independent living would have made a qualitative difference. It was not until 1972, however, that the idea of rehabilitation for independent living was brought to the attention of Congress. In that year, Congress passed H.R. 8395, which declared for the first time that employability could no longer be the only criterion for the delivery of rehabilitation services. Unfortunately, President Richard Nixon pocket-vetoed the bill. Nixon opposed the independent living provisions on the grounds that they would move the federal-state rehabilitation program away from its basic vocational objectives and "toward more ill-defined medical care welfare goals" (DeJong, 1979). The bill continually failed to get through Congress after reintroduction by Congressman Carl Perkins and Senator Jennings Randolph. Had this legislation been enacted, older persons, who were already becoming a large percentage of the population of blind persons in this country, would have had access to rehabilitation services for independent living in the 1970s.

In 1973, Congress passed the Rehabilitation Act (P.L. 93-112), referred to as the "billion dollar program," which required state matching funds to be added to the $650 million federal appropriation for 1974. The 1973 legislation reflected major congressional commitment to the rehabilitation of disabled persons. Greater emphasis was focused on target groups and targeted services. The 1974 and 1976 amendments extended the authorizations for rehabilitation, but the 1978 amendments were most noteworthy in that they established an independent living program for disabled persons without work potential who could be brought to independent living status through the provision of rehabilitation services.

Title VII of the Rehabilitation Act, established by the 1978 amendments to the act, authorized the addition of an independent living rehabilitation program to the federal-state rehabilitation program. Part A of Title VII authorized comprehensive services to severely disabled individuals whose ability to engage or continue in employment or whose ability to function independently in a family or community was limited. Part B authorized the commissioner of the Rehabilitation Services Administration (RSA) to make grants to state rehabilitation agencies for the establishment and operation of independent living centers located throughout the country.

Part C authorized program funds from which the commissioner of the RSA could make grants to state vocational rehabilitation agencies to provide independent living skills training to older blind and visually impaired persons in order for them to continue to live independently in their own communities. However, funds were not allocated for Title VII, Part C until 1986, after the House Select Committee on Aging held hearings in 1985 concerning services to older blind individuals. In 1986, 24 grants were made to 23 states at approximately $200,000 per grant.

Therefore, although Title VII, Part C was a major breakthrough in rehabilitation for independent living for elderly people, its limited allocation of funds and its funding process have decreased its impact on older visually impaired persons nationwide. The first set of grants were made through a competitive process on a discretionary basis and for only one year. This limited amount of time and limited service dollars, compared to the total number of older persons in need of services and the extent of their need, gave agencies just enough time to get their programs in full operation before the year was over. Open submissions were made for three-year funding in the next round.

Although some of the originally funded agencies received money through the next round, others did not, leaving them without the financial backing to maintain their innovative programming on behalf of older visually impaired persons in their states. Five million dollars were allocated in 1986, and by 1991, only $1.1 million of additional funds had been added to Title VII, Part C. In 1991, only 28 states had Title VII, Part C funds.

Some states have never been successful in obtaining a grant. Ironically, the two states with the largest number of older persons, California and Florida, have been unsuccessful in receiving funding. Unfortunately, over half the older visually impaired elderly population in the country have no access to independent living skills training through Title VII, Part C. Even in funded states, the $200,000 allocation does not provide for service to all eligible visually impaired older persons and is insufficient to provide service at the level needed. However, there have been exemplary services provided through Title VII, Part C. For example, in North Carolina, 653 older persons were served from July 1, 1988, through June 30, 1989. These older persons received medical restoration and low vision services; training in O&M, communication, and daily living skills; training in the use of low vision devices; and counseling. An even further benefit was that these services were provided through program centers throughout the state, some located in senior citizens centers, which was a helpful strategy to integrate blind and visually impaired people into the general elderly population.

Title VII, Part C funds have enabled agencies that had not provided services to the elderly population to begin to do so. In some states there had been some service to elderly people through funds that targeted nonvocational rehabilitation. These services are usually supported by nonvocational grants or by state funds that serve as a match to federal funds. Title VII, Part C funds enabled these agencies to expand their services. Some agencies were able to conduct extensive outreach or to begin to serve rural counties that had not been previously served. Others targeted outreach to minority groups, such as Native American elderly people on reservations and Hispanic elderly people who had limited access to rehabilitation services because of language and cultural barriers. Through these funds older people are beginning to recognize that an agency for blind and visually impaired people is not solely for those who are young and employment-bound. That is the positive side of Title VII, Part C; the negative aspect is that even with these funds, many states cannot serve all the eligible older persons in the state, and waiting lists of older visually impaired persons exist.

In the 1990s, current advocates for increased allocation of funds for Title VII, Part C are calling for $26 million to fund each state at the $225,000 level so that services can be made available to older persons throughout the country. An additional appropriation to each state based on the number of older visually impaired persons in that state is also called for. In January 1991, the House Committee on Aging held a hearing in California to hear from professionals and consumers about the extent of the need that still exists for increased Title VII, Part C funds. On May 22, 1991, the committee's chair introduced H.R. 2437, calling for a national Title VII, Part C program funded at $26 million.

SERVICES FOR BLINDED VETERANS

Special note has been made of the impetus caused by the rehabilitation needs of veterans blinded in service to their country. The number of servicemen blinded in the four wars fought by the United States in the twentieth century is relatively small—almost 400 in World War I, 1,400 in World War II, 500 in the Korean action, and about the same number in Vietnam. However, the effect of these numbers on services for blind persons is considerable. After World War I, a demonstration program for the rehabilitation of blinded soldiers was established by the army at Evergreen, Maryland, near Baltimore. This program was known as the Evergreen Program, and although it had flaws, it demonstrated rehabilitation techniques that were later adapted for work with blind civilians. The rehabilitation programs established after World War II had a greater impact on the development of rehabilitation services. These services were set up at army and navy hospitals, at the rehabilitation center at Avon Old Farms run by the army in Connecticut, and later at the U.S. Veterans Administration (VA) Hospital in Hines, Illinois, where the VA's first Blind Rehabilitation Center was established. There are now three additional centers located across the country. The VA (now the U.S. Department of Veterans Affairs) operates long-term care domiciliary facilities and adult day care programs for frail elderly veterans. Many older blind veterans reside in and utilize these facilities.

The VA was responsible for developing the systematic use of a cane for independent mobility. Although blind persons from the earliest times have developed ways to travel from place to place using staffs, canes, and dogs, it was not until the demands made by the veterans of World War II that instruction in the use of the long cane was initiated in the Valley Forge Army Hospital and later at the Central Blind Rehabilitation Center at Hines Veterans Administration Hospital. When the value of the long cane as a travel device was well demonstrated and documented, a master's degree in the Peripatology Program at Boston College was inaugurated in June 1960 with strong support from the U.S. Office of Vocational Rehabilitation, now the RSA. The Boston program was soon followed by the establishment of the Department of Blind Rehabilitation and Mobility at Western Michigan University in July 1961. At present 16 college and university programs in O&M exist throughout the country and are listed in the *Directory of Services for Blind and Visually Impaired Persons in the United States* (AFB, 1988).

The Blinded Veterans Association (BVA) is a national organization, headquartered in Washington, DC, that functions as both a service and an advocacy organization for its members. BVA is authorized by the VA to represent blind veterans in formal appeals and claims and works with other organizations of and for blind persons to monitor and promote legislation related to the delivery of services. Through its outreach program, veterans with eye injuries are informed about rehabilitation services, vocational training, and job-placement benefits. It has 37 regional affiliates that operate volunteer service programs throughout the country.

Service Delivery Structure

In the aging field, funds, policies, and programs descend in a straight line from national to state, area, and local agencies. Service delivery in the field of blindness is less uniformly structured, but parallels be-tween the two service delivery systems can be drawn. In the aging system, funds provided for by the Older Americans Act (OAA) are administered by the U.S. Administration on Aging; in the blindness system, the RSA administers federal funds provided for by the Rehabilitation Act. At the state level, there is a state unit on aging and a state commission for the blind or a generic rehabilitation agency encompassing all disabilities, with a unit on blind rehabilitation. In the aging field, there is a county or multicounty agency for elderly persons (the area agency on aging), and in the blindness field, there are local offices of the state agency for the blind as well as private agencies. All agencies serving the elderly population receive funds through the OAA and may also receive private funds.

Services for blind and visually impaired persons are delivered by numerous private voluntary agencies as well as 50 state agencies providing such services. The private, voluntary agencies for blind persons are independent and freestanding organizations. They are funded by private contributions and endowments, purchase-of-service contracts from state vocational rehabilitation agencies, federal or state research or demonstration grants, and, in some instances, agency workshops that result in income for the agency. Voluntary agencies vary greatly in size, budget, and scope and in the nature of their programs. Some make use of volunteers to provide nonrehabilitation services. Some are beginning to work cooperatively with agencies for elderly persons, for example, in broadening their base of services to older visually impaired persons and pooling their resources in an era of economic scarcity.

Service delivery for blind persons differs greatly from one state or community to another. One of the simplest ways to identify services for a blind person is to consult AFB's *Directory of Services* (1988). Using the directory, service providers in the aging network, for example, can identify appropriate services for visually impaired clients, and a senior citizens center can find a local agency that will provide rehabilitation services for a visually impaired older person or an agency for the blind that can also provide in-service training to agency staff and members of a senior citizens center.

Because of the growing numbers of older visually impaired persons in every community throughout the country, it is important for agencies for blind persons and agencies for elderly persons to collaborate both in planning and service delivery and to make maximum use of their resources on behalf of their mutual clients. An agency for blind persons can coordinate a vision screening program in a senior citizens center or nursing home and make needed referrals for eye care, including referrals to a low vision clinic. Directors of nursing homes can work with agencies for blind persons to receive in-service training to assist staff members in working more effectively with visually impaired residents. They can also arrange with local or regional libraries that are part of NLS to introduce residents to Talking Books. Other options open to workers in the aging field also include joint program planning for the successful integration of older visually impaired persons into services and activities for the elderly population in general.

An example of collaborative planning at the national level exists between two organizations in the blindness and the aging field. The National Council of State Agencies for the Blind (NCSAB) represents state agencies for blind people. It works to improve service delivery to blind persons and to advocate for improvements in the field. NCSAB has entered into a written working agreement with the National Association of State Units on Aging to coordinate service delivery between the two fields.

National Organizations in the Blindness Field

Information about various organizations of and for blind persons may be useful to service providers, particularly those in the field of aging. In addition to the organizations described below are also many national organizations focused on particular eye diseases, such as retinitis pigmentosa (RP), macular degeneration, glaucoma, and diabetic retinopathy. These organizations serve to heighten the level of awareness about the eye conditions and their prevalence and many provide support groups and newsletters for their membership and the general public.

AMERICAN FOUNDATION FOR THE BLIND

AFB is a national organization established in 1921 to make blindness and visual impairment a national concern. AFB's mission is to enable persons who are blind or visually impaired to achieve equality of access and opportunity that will ensure freedom of choice in their lives. AFB accomplishes this mission by taking a national leadership role in the development and implementation of public policy and legislation, informational and educational programs, diversified products, and quality services. It serves as a clearinghouse for information about blindness and visual impairment; provides professional consultation in the areas of aging, employment, and education; conducts research on issues related to vision loss; operates an active public and professional education program through its publication of books, monographs, and brochures; records Talking Books; and provides technology information and evaluation. It also publishes the leading professional journal in the field, the *Journal of Visual Impairment & Blindness.*

AFB's M.C. Migel Memorial Library and Information Center is the nation's largest lending library on the subjects of blindness and visual impairment and contains the Helen Keller Archives. It also serves as a demonstration center for a variety of high-technology devices that provide blind and visually impaired users of the library with access to the print collection. In 1985, a National Technology Center, a technology evaluation center for assessing concepts, prototypes, and commercially available sensory devices, was established. The center works to maximize the number of appropriate devices available to blind people while providing valuable information for providers and users. In addition, AFB's Product Center sells a wide range of adaptive devices and appliances designed for use by blind and visually impaired persons. AFB also manufactures Talking Books and operates a toll-free national information hotline. (See "Resources" for information on AFB and many of the organizations discussed in this book.)

Headquartered in New York City, AFB maintains a Government Relations Department in Washington, DC, and five regional centers staffed by professionally trained consultants who provide consultation, training, and information and referral services to state and local agencies and consumers. The regional centers are located in Atlanta, Chicago, Dallas, San Francisco, and Washington, DC.

ASSOCIATION FOR EDUCATION AND REHABILITATION OF THE BLIND AND VISUALLY IMPAIRED

The Association for Education and Rehabilitation of the Blind and Visually Impaired (AER) is a professional membership organization that promotes education and work with blind and visually impaired persons of all ages. AER was established in 1984 as a result of the merger of two formerly independent professional membership associations— the American Association of Workers for the Blind, establsihed in 1905 after evolving from its origins as the National College Association for the Blind in 1895, and the Association for Education of the Visually Handicapped, established in 1852 originally as the American Association of Instructors of the Blind. AER conducts conferences and publishes a newsletter and a journal. It also conducts legislative advocacy and certifies programs for rehabilitation teachers and O&M specialists. It operates a job exchange and a reference information center. Its membership consists of professionals concerned with educational guidance and vocational rehabilitation of both children and adults.

NATIONAL ACCREDITATION COUNCIL FOR AGENCIES SERVING THE BLIND AND VISUALLY HANDICAPPED

The National Accreditation Council for Agencies Serving the Blind and Visually Handicapped (NAC), founded in 1966, is the blindness field's accrediting body for agencies and schools. It establishes and regularly updates standards for management functions and for specific types of service programs. It publishes these standards in the form of self-study guides that organizations use when seeking accreditation to measure and improve their performance. Teams of volunteer professionals conduct on-site reviews of agencies seeking accreditation or reaccreditation and prepare reports for NAC. Accreditation is granted by NAC commissioners.

NATIONAL INDUSTRIES FOR THE BLIND

NIB was established in 1938 to coordinate the production of 100 workshops for blind persons and to allocate purchase orders of the federal government for approved goods and services to these work-shops. It also works closely with the President's Committee for Purchase from the Blind and Other Severely Handicapped for the purpose of researching and recommending new types of products to be manufactured by workshops, and it proposes prices and price revision of products, as needed. In addition, it works toward improving the efficiency of plants and quality control by conducting management and technical training programs for workshop personnel. Evaluation and training programs for the employment of multiply disabled persons in workshops are established by its Division of Rehabilitation Services.

NATIONAL SOCIETY TO PREVENT BLINDNESS

The National Society to Prevent Blindness (NSPB) was established in 1908 in New York City and is now located in Chicago. The society conducts programs of public and professional education, research, and industrial and community services related to the prevention of blindness. It has a network of state affiliates through which it promotes and supports local glaucoma and preschool vision screening programs and industrial eye safety measures. It works to improve environmental conditions affecting eye health in schools and public facilities. The society also collects national statistical data on the incidence, prevalence, types, and causes of blindness.

MISSISSIPPI STATE REHABILITATION RESEARCH AND TRAINING CENTER IN BLINDNESS AND LOW VISION

The Mississippi State Rehabilitation Research and Training Center in Blindness and Low Vision is a federally funded organization established in the mid-1980s. It is the country's only research and training center in the field of blindness, and it conducts research on all aspects of blindness and low vision. It has collected, analyzed, and published data on the programs and services provided to blind and visually impaired older persons through Title VII, Part C funds.

Services for Deaf-Blind Persons

Individuals who are both deaf and blind or severely hearing and visually impaired have very special needs and require specialized forms of assistance. The Helen Keller National Center for Deaf-Blind Youths and Adults (HKNC) is the leading national organization focusing on the needs of these individuals. HKNC is headquartered in Sands Point, New York, and has six regional offices throughout the country. It was funded by the U.S. Department of Education in 1969. The Sands Point location offers residential rehabilitation and vocational training programs for deaf-blind persons from all parts of the United States. It also provides rehabilitation training and job placement services and conducts research programs.

HKNC's six regional centers work to improve the capability of state agencies to assist deaf-blind persons. The regional centers provide direct diagnostic and evaluation services, adjustment programs, and consultation for parents and teachers. A specialist in aging is located in the Dallas Center and serves as a resource to service providers of the elderly population on service delivery to older persons experiencing hearing and visual impairments.

Educational and Reading Resources

THE NATIONAL LIBRARY SERVICE (NLS) FOR THE BLIND AND PHYSICALLY HANDICAPPED

NLS conducts a national program to distribute free reading materials, including classics, current fiction, and general nonfiction in braille and on recorded disks and cassettes to visually impaired and physically disabled persons who cannot utilize ordinary printed materials. Reading materials and playback equipment are distributed on loan free of charge through a network of regional and subregional libraries and machine-lending agencies. In addition, the service operates a reference information section on all aspects of blindness and other physical disabilities that affect reading. It functions as a bibliographic center on reading materials for disabled people and referral agency to organizations that provide reading materials in special media on loan.

RADIO READING SERVICES

Radio reading services are in operation in 92 cities across the nation, and their numbers are growing steadily. These locally organized and funded units broadcast on regular and subcarrier radio channels, using volunteers to read newspapers, magazines, and books. In areas where subcarrier channels are used, listeners are supplied with special receivers. Radio reading services are used widely and are a favorite of older persons experiencing vision loss who rely on these services as a major source of information.

RECORDING FOR THE BLIND
Recording for the Blind (RFB) was established in 1948 to tape textbooks and other educational materials for students and materials for professionals and blind persons who need to have access to specialized professional and technical literature. It has a collection of 60,000 master tapes of recorded books, and approximately 4,000 titles are added each year based on requests from students and professionals. Recordings are made by volunteers in 29 studios across the country.

THE HADLEY SCHOOL FOR THE BLIND
The Hadley School for the Blind was established in 1920 in Winnetka, Illinois. The school offers 125 correspondence courses in braille and on cassette for legally blind persons. Courses include special programs in independent living for elderly blind and visually impaired persons, in addition to accredited academic and vocational education. The courses cover subjects in the upper elementary school, high school, and college levels, as well as in vocational and avocational areas of interest. The Hadley School also operates overseas offices through which English is taught as a second language in braille.

ADDITIONAL READING RESOURCES
Specialized reading materials in braille, tape, and large type are provided by a number of sectarian groups. A complete listing of them can be obtained through NLS, which also maintains lists of transcribing services through its "Volunteers Who Produce Books" listing. There are three periodicals in braille and recorded form available to blind and visually impaired persons that are independent of the NLS network— the *Matilda Ziegler Magazine for the Blind, Choice Magazine Listening,* and *Dialogue.*

Organizations of Blind Persons

The two major national membership organizations of blind and visually impaired persons are the American Council of the Blind (ACB) and the National Federation of the Blind (NFB). ACB was established in 1961 and has its national headquarters in Washington, DC. NFB was established in 1940 and is headquartered in Baltimore. Both organizations work toward similar goals, primarily to improve the social and economic conditions of blind persons through legislative advocacy. The organizations provide legal services to their members and serve as spokespersons on national and local issues affecting visually impaired persons. They also monitor existing services and advocate for new services to meet the changing needs of the population of blind and visually impaired persons. Both organizations have state and local chapters and special-interest affiliates. They conduct active public education programs, provide scholarships, and publish monthly magazines. Another more recent consumer organization, the Council of Citizens with Low Vision, was organized for similar purposes and is composed of persons who are severely visually impaired.

Parent groups are also a relatively recent development. The National Association of Parents of the Visually Impaired (NAPVI) publishes a newsletter and holds conferences for the exchange of ideas and experiences related to raising and educating blind and visually impaired children. Both NFB and ACB also have parent group affiliates that serve similar functions.

Professional Preparation Programs

Professional preparation programs for training personnel to serve blind and visually impaired persons have developed into formal college or university preparation disciplines. At present, undergraduate and graduate degrees can be earned in the fields of special education of blind children, rehabilitation teaching, and O&M.

The first formal program for the preparation of teachers of blind children was inaugurated in 1921, when the Perkins School for the Blind established a six-month program at the Harvard University Graduate School of Education. A complete listing of the schools offering programs in teaching visually impaired children can be found in the AFB *Directory of Services* (1988).

Rehabilitation teachers, originally referred to as home teachers, began what was a voluntary service in the United States in the 1880s. Services were provided by blind persons who taught other blind persons independent living skills that they had acquired. Their original purpose is significant in that they wanted to teach blind persons to read the scriptures and to be literate. Professional preparation was first attempted in a program established in 1922 by Olin H. Burritt, principal of the Overbrook School for the Blind in Philadelphia, in conjunction with the Pennsylvania School of Social Work and Health.

The first master's degree program in rehabilitation teaching was established at Western Michigan University in Kalamazoo in 1963. At present there are seven graduate and one undergraduate university programs in rehabilitation teaching. Other specializations in the field are developing to keep pace with the needs of blind persons. For example, the Pennsylvania College of Optometry in Philadelphia now offers a master's degree program in vision rehabilitation.

Rehabilitation in the 1990s: Current Issues

In the 1990s, the blindness field faces a shortage of personnel, particularly in the disciplines of O&M and rehabilitation teaching. Considerable efforts are taking place to encourage people to enter these fields. Although university programs have been underenrolled, O&M programs have been attracting more students in recent years. Various paraprofessional training programs are emerging in order to fill the gaps in availability of service to blind and visually impaired persons, particularly elderly persons. Considerable efforts are also underway to recruit various minority group members into the field because of the limited number of minority professionals currently working in blind rehabilitation. Employment of black and Hispanic rehabilitation teachers and O&M specialists may help reduce the language and cultural barriers that can seriously limit access to services, particularly for older persons.

The field is also working toward licensure of these two disciplines, as well as national certification standards for rehabilitation teachers. Such efforts are essential if these service providers are to move out of the realm of blindness agencies and provide services in other service arenas, such as medical settings. Their doing so would help professionals outside the blindness field become more familiar with the two disciplines, would in all likelihood help increase referrals for their services on behalf of clients, and would promote the reimbursement of rehabilitation services through third-party payments such as Medicare and Medicaid. Reimbursement would, in turn, help expand service delivery and promote awareness of such services. Certification and licensure are required for third-party reimbursement, just as they are for other rehabilitation and therapeutic disciplines, such as physical therapy.

The greatest need and challenge for the next decades is to serve the growing population of older persons and to serve them through collaborative efforts with the aging service delivery system. In light of this increasing need, the disciplines of O&M and rehabilitation teaching may be in greater demand, and additional university programs may be necessary. University guidelines for starting new programs are already in existence. The importance of collaboration will increase in the coming years. Services available in the community from the aging network are described in Chapter 9, and efforts toward collaboration between the aging and the blindness systems are described in Chapter 15.

References

American Foundation for the Blind. (1988). *Directory of services for blind and visually impaired persons in the United States* (23rd ed.). New York: Author.

DeJong, G. (1979). Independent living: From social movement to analytic paradigm. *Archives of Physical Medical Rehabilitation, 60:* 435-446.

Lenihan, J. (1977). *Disabled Americans: A history, performance* (Bicentennial issue). Washington, DC: The President's Committee on Employment of the Handicapped.

Levitan, S. A., Magnum, G. L., & Marshall, R. (1976). *Human resources and labor markets.* New York: Harper & Row.

MacDonald, M. E. (1944). *Federal grants for vocational rehabilitation.* Chicago: University of Chicago Press.

Obermann, C. E. (1965). *A history of vocational rehabilitation in America*. Minneapolis: The Dennison Company.

Obermann, C. E. (1967). The limitations of history. In G. N. Wright (Ed.), *Madison lectures on vocational rehabilitation*. Madison, WI: Rehabilitation Counselor Education Program, University of Wisconsin, Madison.

Risley, B., & Hoehne, C. (1970). The vocational rehabilitation act related to the blind. *Journal of Rehabilitation, 36*(5): 26-31.

CHAPTER 9

Community-Based Services for Older Persons

Robert L. Dolsen

In most industrial democracies, one can learn about the delivery of services for older people without straying from one locality. In these countries, the kinds of services that are available and the mechanisms through which clients gain access to them are generally consistent nationwide. Although local governments are most often given the authority to administer programs, the central government mandates services. If private, not-for-profit agencies deliver services, a central authority subsidizes and standardizes the services. But the situation in the United States is quite different.

Diversity of Services in the United States

In the United States, one finds a remarkable variety in local services for aging persons. Some kind of federalism has been a part of the American political landscape since the founding of the republic, and the development of public policy and the implementation of public programs have been the result of the ebb and flow of authority among federal, state, and local governments. The federal government's direct support for the elderly population applies only to solving problems that are extensive enough to be perceived as national crises. The social security retirement program emerged from the belief by the general public during the Great Depression that private pensions were inadequate or unreliable for ensuring basic subsistence. Medicare was a compromise response to the increased costs of health care nationwide.

Although the federal government has assumed primary responsibility for income maintenance and acute health care of elderly people through social security and Medicare, respectively, it has not had the political mandate to provide standardized, direct social and support services for the elderly population. In most instances, Congress has delegated to the states the authority to plan and implement programs, while sharing responsibility for generating the revenue necessary to fund the programs. This shared governmental authority works against the national standardization and universality of community-based programs, which have been shaped primarily by state and local governmental processes.

The voluntary sector, a primary mechanism for local initiatives in the delivery of human services, contributes to the diversity. In any state, any group wishing to address a human need may establish for a modest fee a not-for-profit private corporation for educational or charitable purposes. The group appoints its own board, delineates its purposes, and chooses its clientele. The result is a variety of services under a variety of auspices that reflect the competitive, private, for-profit market more than the developed welfare state. One may find a council on aging, usually private not-for-profit; a commission on aging, usually public; and a public or private neighborhood committee on aging coexisting amid a larger, equally complex milieu of other service agencies. All these groups try to provide similar services to similar clientele. In searching for appropriate help, a needy older person may find frustrating gaps or duplication along with refreshing flexibility and creativity in services afforded by the involvement of grass-roots organizations.

Another significant factor fostering the fragmentation of services for elderly people is the composition of the aging population itself. In the 1970s, an important issue debated among advocates for older persons was how older people should best be portrayed—as vital, productive members of society or as vulnerable, dependent persons. The political and social consequences of each portrayal are obvious. One portrayal may lead policymakers to ignore the critical needs of the frail while they focus on the frisky; the other may lead to a demeaning stereotype depicting all elderly persons as frail, dependent, and needing assistance. Both views capture parts of the total profile. Older persons in an age group that spans as many as 40 years, and with varied social, economic, and environmental circumstances and physical conditions, are more diverse than the numbers of any other age group. It is therefore impossible to design one set of services for them all simultaneously. Instead, services must be designed along a continuum of care.

However, older people can be grouped loosely in terms of their needs. Although needs develop at different chronological ages among the older population, and on an individual basis, there is enough evidence to predict that particular problems will develop at higher rates at different stages of later life. We know, for example, that the average age for widowhood is in the 50s, that the average age for retirement is in the early to mid-60s, and that the incidence of frailty remains relatively low before age 75. Although somewhat simplistic, a perspective based on needs triggered by later life events helps explain the seemingly segmented services for the aging population.

Many different pieces of federal legislation in regard to housing, health care coverage, income, energy, transportation, and social services address the needs of elderly people. Because of the design of the legislative system, however, these pieces of legislation tend to be enacted with minimal coordination. Hence, gaps and overlaps in services occur. Consequently, in the 1973 amendments to the Older Americans Act (OAA), Congress provided the mechanism—the Area Agency on Aging (AAA)—to coordinate local services to aging persons (see Chapter 7). The structure that many AAAs use to plan systems of services is a "continuum of care," a configuration of services ranging from those that are appropriate for active, independent elderly people to those for frail and homebound elderly individuals.

An examination of this continuum of care reveals not one service system but several different independent systems. Agencies for the elderly predominate in the provision of services for active, independent elderly people. But when health problems or sensory loss restricts activity and the services needed become more intensive and complex, such as those in the health care field, professional organizations outside the aging system are also essential. It is worth noting that the kinds of professional care traditionally viewed as institutionally based are now extended into community-based systems; the home has reemerged as often the most appropriate place in which to provide care. Family caregivers are once again the primary source of care and support. It is conceivable that we may again see physicians making house calls as a regular practice, which would make the home a common center for all kinds of care.

Programs for the Post-Middle Aged

People in the post-middle-aged generation, those in their 50s and early 60s, may be beginning to feel some of the vagaries of the aging process. Nevertheless, they are relatively untouched by debilitation as a group. In general, they enjoy good health, live in their own homes, manage their own affairs, and, often, are at the peak of their earning power. Their children have probably left home, and they are changing their family roles and reshaping their activities. Most recently, however, society has witnessed a trend in which adult children in their 20s are staying at home longer than did their previous cohort. This phenomenon continues to reshape roles and responsibilities of many individuals in their 50s. Most people in this generation see their stage of life as replete with opportunities for growth, fulfillment, and increased life satisfaction.

Senior membership organizations have much to offer this constituency—low-cost insurance and financial services; travel tours; discounts on drugs, hotel stays, and other items; and a wealth of educational materials and practical information. The American Association of Retired Persons (AARP) publishes a monthly newsletter and a magazine, *Modern Maturity*, and also offers short courses from its Lifetime Learning Program. On the local level, there are over 4,500 AARP chapters and a variety of educational programs and volunteer opportunities. The National Council of Senior Citizens (NCSC), a membership organization for older persons that has roots in the labor union movement, sponsors local chapters and publishes a newsletter as well.

Learning continues throughout life, and many older persons seek out new educational experiences. Local high schools frequently sponsor adult education courses and offer people over age 60 free passes to school events. Many colleges and universities offer free or reduced tuition to senior citizens who attend regular academic classes. Continuing education departments in universities often develop special non-credit courses aimed at the interests of older persons. These courses are usually held where older people congregate—senior citizens centers, churches, and retirement communities. The elder hostel movement has flourished over the last decade, providing older persons opportunities to take courses while residing at a university for brief periods.

It is important to note that although the literacy rate of the present cohorts of older persons has increased dramatically over previous cohorts, the issue of illiteracy among older persons does not receive adequate attention. It is a critical issue in the 1990s that is being recognized at the federal level. The National Council on the Aging (NCOA) has advocated to Congress that the National Adult Literacy Survey conducted by the National Center for Education Statistics should include elderly people. The survey's results would have the potential to influence future priorities at the federal level regarding literacy. The issue of literacy among blind persons is a priority for the American Foundation for the Blind (AFB) in the 1990s in regard to increasing people's access to reading methods, including braille, large-print, and recorded materials. The issue of literacy among older blind and visually impaired persons is also being explored.

Preretirement planning has emerged full scale in the past decade. Many employers, especially larger corporations, provide employees with preretirement planning assistance to prepare them for successful retirement. For other preretirees, AAAs or other community agencies may offer such training.

Those who find that the press of work and raising children has subsided somewhat and that they have increased free time may wish to help others. If so, they can choose from a wide variety of volunteer activities. Most communities have voluntary action centers, which bring together willing volunteers and needy community agencies. The federal government promotes volunteerism through its locally operated Older Americans Volunteer Programs administered by ACTION, as described in Chapter 7. The Small Business Administration's Senior Corps of Retired Executives utilizes the talents of retired professionals who consult with persons who are starting their own businesses or with community agencies beginning a new enterprise. AARP and local service providers serving aging persons use senior volunteers extensively.

EMPLOYMENT AND TRAINING PROGRAMS

People in their 50s and 60s who lose jobs that provided a livelihood may be devastated. The passage of the Age Discrimination and Employment Act protects the older worker from discrimination in hiring and promotion. A job loss at this age, however, still may mean an agonizing confrontation with age discrimination and, if another job is found, possibly less income and decreased self-esteem. If the person is a member of a minority group, the struggle can be doubly difficult.

The experience of having to find a new job relatively late in life is particularly devastating for the older worker who begins to experience vision loss. Often, neither the older visually impaired employee nor the prospective employer has any idea how to help the employee to continue working. However, it is quite possible to continue employment through vocational rehabilitation and the use of adapted equipment, job modification of tasks, or environmental modification. Minor environmental modification, for example, can create a physical environment that allows the older person to make maximum use of remaining vision through improved lighting, reduction of glare, and the use of color contrast. Large-print materials and equipment like computers with speech output also make continued employment possible.

According to a national survey conducted by the Commonwealth Fund, more than 1.9 million older Americans age 50 to 63 are ready and able to return to work (AARP, 1991). This figure includes women who have not been employed outside the home during child-rearing years, persons who have been out of work because of disability, and individuals who retired early but who wish employment, particularly part-time work. This finding has major significance for labor shortages anticipated for the year 2000 and after. Demographic trends seem to indicate that employers are likely to recruit older, more mature workers during the coming decades because this pool of available employees will consist of experienced individuals. Disincentives to continuation of employment or reentry into the work force must be overcome, however, including employer attitudes steering older workers to lower-level positions and a lack of sensitivity to the need for a supportive work environment. This is particularly true for the older worker with vision loss.

In recognition of the importance of work incentives, the Administration on Aging (AOA) established the Business and Aging Leadership Awards to honor companies that develop policies and programs of mutual benefit to business and older Americans. Awards focus on the areas of employment and training, including the following:

- hiring, retention, training, and flexible work scheduling programs that promote full and protective utilization of older employees in the work force;
- work and family issues, including programs helping employees to balance work and caregiving responsibilities;
- health promotion, volunteerism, and community initiatives, including programs to strengthen the capacity of public organizations to arrange needed services through the volunteer efforts of employees and retirees.

The most visible and successful public effort to help unemployed older persons is Title V of the OAA, the federally funded Senior Community Services Employment Program. This program subsidizes part-time employment for low-income persons aged 55 and over until they obtain permanent employment. With locally operated projects in communities across the nation, the program is partly administered by state units and AAAs and partly by national contractors such as AARP, NCSC, NCOA, the U.S. Forestry Service, and the National Farmers Organization. Other contractors are national organizations for minority older persons, representing such groups as blacks, Hispanics, Pacific Asians, and Native Americans.

Positions funded by Title V that are in-service organizations meeting the needs of older people are ideal for many older visually impaired persons, who are eager to be productive and gainfully employed. Although such placements have so far occurred on an extremely limited basis, there is opportunity for growth in the near future. The primary stumbling block is the need to educate directors of agencies with Title

V positions, about the capabilities of older visually impaired persons and the minor modifications or adaptations that enable the older visually impaired person to be successful in these positions. The Job Training Partnership Act, which funds employment training and placement projects, allocates funds for special projects to train persons aged 55 and over. Administered by the states, these training and placement projects may be operated by AAAs, private industry councils, or any of several other kinds of agencies. These funds provide yet another opportunity for older visually impaired persons to become trained for reentering the job market. The passage of the Americans with Disabilities Act of 1991 will also have a positive and powerful impact on improving employment opportunities for older visually impaired workers.

ASSISTANCE FOR WIDOWS

A woman who loses a husband who was the sole family breadwinner will not only be struck by grief and the loss of emotional support but will also suffer a substantial loss of income. All too often, she is prepared neither to enter the job market nor to manage the family's financial affairs (Fenano & Banesi, 1982). As increasing numbers of women work because of the need for two incomes and the higher divorce rate, this lack of experience in employment and in financial management among many women will change, and change even more dramatically as the baby boom generation ages.

A widow may find immediate help in a widows' peer counseling group, usually directed by a community mental health center, religious organization, senior center, or local membership organization. AARP's Widowed Persons Service provides materials and directions for community organizations seeking to develop such a group. For help in earning an income and taking charge of personal affairs, universities and community colleges frequently sponsor women's centers and displaced homemakers' programs, which can give widows needed support and advice.

CAREGIVING

One other issue pervasive for people in their 50s and 60s is the responsibility of caring for an aging parent. This responsibility is typically assumed by daughters, daughters-in-law, or other female family members. Sometimes referred to as the "sandwich generation" caring for children and aged parents, people in this age group often stretch their financial and emotional resources at the risk of their own well-being. The number of available respite programs, support groups, and publications for caregivers is growing rapidly to respond to this enormous need. As people live longer, the incidence of Alzheimer's disease and other physical conditions and disabilities has helped create the "sandwiching" phenomenon experienced by this generation. By necessity, employers are becoming more flexible about work hours for women who must work part time to provide care for a parent. (The issue of caregiving in the 1990s is discussed in greater detail in Chapter 13.)

Services to the Young-Old

With aging come new opportunities for personal growth, friendship, leisure pursuits, volunteerism, and employment. But the aging process has also been described as a series of losses—losses of income, friends and loved ones, mobility, vision and hearing, physical strength, and productive pursuits. Successful aging—"aging well"—is essentially the best use of one's remaining resources to maintain one's independence and quality of life. The young-old, those 65 to 74, begin to face a series of losses and to require formal support services to complement or enhance remaining personal resources. Although they generally retain much of their vigor, most young-old persons experience a substantial loss of income in retirement, a loss invariably exacerbated over time because of inflation. The young-old also begin to experience chronic illnesses that limit mobility, see many close friends die, and, if they are women, become widowed.

At this stage in life, problems begin to occur concurrently, each deepening the impact of the others. For example, the widow who loses her husband and consequently her income may find that modest earnings and social security checks do not meet her steadily increasing health care bills. Her home, far larger than she requires, may need structural repairs. The onset of vision loss can further limit her ability to do daily tasks. With the loss of some close friends, her loneliness may deepen into social isolation and occasional deep depression. She may no longer bother to prepare complete meals for herself, may leave the house less and less, and may lack the energy to keep herself and her home in order.

Although most young-old people cope successfully, the widow just described is not atypical. People in such circumstances can take advantage of services for aging persons. Although there are no guarantees, elderly people who strengthen and preserve their personal resources are best able to delay or prevent the debilitating conditions that strike with greater prevalence in the later stages of aging.

FINANCIAL SERVICES

For financially needy persons who are elderly, blind, or disabled and whose incomes including social security are inadequate, Supplemental Security Income (SSI) is available. Eligibility for SSI is based on stringent and demonstrable low-income levels. Recipients must be at least age 65 or must be disabled. One applies for SSI at local social security offices. The Social Security Administration estimates that a significant number of eligible persons have not applied for SSI benefits. A percentage as high as 35 to 50 percent of eligible elderly persons is not currently participating in the program (Delfico, 1990). In addition, the SSI program is particularly inadequate in serving the needs of non-English-speaking persons. This is because public information and outreach materials traditionally have not been widely available in Spanish and other languages. As a result, persons who do not read English have not been made aware of the eligibility criteria and have not applied for assistance. Over 30 SSI outreach demonstration projects were funded in 1990 to develop targeted outreach strategies for the hard-to-reach, potentially eligible population, including blind and visually impaired older persons.

Other federal income-maintenance programs that have no age requirements include those providing food stamps and low-income energy assistance. Both programs have income requirements and serve a disproportionately high percentage of elderly clients, and they operate through county departments of social services or welfare offices.

Although the federal government has been predominant in income-maintenance programs, state governments have also played significant roles. Some states with income taxes honor the extra exemptions for elderly and blind people in the federal income tax code. Some enacted extensive programs for property tax relief for elderly and disabled people and developed home-heating energy assistance programs for elderly individuals. Help in understanding and applying for these income programs can usually be found at senior centers or through AARP's local Tax-Aide services.

Other income extenders include many discount programs for older persons. In every community, local merchants advertise discounts for senior citizens, and some states have encouraged statewide discount programs such as that distributing the Golden Buckeye Discount Card in Ohio. Southwestern Bell, in conjunction with the National Association of Area Agencies on Aging (NAAAA), initiated a national effort with its "Silver Pages," which provides telephone listings of establishments offering senior discounts in each community. National membership organizations are also sources of discounts. One example is the AARP Pharmacy Service, which sells nonprescription drugs at reduced prices.

OUTREACH

Services are only as good as the extent to which possible recipients are aware of them and know how to access them. In light of the increasing diversification of the aging population, special needs groups, and programs to meet current needs, greater outreach efforts are being developed to identify and inform targeted groups. Of particular importance are appropriate strategies to identify minority elderly persons who, for reasons of language and because of cultural barriers, are out of the mainstream of aging services utilization. Other outreach methods identify and make services accessible to older persons who have physical or sensory impairments or who are developmentally disabled. Considerable outreach activities are also needed to identify and inform older persons in rural areas who are unaware of services.

The use of bilingual-bicultural outreach workers is essential to help older minority-group persons feel comfortable in seeking out and accepting services. Outreach strategies can take the form of disseminating information in print through fliers, posters, and newsletter or newspaper articles and through radio and public service announcements, door-to-door efforts, and educational programs at senior centers. In-service staff training supplements these strategies. Particular attention should be paid to sensory-impaired older persons during outreach. Increasingly, outreach components are a critical part of new services or of revitalizing underutilized services.

SOCIAL PROGRAMS

Problems associated with social isolation are generally not remedied with increased income alone. Lost friends and abandoned social activities often lead to ennui and a diminished quality of life, which can be relieved only by a social milieu and new or renewed activities. Such activities are best made available in group settings, such as senior centers and nutrition sites, where social opportunities are most likely to be found.

Senior centers take many forms, ranging from simple storefront operations to large complexes that include auditoriums, gymnasiums, and swimming pools. The centers may be located in schools, churches or synagogues, or senior housing or may be freestanding. All, however, provide a space in which people can gather for educational and recreational activities and for informal socializing. Most centers provide information on community services and offer transportation for mobility-impaired older persons. Most serve as nutrition sites. They may be run by professionals or volunteers, but most draw on community resources, such as schools, membership groups, social agencies, and professionals, to provide services to their participants.

For seniors, nutrition sites rekindle dining as a social event. Funded through the AAAs from federal appropriations under Title III of the OAA, these nutrition programs may provide meals at a senior center, an American Legion hall, a township hall, or any number of places where people gather. Targeted toward elderly people of all income groups who have lost the ability or the interest to make well-balanced meals, nutrition programs also try to encourage good eating habits for their participants through nutrition education.

The senior center is continuously challenged to change and expand to meet the diverse emerging requirements of an aging society consisting of well and frail elderly individuals. Centers must exert considerable effort to reach out to underserved, low-income, and minority elderly people as well as sensory-impaired older persons. To assist centers, NCOA (1990) has developed a set of guidelines called *The Senior Center Standards and Self-Assessment Workbook: Guidelines for Practice.*

TRANSPORTATION

Transportation is one of the key access services that enables older persons to obtain the other services they need. Other access services include outreach, information and referral, escort, and advocacy services. Transportation services for the elderly population may include the rerouting of buses, the use of accessible vehicles, and the provision of door-to-door transportation. A survey conducted by NAAAA revealed that transportation was among the top two unmet needs of elderly people ("NAAAA transportation," 1990). AOA reports that transportation is the third largest consumer of OAA dollars, following congregate and home-delivered meals ("Transportation," 1991). Not only is transportation crucial to the independence of elderly individuals, but other Title III services are dependent on it. The lack of adequate transportation for rural elderly persons is a critical service issue of the 1990s. For the older visually impaired person, door-to-door transportation is the key to keeping appointments for social, medical, and legal services. Currently, 3,500 organizations provide services to elderly and disabled people via 11,000 vehicles funded by the Urban Mass Transportation Administration (UMTA) through its Section 16(b)(2) program. UMTA is the federal organization that provides subsidized purchase of accessible vehicles to organizations serving elderly and disabled people. Needs for transportation services will continue to increase as people live longer and larger numbers grow increasingly frail.

LEGAL SERVICES AND PERSONAL COUNSELING

Two needs common among young-old people are help with wills and estates and personal counseling to assist with family problems or to overcome depression. Legal services bureaus offer legal assistance to low-income persons, and AAAs frequently fund positions for senior law specialists in the bureaus. Also, some local bar associations provide pro bono services to older persons regularly.

Community mental health centers are increasingly sensitive to the needs of older persons and are making concerted efforts to address the problems of depression and loss by setting up appointments at seniors' gathering places or even by visiting people's homes. The clergy, frequently the preferred source of solace and counsel for older persons, remains a valuable resource for those elderly people experiencing losses. With regard to visually impaired persons, many social workers and other professionals in counseling roles, including members of the clergy, are initially uncertain about their ability to handle the psychosocial issues of aging and vision loss. For this reason, in-service training from agencies for blind and visually impaired persons helps the service provider understand the issues and gives them a degree of comfort in responding effectively to this special population. Both legal services and counseling are frequently available at senior centers and nutrition sites.

HOUSING

It is at the young-old stage that many persons take stock of their housing needs. Their homes may be too large, too difficult to maintain, or too difficult to maneuver in or may represent equity not readily available to them as owners. Essentially, their option is to move if other available housing is better suited to their circumstances or to make their current homes secure and manageable.

Retirement Housing

Persons who wish to move from their own homes and who are ambulatory and independent may first consider retirement housing. There is a wide variety of choices, ranging from publicly funded apartment complexes to luxurious leisure communities developed with private funds. Retirement housing generally enables older persons to be free of costly, time-consuming home maintenance; to be secure from crime; and to scale down their living space.

Private developers tend to reach those with middle or higher incomes. Depending on their needs and their degree of independence, these individuals might buy a small house or a self-contained apartment in a retirement community, prepare all their meals at home, and participate in recreation activities. Or they might choose a facility that supplies smaller living quarters, provides all meals in a group setting, and offers maid and chore services as well as other assistance. A new trend in retirement housing is "life care." It gives older persons the opportunity to live independently in an apartment, knowing that if health deteriorates, they will be guaranteed long-term care at no extra cost. Generally, people who live in life-care facilities must buy apartments or homes. Often the purchase price is retained by the facility when the individual dies. The option of retirement community living is available only to older persons of middle incomes or above.

Senior housing apartments that are part of public housing are available to older persons with low incomes. Public housing complexes are often connected to social service agencies that help senior citizens. They encourage the residents to participate in social activities and a variety of social services. Many senior centers are located in public housing complexes. Some public housing programs offer rent subsidies through the U.S. Department of Housing and Urban Development for elderly people who meet the income requirements. Unfortunately, most publicly subsidized retirement housing sites have long waiting lists.

Alternative Housing

For elderly people who need to draw income from their homes but who prefer to continue living in them, a few enterprising communities have established home-equity conversion or shared housing projects. Usually incorporated privately, a home-equity conversion agency purchases the elderly person's home and maintains it while providing monthly payments to the person. When the person dies, the agency will own the home. Shared housing brings together two or more elderly people who need a home with people who are willing to share homes too large for their individual needs. The agencies involved sometimes provide necessary restructuring of the homes to prepare them for multiple occupancy. State and municipal housing commissions are good sources of information on alternative housing arrangements.

Repair and Maintenance

For those whose physical and financial resources are too stretched to maintain the homes in which they live, community-based agencies may provide assistance. AAAs fund minor home repair projects, handyman services, and chore services to keep the homes of needy elderly people in decent repair. Some agencies provide heavy cleaning services for older persons who cannot clean their homes. There is usually a dollar limit on repairs for each home, but occasionally roof and furnace replacements are permitted. For older persons who can afford small repairs but are unable to perform them personally, senior centers often sponsor handyman services for a low fee. Local community action agencies weatherproof the homes of low-income elderly people, providing insulation and storm windows. Some state funds provide loans and grants for these purposes.

The coordination of housing repair and maintenance and of housing placement programs is particularly difficult because of the multiplicity of agencies that provide these services. Some senior-oriented agencies have established advocates to help older persons negotiate the systems involved. For example, each AAA in Michigan has a shelter adviser who is knowledgeable about housing and energy programs and is available to help elderly people sort out housing choices. These services are extremely important for older persons who have lost their vision and who do not have the resources to obtain this needed assistance. All services relating to housing repair and maintenance are intended to help the older person to "age in place" and to age well.

HEALTH SCREENING

Finally, with the onset of chronic illness, older persons often recognize how necessary preventive measures can be in maintaining normal activities. Local health departments may offer blood pressure checks, cholesterol tests, and influenza immunization clinics in convenient locations for elderly people. In some instances, an AAA may fund full-scale health screening and dental checks, hearing tests, and vision screenings through health-related agencies. Swimming for those with arthritis and senior physical fitness sessions may be offered by community centers, schools, or senior centers or may be available at reduced rates in private fitness centers. Physical activity at a level appropriate to the individual is extremely helpful in maintaining optimum health and functioning.

Services to the Old-Old

All the services described thus far continue to be useful, if not essential, to those age 75 and over. However, in the later stages of life, when older persons experience the highest incidence of chronic illness and physical frailty, the need for care becomes most urgent. The sites for service delivery often shift from social and recreational facilities to homes and health-related facilities, where personal security is greater. Environments once easily managed may become potentially threatening, and delays in services, once mere inconveniences, can become crises.

The widow who went to work in her mid-50s to support herself, who later visited the senior center and met new friends while having lunch there, and who chose to stay in her own home because chore and minor home-repair services kept it livable is now 25 years older than she was when her husband died. Her health may be much more precarious and her constitution more frail. She may suffer severe arthritis, congestive heart failure, or mild strokes, and some loss of vision and hearing may restrict her mobility profoundly. The number of balanced meals she makes is small, not because of a lack of enthusiasm but because of the difficulties involved. Her frailty and difficulty with mobility make visiting her friends an energy-sapping or impossible task, and her physical fragility makes living alone risky. Although chore services continue to help maintain her house, she may now need assistance in simple activities of daily living.

Her income, depleted by increasing health care bills and inflation, is clearly inadequate, and most of the personal help she gets is from her daughter. Adult day care may provide the rehabilitation, socialization, and motivation she needs and at the same time provide respite to her daughter or allow her daughter to continue to work. Adult day care represents one of the services along the continuum ranging from community-based to residential long-term care. A review of care along the continuum follows.

LONG-TERM CARE SERVICES

The effectiveness of long-term care services that provide treatment of chronic conditions and support for activities of daily living depends largely on the residential environments involved. For the most appropriate environment, services should be provided in the least restrictive setting, but one that can continue to maximize physical and psychological well-being. An appropriate environment is one that provides security and enables the older person to maintain the greatest degree of independence, autonomy, and control given his or her available resources, both personal and supportive.

The fundamental decision facing functionally disabled older persons and their families is whether assistance is more appropriately offered in a facility or in the home. A facility offers a professionally managed environment with continual surveillance and various degrees of health and personal care. For a functionally disabled older person whose health and safety can be made secure at home and who, with help from family members and support services, can perform activities of daily living or be assisted with these activities at home, the home is the optimum choice. The availability of resources, the life-style of the older person, and the family's preferences are often factors in the older person's decision. All too frequently, though, the availability of reimbursement becomes the predominant factor. The cost of home care is enormously expensive for those over the Medicaid eligibility level.

The federal Medicaid health care program for below-poverty persons is the largest source of reimbursement for nursing home care. Older chronically ill or disabled persons whose incomes exceed poverty guidelines cannot be reimbursed for custodial nursing home care through Medicaid or Medicare. Consequently, many such older persons "spend down" their assets to the poverty level to become eligible for

Medicaid reimbursement. If the need for care in the home exceeds Medicaid's limits for home care, the older person's only option is nursing home care, for which Medicaid limits are much higher. A few states have received waivers to provide Medicaid reimbursement for comprehensive home care, but the practice is uncommon.

It is important to note that most older persons want to remain in their own homes for as long as possible with whatever health care and support services are available. Familiarity and continuity help stabilize the most difficult situations. Changes in living environments are most successful when the older person makes the decisions or is a full participant in decision making. If care is not needed and social isolation exists, many older people choose congregate living arrangements to meet their needs for socialization and communal well-being. But even these changes are compromises requiring some period of adjustment for successful resolution. If moves to nursing homes occur under stress, morbidity and mortality rates increase dramatically.

HOME CARE

Facilities work to mold the older person into the structured life of the institution. In contrast, the home setting provides for individual differences to a greater extent and is strongly responsive to the individual's needs and abilities. Maintaining a home as a long-term care site demands ingenuity, coordination, and continual adjustments in services on the part of family caregivers and service providers. Long-term home care can be less expensive than nursing home care if care is needed much less frequently than the continual care provided in a nursing home or if the level of care involved is not the skilled care provided in a nursing home. Home care can also be less expensive if the cost of managing the home is fixed and would be paid anyway or if informal helpers—family and friends—are willing to perform personal services. For not only are services relating to income, energy, home repair, and chores still necessary to keep the home in working order, but now the inside of the home must be made secure and safe for the older person. An environmental review of the home may reveal that throw rugs must be picked up or tacked down, furniture must be moved to accommodate a walker or a wheelchair, grab rails are needed in the bathroom, food in upper shelves of cupboards must be made more accessible, and so on. Case managers, community nurses, or public health nurses may assist in environmental reviews. (A review of issues in environmental design and modification is in Chapter 13.)

If the client's conditions are precarious, measures must be taken to ensure periodic or constant surveillance to alert emergency care agencies when help is needed. For a person whose condition does not necessitate surveillance related to instantaneous response, senior centers or religious groups may offer telephone reassurance or a daily call by a friendly visitor. In some local communities, mail carriers have arranged to call a designated agency if mail delivered to a person's home is not picked up. In cases involving conditions that may require a medical emergency response, local agencies can install an electronic emergency alert system activated at the touch of a button. With such a system, the older person can signal the need for emergency help, and in addition the agency checks in with the person at a preset time each day. If the button is touched before the preset time, a telephone signal is sent to an emergency health facility telling an ambulance unit where to go and what emergency to expect.

The services that allow older persons to function in their homes are primarily personal care and support services, which restore people's capabilities or compensate for the loss of these abilities. Older persons can receive skilled nursing, health aide services, physical therapy, occupational therapy, speech therapy, and so on from a home health agency as they would in a hospital. They can also receive homemaker services from a home care agency; daily home-delivered meals for special diets from a nutrition project; and telephone reassurance calls, friendly visitors, or senior companion services. In addition, some older persons may receive oxygen from a medical equipment agency. Or they may receive all these services from a single agency.

The home care market, which serves those with the least time and resources to make informed consumer decisions, is unfortunately confusing. Deregulation and competition have precipitated hospitals, nursing homes, and for-profit agencies into an arena dominated by not-for-profit home health agencies and public health departments. Agencies offer different combinations of services at different rates with different levels of quality. Although competition has driven costs down, in some instances, physicians, nurses, and discharge planners, as well as their patients, struggle to cope with the constantly changing market.

In a growing number of states, case management or care management systems have emerged to provide assistance to home care consumers. Often operated by an AAA in its role as a local advocate for older persons, case management projects conduct comprehensive assessments of the needs and resources of older people who are at risk, including a home environment review. The projects develop care plans with services to enable persons to remain in their own homes and monitor the delivery of community-based services. Totally client focused, case management helps families assume reasonable responsibilities for their aging relatives and arranges counseling to clarify family roles. A case management project may conduct readmission testing, a mandatory service for applicants to nursing homes to screen out those who may be able to stay at home. (A review of long-term care options as well as issues in long-term care is presented in Chapter 13.)

Despite the losses associated with the aging process, it is important to remember that opportunities for growth, learning, and personal development continue until the last days of life. Older persons 60 and over need to remain physically and mentally active. They can take advantage of social, recreational, and educational programs; educational programs are sometimes offered in long-term care facilities as well. Intergenerational programs that bring young visitors into senior centers and nursing homes for conversation and friendship and joint activities enhance the emotional well-being of older persons. Recreational activities and opportunities to socialize make life worth living for those at any age, particularly those who are frail and vulnerable.

Targeting and Cost Sharing

Because of the enormous cost of providing services to older persons, the issue of "cost sharing"—the sharing of costs between the federal government and the older consumer—for Title III programs and services is under considerable debate. Targeting of services, in which funds and programs are directed specifically at certain subpopulations, is also a focus of attention. At forums held by AOA in five cities in 1990, service providers testifying about the reauthorization of the OAA identified cost sharing and the targeting of services as the two main issues of concern ("AOA forums," 1990). There is currently a voluntary cost-sharing policy. For example, older persons contribute one dollar for hot lunch or for home-delivered meals and a dollar or two for door-to-door transportation or for chore services. Although a more intensive cost-sharing structure is a future possibility and the implementation of cost sharing could be viewed as "fee for service," under current proposals all those unable to share the cost might be exempt.

Under proposed funding schemes, cost sharing could apply to adult day care, legal services, homemaker services, home-repair programs, respite care, and counseling, in addition to meals and transportation. In addition, the targeting of support services to special groups of older persons is considered increasingly essential as the older population becomes more diversified and requires special attention and accessibility to services. This is true in regard to older minority persons as well as disability groups in need of equal access to generic aging services ("AOA forums," 1990).

Access and Advocacy Systems

Planners and coordinators of service systems for older persons continually work to improve services along a continuum of care so that kinds and levels of services are appropriate to the various losses suffered by elderly people. But even as the ideal emerges, given the diverse patterns of local service delivery, the keys to helping older people find appropriate paths to services are the community access and advocacy systems, especially for vulnerable elderly people. AAAs, mandated to maintain a comprehensive inventory of resources and to advocate on behalf of elderly people, place considerable emphasis on making community service systems responsive to older people. Almost all the agencies provide information and referral, outreach, and transportation services, often through visible senior citizens agencies, such as senior centers and councils on aging. Various community agencies may provide housing or nursing home placement services, shopping assistance, or escort services. Senior legal services provide advice and advocacy to ensure that authorized entitlement services for elderly people are delivered appropriately.

Effective access systems that target areas in which minority and low-income persons reside and focus on them with concentrated information, outreach, and transportation efforts are the most effective mechanisms of ensuring service to those in greatest social and economic need. The primary mechanism for reaching isolated, impaired elderly people is an information program that keeps those who are in a position to know about these people—physicians and their staffs, hospital discharge planners and medical social workers, counselors, religious leaders, and adult public service workers—aware of the available services. For both professionals and consumers, the key to discovering what services are available and to negotiating the service system is successfully knowing where to find information. AAAs, found in every part of the country, are listed in the Yellow Pages or in the city government pages of the local telephone directory. These offices have an information and referral service to direct older persons and those working with them to agencies providing direct services. Membership organizations for seniors, such as AARP and NCSC, have local chapters that provide information about their services. Most service and membership organizations for aging persons also have newsletters with information about new services and programs for elderly people in the community.

Advocates for older people in the United States who work toward a more manageable system of services may lament how far this country is from having an ideal service system for the elderly population. Nevertheless, accessible and rational systems of decent and appropriate care for elderly people do continue to emerge, expand, and improve. As the understanding of the needs of older people grows and keeps pace with the growing and diversifying population of older persons, planners and service providers will continue to create improved service delivery structures and systems.

References

American Association of Retired Persons. (1991). Number of older Americans ready and able to work larger than anticipated. *Working Age, 6*(4): 1.

AOA forums focus on reauthorization of the Older Americans Act. (1990). *Older Americans Report,* p. 173.

Delfico, J. F. (1990). Testimony before the Joint Hearing of the House of Representatives Select Committee on Aging and the Subcommittee on Retirement Income and Employment: April 6, 1990. Washington, DC: U.S. General Accounting Office.

Fenano, K., & Banesi, C. (1982). The impact of widowhood on the social relations of older persons. *Research in Aging, 14:* 227-247.

NAAAA transportation report. (1990). *Older Americans Report,* p. 123.

National Council on the Aging. (1990). *The senior center standards and self-assessment workbook: Guidelines for practice.* Washington, DC: Author.

Transportation will be the focus of OAA priorities. (1991). *Older Americans Report,* p. 42.

CHAPTER 10

Low Vision Services

Randall T. Jose

Visual impairment is a common problem associated with aging and can mean a difficult adjustment for the older person and his or her family members. Because vision loss is a problem that many older people accept as a normal part of aging, they do not seek assistance or services to improve their visual functioning. Many older persons are unaware of the kinds of services that exist. Many do not visit an eye care specialist regularly, and most have never even heard of a low vision evaluation and low vision services. In addition to helping older visually impaired persons handle their loss of vision, it is important for other service providers to inform newly visually impaired persons about available low vision and rehabilitation services and to encourage them to use these services.

Background and Definitions

"Low vision" is defined as a vision loss that is severe enough to inter-fere with the ability to perform everyday tasks or activities and that cannot be corrected to normal by conventional eyeglasses or contact lenses. The prevalent causes of low vision among elderly persons in the United States are macular degeneration, glaucoma, and diabetic retinopathy (National Society to Prevent Blindness, 1980). These eye diseases and cataracts, described in Chapter 3, are associated with the aging process. It is not surprising, then, that 70 percent of the visually impaired population in this country is over the age of 60. It is also not surprising that in most low vision clinics across the country over half the patients are age 50 or older.

In spite of these statistics, not enough low vision clinics offer services that are specific to the needs of older people. This lack of special services for older persons will become an even greater problem in the year 2000. It is predicted that the number of persons age 65 and over will be 32 million, compared to 23 million in 1977 (Lowman & Kirchner, 1988). Because the number of older persons with low vision will also grow dramatically and less than half of the people with low vision in the United States are now receiving services, this prediction mandates an expansion of low vision rehabilitation services and suggests that the emphasis in the delivery of these services must be changed (Kirchner & Phillips, 1988).

Visual impairments are measured in the office of the ophthalmologist or optometrist. Loss of acuity, central scotoma (blind spot), loss of peripheral (side) vision, hazy or blurry vision, photophobia (sensitivity to light), night blindness, and difficulties with color vision are all types of visual impairments. The determination of the extent of a visual impairment is but one aspect of a low vision care program. Another essential aspect is the determination of the impact of the impairment on the individual and on his or her visual functioning. How a particular impairment (for example, central blind spot) impedes a person's ability to maintain his or her habitual life-style is the handicapping effect of the impairment, referred to as "visual handicap" (Colenbrander, 1977). Visual handicap or functional impairment is a more difficult parameter to measure than visual impairment and probably is less likely to be ascertained accurately.

The goal of a low vision program is to minimize the disabling effect of a visual impairment through the use of specialized optical devices, instructional programs for their use, and coordinated rehabilitation services. However, there is such a broad range of visual impairments and an even greater range of problems created by these impairments that it is difficult to establish a technically proficient and cost-effective system of providing services. For example, how does one provide services to both a person with 20/70 vision who is severely functionally impaired and another person with 20/200 vision who denies having a visual problem? (For a discussion of these measurements of acuity, see Chapter

3.) It is a dilemma faced by low vision practitioners daily. Practitioners who provide low vision care for visually impaired persons must organize a systematic program of examinations and evaluations that measures the individual's impairment, describes the functional impairment, correlates the visual impairment with the degree of functional impairment, suggests optical and rehabilitative intervention, provides or coordinates appropriate optical training and rehabilitation instruction, and monitors the extent to which the disabling condition is reduced by the provision of low vision services.

The Low Vision Service

Low vision services are designed to help a visually impaired person use his or her remaining vision most efficiently and effectively. They are provided by a coordinated team of professionals who evaluate a person's vision and the way the person uses vision in various aspects of life. Services are found in such settings as colleges of optometry, hospitals, departments of ophthalmology at medical schools, private practices, and agencies for blind and visually impaired persons.

Low vision services should not be initiated until the appropriate medical or surgical care has been provided for the individual. The optometrist or ophthalmologist who is providing the person's low vision care is responsible for evaluating the medical care received and for examining the ocular health of the person to determine the need for additional medical services. These services can then be provided prior to or in conjunction with low vision care. It is important to remember that individuals can have more than one kind of visual impairment; for example, someone with cataracts may also have glaucoma. It is important for the eye care specialist to explain the eye condition to the patient and to make certain that the patient has a good understanding of the disease process.

Ninety percent of persons who are visually impaired can be helped by low vision services. Because statistical data are difficult to collect and interpret, this statement is based on the author's clinical experiences in six different settings, rather than on a statistical analysis. The major problem in conducting such an analysis is how to determine who has been helped and how successful the low vision service has been. For the purposes of this discussion, the low vision rehabilitation process is considered successful if a patient receives a low vision device (optical or nonoptical) after an evaluation and uses the device several times a week to perform a task she or he could not have performed without the device.

One problem encountered by eye care specialists is the large number of patients, especially elderly patients, who can be helped by low vision rehabilitation but who are not ready to seek services or accept the services offered. Many older patients who are seen in clinics could benefit from the use of low vision devices if they were receptive to using a device. Frequently, the older person goes to the low vision evaluation desiring a stronger pair of eyeglasses that will correct vision almost back to normal. However, providing this kind of correction is not always possible. Even after the introduction of a low vision device, many older patients are discouraged because the device does not enable them to see as they did before the vision loss. Older persons may require more instruction over a longer period of time than younger persons to adjust to the way the low vision device helps. It is an important issue for low vision specialists to know and understand in their work with older people.

In essence, a low vision service represents a problem-solving endeavor to improve the individual's independence and self-reliance. The collaboration between the low vision clinician and other service providers working with the older person is what differentiates low vision services from low vision examinations. Service providers in the field of aging can make their most significant contribution to elderly persons with low vision through low vision services. The functional aspect of a visual impairment is best measured outside the clinic, and some system for doing so needs to be built into every service program organized and developed for older people. With the help of various service providers, the typical low vision examination and resulting optical prescription can be modified into a low vision service that better reflects the needs of older visually impaired persons. A description of the steps involved in consultation with a low vision service follows.

REFERRAL

The majority of referrals to low vision clinics are made by primary-care ophthalmologists and optometrists after initial eye examinations result in a diagnosis of vision loss due to pathology or trauma and after it is determined that low vision devices may be helpful. Referrals may also come from rehabilitation counselors or teachers and orientation and mobility (O&M) specialists who are working with visually impaired clients. Because the general public does not usually know about low vision services, self-referral is less likely. Other referrals may come from physicians, social workers, or teachers of visually impaired students.

INTAKE

Intake is the first step in providing low vision care. Before patients are actually examined, it is valuable to know what they would like to be able to do visually and what they at present are unable to do (sew, read, watch television, for example) because of the onset of vision loss. The more important a task is to the individual, the more likely he or she will do what is necessary to maintain the ability to perform it, such as working at closer distances and with limited visual fields, showing interest in the use of low vision devices, and coping with the perceived stigma of being visually impaired and having to use the devices in public. Success for an older person is unlikely if an eye specialist tries to prescribe a low vision device for a task of little importance to the individual throughout his or her life. For example, a device prescribed for reading will not often be used by a woman who has never been an avid reader but whose most significant pastime is knitting. Unfortunately, this mismatch occurs in many examination rooms when insufficient time is spent learning about the older person's current needs and interests. The identification of valued activities and desired goals is therefore the first step in a comprehensive low vision evaluation and an important part of the intake process.

Intake Questions

The questions asked during intake are essential in obtaining vital information, and some representative questions to be used during intake are presented below. The person's low vision clinician or other service provider can use this format, or it can be used when the low vision clinic is located at the agency for the blind. In this case, a rehabilitation teacher or agency social worker can gather this information for the low vision clinician. In either case, the visually impaired person can be asked the following general questions directly:

- How active are you, and in what activities are you involved?
- Are there any activities that you cannot perform that you would like to be able to do?
- How are you feeling about your visual impairment?

It will significantly improve the likelihood that the person will receive effective services if the low vision clinician knows this basic information. Based on this open-ended format, a 10-page report can be compiled on one client or a two-paragraph report on another. Each report may accurately reflect the person's needs and the extent of the visual impairment. The two parameters the clinician needs to ascertain before the completion of the low vision examination are:

- How does the functional vision loss compare with the visual impairment (i.e., the clinically measured loss)?
- What tasks are most likely to motivate the person to use a low vision device?

The information gathered during the intake and case history processes will assist the eye care clinician in determining the best low vision device or devices for the patient.

Taking a Case History

In addition to asking the intake questions, assembling a case history on a patient is an integral part of the information-collecting process. Typical questions on previous medical and vision care need to be asked. In addition, it is most important for the clinician to read any reports that have been sent to the low vision clinic and to speak to any family member, friend, or professional who accompanies the older person to the low vision evaluation.

After the formal case history is taken, the clinician and the patient should have an informal discussion to establish a working relationship.

As indicated earlier, many patients come to the low vision clinic with the hope of getting a regular pair of eyeglasses that are "stronger" and that will let them see as they did when they had 20/20 vision. They must be informed from the start that regular eyeglasses are not sufficient to help them and that there is no miracle cure for low vision. Even older patients who indicate they know what low vision devices are often hope for restored vision. Thus, an intake protocol that educates patients about the benefits as well as limitations of low vision devices has a higher success rate.

O&M specialists and rehabilitation counselors or teachers who may be serving the elderly visually impaired person may be able to help develop a list of areas of difficulty in visual functioning. If possible, this professional should accompany the person to the examination. If the older visually impaired person is not working with these professionals, the eye care specialist must determine both the visual impairment and the functional aspects of the impairment during the low vision examination. A family member or friend can provide information to supplement what the patient reports. For this reason, it is critical that low vision specialists take the time to solicit complete information from the elderly patient.

It is helpful for service providers to attend at least one examination, if possible; doing so will help them write future reports on the client, prepare other clients for low vision examinations, and determine which clients may benefit from low vision care. Often during a meeting with a patient, the clinician will ask a question whose answer can be found in a report already sent. This repetition is intentional: A patient may not provide the clinician with the same details presented by a service provider or friend because of anxiety surrounding the examination, and information gathered in different instances should be compared and reviewed to compile a complete picture.

The Low Vision Examination

Most low vision examinations are conducted in a series of two or three visits with the following components: (1) the initial examination, which includes intake, (2) a loaner or home training period in which the patient borrows low vision devices and tries them at home or in the environment in which they will be used, (3) a follow-up visit that usually consists primarily of training, and (4) a final dispensing and training visit. If problems with use of a prescribed device exist, more visits to the clinic may be needed before optimum proficiency and comfort with the device are achieved. The initial examination usually consists of the following: (1) intake and the compiling of a case history, (2) acuity evaluation, (3) refraction, (4) visual field evaluation, and (5) binocular vision assessment. In addition, the patient undergoes color vision evaluations, contrast sensitivity testing, and a magnification assessment.

ACUITY EVALUATION

Acuity tests can set a positive mood for the low vision examination, if done correctly. A patient with low vision is probably used to being able to read only one or two letters on a regular eye chart or being told to count fingers, that is, to tell the examiner how many fingers he or she is holding up near the patient's face. However, special low vision charts have large numbers and letters, sometimes beginning with one very large number on the first page, with the numbers decreasing in size through several pages of the chart. The person who reads one letter on a regular chart will read all but the last two pages on a low vision chart. Thus, the low vision chart demonstrates to patients that even though they have been told they are legally blind or have only 10 percent vision, they do have functional vision that can be maximized by low vision devices. Without even picking up an optical device, in such instances, the low vision clinician has already improved the patient's perception of his or her vision and has instilled a positive attitude toward the rest of the examination. The patient's acuity is also checked at near distance during the examination, and special charts are used with large letters and numbers with high contrast and appropriate spacing.

It is important to remember that 20/200 vision is a criterion for legal blindness, not total blindness. A person who is legally blind may still be able to see faces at 3 to 5 feet, watch television at 5 feet, move easily through familiar areas, and probably move independently in unfamiliar areas. Numerous persons who come to the low vision clinic with 20/200 vision still drive automobiles. Although driving in such cases is illegal, that some individuals with 20/200 acuity attempt to drive demonstrates that a legally blind person still has a significant amount of functional vision. It is important that eye care specialists and service providers convey this information about legal blindness to help older visually impaired patients understand that they can usually benefit from the use of low vision devices.

The acuities measured are written as part of a low vision examination, with the test distance first and the size of the letter or number second. The size of the letter or number represents the distance at which an individual with 20/20 acuity would see. Thus, a 10/100 acuity means that the person was tested at 10 feet (more common for a low vision patient than the typical 20-foot test distance) and that he or she sees a letter at 10 feet that a person with 20/20 vision sees at 100 feet. It is helpful not only to know that a patient has 20/200 vision but to understand the functional definition of this acuity. It is particularly important for rehabilitation professionals working with visually impaired clients.

Rehabilitation counselors or teachers, O&M specialists, and other service providers working with older persons may find that the best way to start developing a mental picture or definition of an acuity measurement is to observe people with different acuities to see what they can and cannot do. It also helps these professionals assess the person's performance in light of vision that is measured. If the client with 20/50 vision says she cannot see the television screen at 5 feet, this information indicates that more important factors than acuity may be contributing to this individual's impairment.

REFRACTION

Refraction is the process by which the eye care specialist determines if the eye is out of focus and if a prescription is needed to improve vision. During this process, the specialist determines the "refractive error" or optics of the eye that prevents light from being brought to a single focus exactly on the retina. Typical refractive errors are nearsightedness (the ability to see at near distances but difficulty seeing at far distances), farsightedness (the ability to see at far distances but difficulty seeing at near distances), and astigmatism (in which rays of light do not come to a single focal point on the retina as they should). The clinician determines the power of regular glasses that will bring light to a focus on the retina.

There are two mechanisms by which a person can suffer a loss of visual acuity. One is to have the eye out of focus (optical); the other is through disease or trauma (pathological). It is important to rule out optical problems (and the need for regular eyeglasses) as a cause of reduced acuity before proceeding to the determination of magnification. If it is determined through refraction that conventional eyeglasses can improve acuity, then less magnification will be needed in the optical device being considered as a prescription.

Typically, the lower the magnification, the more options there are for prescribing a device and the easier it will be for the patient to adapt to its use. For instance, a person with 10/200 (20/400) vision needs 10x magnification to read; 10x magnification requires that reading material be held at a work distance of 1 inch. If a regular pair of eyeglasses improves the person's acuity to 10/60 (20/120), then only 3x magnification is needed, which allows a 3-1/2-inch work distance and a significantly greater number of options for devices, such as bifocals for persons who do not want to use conspicuous devices or a telemicroscope to increase the work distance.

It is difficult to explain to patients in low vision clinics why simply giving them a stronger pair of eyeglasses will not restore their visual acuity. Two important concepts must be outlined to minimize unrealistic expectations—the nature of the pathology and the difference between conventional lenses and optical devices. The concept of pathology can be broached by first asking patients what caused their low vision. In the ensuing discussion, patients can be encouraged to ask the clinician about the disease. A service provider or family member who is present can also remind or encourage the clinician to have this discussion with the patient if the clinician has forgotten to do so during the examination. No one should be reluctant to ask questions about the patient's eye condition or disease and its functional implications.

The difference between conventional lenses and optical devices should also be explained. Patients can be informed that regular eyeglasses simply focus light on the retina at the back of the eye. The light focuses at a central point (the macula) where all the 20/20 cells (the cones), which allow a person to see fine detail and differentiate color, are located. However, in the case of a pathological disease, wherein the special 20/20 cells are nonfunctional, regular eyeglasses cannot improve vision. To see detail, the person must move closer to the object or use optical devices that will magnify the object so that the image projected to the retina is enlarged.

Even though most older visually impaired patients will not benefit from a refraction because of eye pathology that cannot be optically corrected, it is important that the need for a change in conventional lenses be investigated. The clinician will use both subjective and objective techniques for determining the need for a new correction.

In the objective technique (retinoscopy), the patient looks through various hand-held lenses while the clinician shines a light into his or her eye to see which lens allows the light to focus on the retina. When the correct lens is determined, the amount of nearsightedness, farsightedness, and astigmatism can be accurately measured without the person's having to make any choices of lenses. It is a particularly valuable test for those patients who have difficulty selecting the better lens during the subjective test.

In the subjective technique, patients are shown various lenses until they determine which one allows them to see most clearly. The results should agree closely with the results of the objective test. With all low vision patients, hand-held lenses are used instead of those attached to machines (phoropters). This allows them to look around blind spots, provides maximum lighting, and gives the older patients more time to determine which lenses are appropriate.

Family members and service providers sometimes hear patients, especially older ones, lament the decisions they had to make during the subjective part of the refraction examination. People are often anxious about having made a mistake on one of the choices. To allay their fears, it can be explained that the clinician checks every decision on a lens two or three times, and their uncertainty will not affect the accuracy of the lenses that are prescribed. Once the refraction is finished, the clinician is assured that whatever acuity loss is present is the result of pathology and not of the patient's need for a new pair of conventional eyeglasses.

VISUAL FIELD EVALUATION

"Visual field," the area of physical space visible to the eye, is measured in degrees as an angle. To determine the extent of a person's visual field, it is necessary to know how much intact retina the patient has as well as the location, extent, and density of any blind spots (scotomas). This assessment is important for determining which optical device and training program to use (Jose & Ferraro, 1983).

There are two basic types of visual field losses. The first is central field loss, caused by central scotoma or central blind spot, which is most prevalent in older people (see Figure 1). This loss is usually the result of macular degeneration, sometimes referred to as "age-related

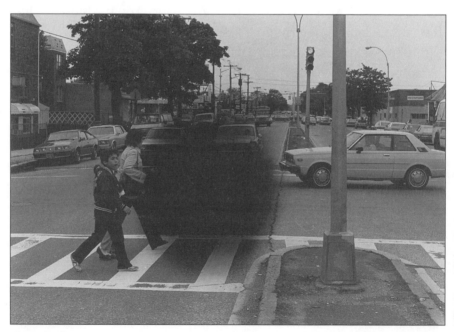

Figure 1: Vision characterized by central field loss, often the result of macular degeneration.

macular degeneration." Initially, there may be only distortion instead of a blind spot. Distortion is measured with the Amsler Grid, which is made up of a regular pattern of intersecting vertical and horizontal lines. Even though the acuities may still be 20/20, it is usually more difficult to manage and prescribe for this loss than the absolute blind spot of more advanced macular degeneration.

The second category of visual field loss is peripheral loss. This type frequently exists in the beginning stages of retinitis pigmentosa or glaucoma. Another type of visual field loss is a mixed field loss, a combination of the first two categories. There are also sector field losses, such as a loss of interior field due to retinal detachment.

BINOCULARITY ASSESSMENT

The clinician needs to evaluate how well the patient's eyes work together. There are limited clinical techniques for evaluating this aspect of vision with low vision patients. Normal or binocular vision involves the simultaneous use of both eyes. Sometimes, an individual with low vision may have binocular vision only when looking at objects from afar, up close, or vice versa. In such cases, optical devices may be prescribed for both eyes to sustain binocular vision. However, most low vision patients are monocular, and the clinician or the service provider must explain that even though the device is used only for one eye, the other will not deteriorate or atrophy. It is a particularly strong concern when the person has to patch one eye temporarily to prevent double vision (diplopia) when using the optical device with the other eye.

In monocular vision, there may be vision in both eyes, but the difference between the acuity of the eyes is great enough so that the brain cannot fuse together the images from both eyes. The image from the eye with the poorer acuity will usually be turned off (suppressed), especially when the individual is trying to see detail. The person still uses both eyes (unless he or she has no light perception) when he or she walks around relying on peripheral vision. Depth perception is still present, and in certain situations, the person may think both eyes are being used even though the brain is suppressing one eye. When devices are prescribed, a patch may still be needed for the poorer eye because of "retinal rivalry," which occurs when the incompletely suppressed poor image degrades the image of the better eye. The person often reports better vision when the poorer eye is closed.

A person with biocular vision does not have binocular vision but has good enough vision in each eye so that one eye is used for distance tasks and the other for near tasks, or one eye starts the reading task and the other takes over after a time and finishes. For this situation, the clinician may prescribe a telescope for one eye and a microscope for the other. It is a little harder for older persons to adapt to this system.

COLOR VISION

Most of the color problems of older persons with visual impairment are associated with the loss of acuity and involve difficulty seeing subtle color changes. A color vision test can provide helpful information to the eye care specialist. When a color defect is detected, the clinician can only report the defect; no specific therapy exists. The awareness of difficulty in color detection is useful in identifying the need for environmental modification in the homes of older persons (Hiatt, 1981). The general remediation is the use of high contrast and good lighting in the living environment.

CONTRAST SENSITIVITY

The test for contrast sensitivity is a new test that is being used fairly routinely in low vision evaluations. The test demonstrates how much acuity a person loses with small changes in contrast. It shows the need for extra light when reading and special filters outdoors. It also helps service providers in designing appropriate living environments for their clients.

MAGNIFICATION ASSESSMENT

The previously described tests provide the clinician with an essential description of the impairment. Information gathered on the patient's need during intake provides some specific objectives for the low vision examination and the subsequent prescription of any devices. The clinician must put this information together and then consider treatment options. Clinicians use the person's distance acuity and the acuity needed to perform a task in question to determine the level of magnification needed to help the person. For example, a person who has 20/200 acuity and must read 20/40 print needs 5x magnification. Then the type of magnifying device that best gives this magnification level must be determined. There are four basic means of magnification—size magnification, distance magnification, angular magnification, and projection magnification.

Size Magnification

In size magnification, the object is simply made larger. The size of the print used in a large-print edition of *Reader's Digest* is an example of size magnification. Using a felt-tip pen instead of a ballpoint to write can provide 5x magnification.

Distance Magnification

In a sense, everyone uses distance magnification daily. If you cannot see a sign at 10 feet, you move closer to read it. As you move closer to the object, its image is enlarged on the retina until it becomes visible or readable. A person with low vision enlarges reading material by moving it from a conventional 13-inch work distance to 2 or 3 inches. A lens is used (usually as eyeglasses) to bring the enlarged retinal image into focus. It may be helpful to remember that the lenses prescribed for reading do not magnify. They simply put the magnified image into focus on the retina. A nearsighted person may accomplish this task by removing his or her eyeglasses—that is, by taking off the myopic distance correction. Young people can often accommodate to focus on pointed material held at a close work distance.

Angular Magnification

Angular magnification is created when binoculars are used. When using binoculars, a person with low vision is able to see distant objects, especially if those objects are too big to move or too far away to walk to. The preferred device is usually a monocular telescope for low vision, which is most effective at a distance of 10 or more feet. For closer distances, the telescope must be focused or an auxiliary lens must be placed on the front of the telescope to keep nearer objects in focus on the retina.

A telescope with a cap (lens) on the front is called a "reading telescope" or "telemicroscope" and actually uses both angular magnification (through the telescope) and distance magnification (through moving the object closer than 20 feet and focusing for that distance or using a focusing cap). The total magnification is the product of the angular magnification and the distance magnification. A 2x telescope with a +8 cap (2x microscope) has a total magnification of 4x.

Projection Magnification

Projection magnification is used when 35 mm slides or 2x2 slides are projected onto a surface. Detail is magnified several times. This kind of magnification for low vision is not commonly used. A special type of magnification is seen in closed-circuit televisions, in which a camera focuses on a page of print and projects it onto a wide television screen. It is an example of an electronically generated size magnification. The letter on the screen is physically larger than the one on the page. To increase magnification, a person with low vision can move closer to the screen, thereby making use of distance magnification. Thus, if a letter is magnified ten times on a screen and is viewed two times closer than normal (typically considered 16 inches), the total magnification is the product of the distance and the size magnification—2x10x=20x. High levels of magnification are easy to obtain with devices utilizing this principle of magnification.

Optimum Solution

After the level of magnification needed for the patient's task requirements and the best corrected acuity are determined, the clinician must consider which type of magnification might best resolve problem areas and then evaluate those specific optical devices representing the optimum solution. (The types of devices available as treatment options are discussed later in the chapter.) At this point in the examination, the clinician determines the prescription most likely to benefit the patient. Once the patient receives the device, he or she must be taught the skills necessary to use the device effectively and practice using it in the environments in which it is needed. It takes place as the training and instructional phases of the clinical examination or may be provided by professionals in a nonclinical setting.

Training and Instruction

Training and instruction are used in slightly different ways. In the training phase, the clinician or office assistant teaches the patient the mechanical skills needed to use the prescribed optical device. Handling the device physically, localizing, and spotting are examples of training. "Localizing" refers to locating the object or area to be viewed with the use of the low vision device. At this training stage, the instructor focuses the device for the visually impaired person, who then attempts to identify the object to be viewed directly in front of him or her. If the visually impaired person has difficulty finding the object, the instructor verbally indicates the direction in which the person should move the device until it is directed squarely at the object. "Spotting" involves finding the object without the device, then holding the device, such as a telescope, aligning it between the eye and the object, and focusing the device until the image is as clear as possible.

The instructional phase is usually supervised by an individual with a specific professional background in rehabilitation, education, or mobility. In this phase, the patient is taught to utilize the device most efficiently in his or her particular environment and life-style. The training phase is typically done in the clinic, and the instructional phase in the clinic or the home or social setting, wherever the device will be used. The goal of the initial visit for the patient is to bring the patient to a level of proficiency with the device that allows him or her to borrow the device and use it in a home training program for two or three weeks.

Follow-up

Follow-up visits and ongoing communication between the patient and the professional are essential for continued successful use of the patient's low vision devices. Even after the instructional phase, patients, particularly elderly patients, may experience difficulty using the devices on their own. They may experience changes in functional vision at different times of the day, in new environments, or in performing tasks over periods of time and may need further assistance beyond the safeguards built into training. It is important for the patient to know that follow-up services are available and that he or she can contact the low vision clinic for additional help at any time.

Optical Devices

It is important for patients, family members, and service providers to realize that low vision devices are not the sole answer to all an individual's visual problems. Much of the individual's success with the optical device and other recommendations depends on the support the older person receives outside the clinic. The more encouragement and monitoring after the examination, the greater the chance that the older person will eventually be able to maintain his or her own personal lifestyle. A service provider or family member can more effectively provide this nonclinic follow-up care if he or she has a good understanding of the examination results and principles of the prescribed devices.

The following section is a brief overview of the kinds of optical devices that are available and their uses and limitations. But it should be noted that many other kinds of nonoptical devices can be prescribed independently or in conjunction with optical devices to enhance visual performance. The categories of nonoptical devices are those that provide comfort (reading stands); control illumination (sunfilters, contrast filters, and reading slits); and offer increased size of objects to be viewed (large print, felt-tip pens, and so on). The simplest of these devices can often make the difference in a patient's success and comfort in performing a visual task.

MICROSCOPES

For the purposes of this discussion, optical devices that are mounted onto frames have been categorized arbitrarily as microscopes. This kind of device usually provides the largest field of view but the shortest working distance. It is the short distance for work (2 to 8 inches) that the older person usually rejects. In addition to the large field of view, the major advantage of this type of system is that the person can function with both hands free. However, the microscope has a critical focal distance, and small movements, such as physical tremors that cause it to move, throw the reading material or other objects being viewed in and out of focus. This unsteadiness is a particularly frustrating problem for older people who cannot maintain a steady fixation point and lose their place as print or other material to be viewed goes in and out of focus. A reading stand is often used to offset this problem. A good stand allows the person to read comfortably at a close work distance, maintain good posture, and move the material on the stand from right to left to minimize distracting head movements.

MAGNIFIERS

Magnifiers are designed to help a person with low vision with near tasks. They are either hand held or mounted on a stand. The simplest magnifier is hand held (see Figure 2), allowing the person to see at a

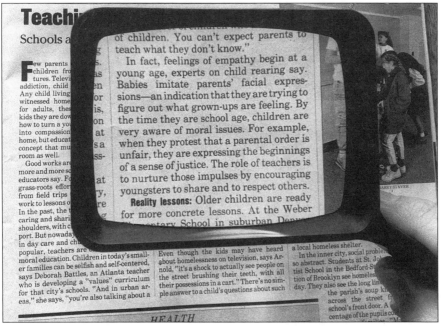

Figure 2: A hand-held magnifier. Source: *Visual Impairment: An Overview.* New York: American Foundation for the Blind, 1990.

normal work distance while providing a moderately acceptable field of view. Because many people use magnifiers, there is no stigma attached to using one in public, and thus many patients prefer this type of device. The disadvantage is that hand-held magnifiers do not allow the person to have both hands free while reading material or viewing an object.

Another problem is that the user must maintain an exact lens-to-object viewing distance to keep a clear image. If the person has tremors or unsteady motor control, the hand-held magnifier can be difficult to use. In this case, a stand magnifier may be considered. Because the stand can be laid on the paper or other surface and the surface remains in focus, the stand significantly reduces the problems of tremors. Although the stand magnifier is more cumbersome to use and carry than is a hand-held magnifier, it is often the preferred device for use in public. Contrary to popular belief, the stand magnifier is a complicated optical device often prescribed in conjunction with bifocals or reading lenses for optimum acuity and field to be maintained.

Both hand-held and stand magnifiers are used for short-term reading or viewing tasks. Each can be dispensed in an illuminated form if extra lighting is needed for such a task as reading a menu in a dimly lighted restaurant.

TELEMICROSCOPES

Telemicroscopes are telescopes that are focused for near work. They can be used for both distant and near work if a special cap is placed on the front of the telescope when the device is used for near activities. When the cap is removed, the telemicroscope becomes a distance telescope to be used for a task such as watching television.

The large field telemicroscope is a compromise between a small telescope (which usually allows for a long working distance and a small field) and a microscope (which gives a short working distance and a large field). A larger telescopic lens system with a full field can be utilized when a task does not require mobility. Older persons usually like the larger system better than the smaller one; it allows them to localize more easily and keep their place more comfortably on a line of print or on a task.

TELESCOPES

As indicated earlier, telescopes are the only devices that provide for distance viewing. Hand-held telescopes often permit an adequate field of view and are cosmetically more acceptable than some other devices because they can be used with discretion (see Figure 3). The telescope is usually for short-term tasks, such as reading signs. If the person requires the use of both hands, such as during work, or needs the telescope for long-term tasks, in the classroom, for instance, then the system can be mounted in a spectacle. As with the telemicroscope, the telescope can be designed as a bioptic so that the patient looks underneath the telescope mounted in the upper position of a spectacle lens when general mobility is needed and then drops the head and looks up into the telescope for seeing objects in the distance.

If the task does not require mobility, a larger field is obtained, and localization problems are minimized when a centrally mounted full-field telescope is used. Many older people cannot use spectacle-mounted telescopes and have difficulty aligning small hand-held telescopes because of tremors and generally poor motor control. Larger,

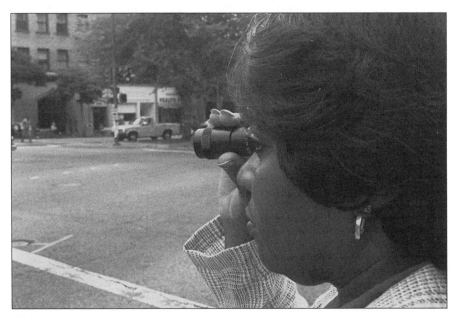

Figure 3: The use of a hand-held telescope. Source: *Visual Impairment: An Overview.* New York: American Foundation for the Blind, 1990.

hand-held monoculars that allow for a firmer grip and provide a larger field often offset this problem. Binoculars are also acceptable devices for individuals with tremor problems, especially if the devices are mounted on a tripod or a stand.

Conclusion

The low vision examination and other related professional services can be provided in a variety of offices, clinics, or centers. The professional and financial resources available dictate the number and training of the people who interact in the care of the visually impaired older person, the extent of their involvement, and the quantity and quality of the equipment and facilities used. The most important characteristic of an effective low vision service is the multidisciplinary approach, in which the examination data are shared among a variety of professionals in a coordinated and cooperative manner. Such professional interaction facilitates more successful rehabilitation of the older visually impaired person.

Because minimal third-party reimbursements are available for low vision services, it is not difficult to understand why there are not yet enough low vision clinics around the country. The provision of excellent low vision care is an expensive endeavor, requiring the cooperation of clinicians, administrators, and other professionals who work with older visually impaired individuals.

Vision loss may be only one of many problems the older person faces. Therefore, those who work in vision care programs need to realize that vision care is often given a lower priority by the older person in relation to the host of other medical, psychological, financial, or social problems he or she may be experiencing. It is essential to encourage older visually impaired persons to make eye care a priority and not just to accept visual impairment as a normal aspect of aging whose disabling effects often cannot be minimized.

Even in cases in which vision care is the patient's lowest priority, a basic low vision evaluation should be offered. The purpose of this basic evaluation is to educate the patient about the possibilities available to maximize vision. If optical devices are demonstrated and improvements in acuity are realized and discussed with the patient, he or she may want to take advantage of these improvements to enhance independent functioning. Often, if success is obtained with an optical device and the person engages in some small activity whose performance has previously not been possible, this success leads to further experimentation and an increased level of activity and independence. Success breeds success, especially in a rehabilitation process.

As more social, recreational, rehabilitation, and educational programs are developed for older visually impaired people, consideration should be given by service providers to the systematic referral for a low vision examination of older people experiencing vision problems. It may be done through a telephone call about the person being referred or through vision screening at a senior citizens center (Jose, 1983). For the older visually impaired person to benefit fully, low vision clinicians and service providers must communicate. Not only will the person receive a better examination, the results of that examination will be more productive.

Through the coordination of clinical and service activities, older visually impaired persons will have greater opportunities to increase their levels of independent functioning and will be able to continue valued activities and to feel as though they are a productive part of family, friends, community, and society. Although low vision devices do not always work miracles, they can be experienced as such through comprehensive vision rehabilitation.

References

Colenbrander, A. (1977). Dimensions of visual performance. *Transactions of the American Academy of Ophthalmology and Otolaryngology, 83:* 332-337.

Hiatt, L. (1981). The color and use of color in environments for older people. *Nursing Homes, 30:* 18-22.

Jose, R. (1983). *Understanding low vision.* New York: American Foundation for the Blind.

Jose, R., & Ferraro, J. (1983). A functional interpretation of the visual fields of low vision patients. *Journal of the American Optometric Association, 54:* 885-893.

Kirchner, C., & Phillips, B. (1988). Report of a survey of U.S. low vision services. In C. Kirchner (Ed.), *Data on blindness and visual impairment in* the U.S. (2nd ed., pp. 285-293). New York: American Foundation for the Blind.

Lowman, C., & Kirchner, C. (1988). Elderly blind and visually impaired persons: Projected numbers in the year 2000. In C. Kirchner (Ed.), *Data on blindness and visual impairment in the U.S.* (2nd ed., pp. 45-52). New York: American Foundation for the Blind.

National Society to Prevent Blindness. (1980). *Vision problems in the United States: Facts and figures.* New York: Author.

CHAPTER 11

Rehabilitation Teaching for Older Adults

John E. Crews and Lynne Luxton

The growth and development of the profession of rehabilitation teaching in many respects mirror the evolution of what we often call the "field of blindness." Rehabilitation teachers emerged from a charity model of services in the 19th century as "home teachers" who provided instruction in reading scripture. Today they constitute a cadre of university-trained professionals who address the broad array of skills needed by individuals who are blind and visually impaired to live independently at home, to obtain employment, and to participate in community life. As a discipline, rehabilitation teaching combines and applies the best principles of adaptive rehabilitation, adult education, and social work to the following broad areas: home management, personal management, communication and education, activities of daily living (ADL), leisure activities, and indoor orientation skills. Outdoor orientation and mobility (O&M) training is provided by an O&M specialist (see Chapter 12).

The demands of rehabilitation teaching often require these professionals to address broad rehabilitation goals and to identify and coordinate an array of community resources. In that challenge lies the joy and satisfaction of the profession. Moreover, rehabilitation teachers who work with older persons must address the very specific circumstances that older people face. For example, older persons who are blind or visually impaired experience other age-related health conditions, such as hearing loss, heart disease, and mobility impairments, at rates at least as great as the general population. Rehabilitation teachers must be prepared to deal with these circumstances, as well as the loss of vision.

Historical Perspective

Rehabilitation teaching evolved from the goodwill and concern of charitable organizations and church groups in the 19th century and the early part of the 20th century. Instruction focused on teaching newly blinded individuals to read religious materials. In England in the 1850s, Dr. William Moon, a blinded minister, developed a system of embossed type (Moon Type) that enabled blind people to read the Bible. In the United States, the Pennsylvania Home Teaching Society and Free Circulating Library for the Blind in Philadelphia was organized in 1892 by John Rhodes of the American Bible Society and William Moon. Training continued to emphasize the reading of religious materials (Koestler, 1976).

The first rehabilitation teachers, most of whom were women who were blind, were called "home teachers." In time, home teachers recognized the necessity of moving beyond instruction in reading the Scriptures to the broader areas of communication skills, daily living skills, and handicrafts. Virtually no formal training was available for these instructors, who assembled an array of adaptive techniques, hints, and "rules of thumb" that helped people who were visually impaired and blind to perform daily tasks.

Connecticut was the first state to fund home teaching in 1893. Koestler (1976) observed that by 1926, 25 states had home teaching programs. Because home teachers attempted to respond to the broad needs of blind people, their efforts continued to expand beyond skills training to case finding, the prevention of blindness, and employment.

In the 1920s and 1930s, efforts were made to professionalize the discipline, but it was not until after World War II that rehabilitation teaching developed as a profession. The world wars had a marked impact on rehabilitation; veterans who were blinded in the wars required rehabilitation. In 1918, the federal Soldiers Rehabilitation Act was enacted, followed in 1920 by P.L. 66-236, the federal Civilian Vocational Rehabilitation Act. The 1920 law was a major step toward recognizing the federal government's responsibility in providing vocational rehabilitation services for all Americans. The federal government continued its leadership role into the 1970s with the passage of the Rehabilitation Act (P.L. 93-112), and the 1978 amendments designated independent living as a viable outcome of rehabilitation. Title VII, Part C, of the Rehabilitation Act recognized the particular independent living needs of older persons who are blind, but funds were not appropriated until 1985. Even then, only $5 million was appropriated, to be awarded in segments of $200,000 to 23 states (one state received two grants) in 1986. Nevertheless, that action was an important legislative and policy step recognizing the needs of older people who are blind and visually impaired.

Cosgrove's (1961) book-length evaluation of rehabilitation teaching was the turning point for the development of the profession. Her study stimulated the federal government to develop university training programs in rehabilitation teaching. In 1963, Dr. Ruth Kaarlela started the first master's degree program in rehabilitation teaching at Western Michigan University in Kalamazoo. There are now six training programs for rehabilitation teaching in the country—five at the graduate and one at the undergraduate level at Western Michigan University, Northern Illinois University, University of Arkansas at Little Rock, San Francisco State University, Hunter College (New York), and Dominican College (undergraduate; New York).

These programs train rehabilitation teachers to understand specialized learning and teaching methodologies, eye pathologies, low vision, the psychosocial aspects of vision loss, the principles of rehabilitation teaching, gerontology, multiple-disability issues, adaptive techniques for ADL, communication skills, and indoor orientation skills.

The Older Blind and Visually Impaired Constituency

Rehabilitation teachers who serve older people who are blind recognize that the circumstances of elderly persons are more complex and more fluid than might be expected. A recent study in Michigan (Crews, 1991) involving 138 older persons revealed that the average age of women served in the state independent living rehabilitation program was 80. The average age for men was 78. Of the women served in that program, only 23 percent were married, whereas 46 percent of the men had spouses. Eighty percent of the individuals served had an onset of vision loss after age 60; in fact, 39 percent lost vision between the ages of 70 and 79, and 23 percent lost vision after age 80. Only 18 percent lost their vision between ages 60 and 69. In the Michigan study, half of the individuals served experienced macular degeneration. In addition, these individuals reported other age-related disabilities at rates equal to or greater than the general older population.

These data begin to define a number of important issues. Older women may find themselves "at risk" because there is no spouse to provide support or caregiving, and the spouse is the most tolerant and resilient caregiver. Yet for men who are married, the loss of a spouse may threaten the loss of independence. Moreover, since elders lose vision in or near retirement, they may not be able to avail themselves of vocational rehabilitation services offered to their younger cohorts. In addition, the onset of other age-related disabilities obviously complicates the rehabilitation process. For those older persons who experience both severe vision and severe hearing loss, progress in rehabilitation may be compromised. The consequence of these circumstances clearly suggests that serving older people who are blind is often extremely complex.

In addition, the situation faced by older persons is fluid. Gerontologists often speak of the "cascade" of traumatic events that compromise independence. Older persons who are blind or visually impaired experience a situation as fluid as any other older person's. For 80-year-old persons who typify the Michigan study, other age-related changes are inevitable. Support systems may change with loss of a spouse or an adult child. The individual who successfully used limited vision may lose remaining vision, thus compromising strategies that preserved independence.

Rehabilitation teachers who work with older persons must be prepared to deal with both the complexities of the situation and the fluid circumstances that aging invites. Rehabilitation teachers must recognize and respect the integrity of an older constituency. Although older persons in the Michigan study presented multiple needs, the elder population is remarkably heterogeneous. Each person's experience is unique and requires an individualized approach to rehabilitation teaching.

Goals of Rehabilitation Teaching

Rehabilitation teaching is defined as "a professional discipline in which instruction and guidance is provided to visually impaired individuals through individualized plans of instruction designed to permit the clients to carry out their daily activities, to manage their lives more efficiently within their environment, and to reach their potential for self-independence, self-esteem, and productivity" (Asenjo, 1975, p. 10). In many respects, the profession of rehabilitation teaching reinforces the powerful dimension of the disability movement—the theme of empowerment. By teaching skills in communication, ADL, and personal management, consumers are empowered and enabled to carry out the activities that they identify as valuable. A successful rehabilitation teacher realizes the empowerment goals identified by younger people in the disability movement and transfers them to older persons.

The most forward thinkers in rehabilitation challenge us to reconsider the outcomes of rehabilitation. Williams (1984) writes:

> Rehabilitation is an approach, a philosophy, and a point of view as much as it is a set of techniques. The aim of rehabilitation, to "restore an individual to his or her former functional environmental status, or, alternatively, to maintain or maximize function" should be at the heart of all care of aging persons in order to help them continue to live as full a life as possible. (p. xiii)

And Fenderson (1986) argues:

> In rehabilitation, the therapeutic goals and emphasis shift from diagnosis and treatment to function and performance. The goals are not limited to physical performance alone. They encompass, as do those of the relatively new medical specialty of family medicine, an "extended boundary" concept of the person in his/her environment. (p. 4)

Williams and Fenderson help to define the goals and outcomes of rehabilitation teaching. Rehabilitation teachers recognize the importance of "small gains" that older people achieve in the rehabilitation process. For example, learning a strategy to set the household thermostat may be a "small gain" that creates significant satisfaction as an older person is able to exercise more control over the environment.

Williams (1984) asserts the concept of "small gains" and argues that such gains can make all the difference between being able to live in one's own home and requiring care in a long-term care institution. Williams cites the example of being able to transfer from wheelchair to commode to bed, but the concept is equally powerful among elders who are visually impaired, as they achieve the small gains that lead to meal preparation and increased communication skills.

A second goal for rehabilitation teaching has to do with sustaining functional ability. All of us can become enamored with the concept of demonstrating "miraculous" increases in a person's capacity to perform certain tasks, but "small gains" also lead to measurable increases in life satisfaction. Moreover, given the nature of an older—sometimes fragile—population, sustaining a level of ability is equally valuable to increasing function. If an older woman can continue to pay bills, prepare meals, and get around the home as her vision declines, then sustaining that level of function is of significant value.

Even though rehabilitation teaching clearly emphasizes teaching skills in such areas as communications, ADL, and household management, rehabilitation professionals recognize that the outcomes of rehabilitation are more than the discrete skills of slicing, chopping, and dicing might suggest. For example, the skills of food preparation lead to the task performance of preparing meals. In addition to the satisfaction of being able to take care of one's self and immediate family, learning meal preparation skills enhances quality of life and provides an important affirmation of a societal role.

A third goal associated with rehabilitation for older persons who are visually impaired has to do with the importance of sustaining active life. Rehabilitation teachers play an important role in this goal. Fulton and Katz (1986) advance the concept of "active" and "dependent" life, and their study makes a powerful argument for the role of rehabilitation teachers. Fulton and Katz studied a large sample of older people, and they noted the life expectancy of various cohorts of elders. For example, they noted that someone aged 60 to 65 has a "life expectancy" of 16.5 additional years. They then classified those years as "active life" and "dependent life." Active life was defined as "being independent in six activities of daily living, including bathing, dressing, transferring, eating, personal grooming, and walking across a small room" (p. 38). Dependent life was defined as needing assistance in any one of these areas. It is worth noting that these six areas define much of what rehabilitation teaching is all about.

According to Fulton and Katz, for the person aged 60-65 who can expect to live 16.5 additional years, 10 years would be classified as active, and 6.5 would be classified as dependent. Persons over the age of 85 can expect 7.3 additional years of life, 2.9 as active and 4.4 as dependent.

This study makes a strong case for rehabilitation teaching. If an older person who is visually impaired can be provided with skills and strategies to remain as productive as possible and to be able to enjoy as many years of life as independently as possible, then rehabilitation has clearly been successful. In many respects, rehabilitation teaching drives a wedge between "active" life and "dependent" life to preserve years of productivity. Rehabilitation teachers help older persons maintain years of active life and adapt successfully to the changes of dependent life. This study makes a compelling argument against the policy of dismissing services to older persons as less "valuable," and it suggests the possibility of cost-benefit arguments for rehabilitation teaching.

Two case examples may serve to demonstrate what rehabilitation teachers do and how the work impacts upon people's lives. Mr. B was 70 when a rehabilitation teacher first visited him. Mr. B had retired from the post office and lived with his wife. He had recently been diagnosed with macular degeneration. He explained that he had been to four different ophthalmologists, and because each had told him the same thing, he concluded "I guess I got it." His health was quite good, and although he was upset with this recent news about his eye condition, he knew that he had coped successfully with other difficulties throughout his life.

Mr. B and the rehabilitation teacher worked toward the goals Mr. B identified. He clearly enjoyed getting out with other people and readily joined and became active in the local peer support group that the rehabilitation teacher had established. There he met an old friend from his post office days, and that eased the transition. He also wanted to continue keeping the family financial records, an important role for him. The rehabilitation teacher helped him create a large-print ledger and by using felt-tip pens, he was able to continue to keep these records. A hand-held magnifier, prescribed for him through the low vision clinic, allowed him to read his bills and statements. Large-print checks from his local bank made check writing easier. The rehabilitation teacher worked with Mr. B to reorganize his work area, creating a large-print filing system and adding lighting to his work area. He had never thought much about lighting before his vision problem, but he learned that it was an important factor to consider. He found that if he worked at the kitchen table with the curtains open and his back to the window, the natural light helped him to see with greater comfort.

Mr. B's wife prepared all the meals, and he was concerned about what he would do if something happened to her. After his success with the financial records, Mr. B had the confidence to try learning basic cooking skills. Because he still had useful vision, the rehabilitation teacher stressed increased illumination and the use of color contrast. She also helped him learn to confirm what he was doing by using tactual cues. He learned to gauge tactually the amount of margarine needed for spreading on his toast. When he made instant coffee, she suggested that he use a white cup, so that he could see the contrast of the coffee against the cup as he poured the water.

The rehabilitation teacher marked the oven at 350 degrees, provided Mr. B with a large-print timer, and gave him instruction in using the oven safely. He enjoyed baking brownies and used long safety oven mitts to take pans in and out of the oven. He also learned how to use the microwave oven.

Outside the home, Mr. B wanted to continue taking care of the lawn and performing some wood-working activities. He found that with a visor over his eyes to avoid glare and careful use of brightly colored targets, he could pretty much keep up with the lawn. The rehabilitation teacher helped Mr. B with increased illumination in his wood shop and encouraged him to use dark markers or tactual markings to mark wood before cutting. These adaptive techniques, combined with a strong support system, allowed Mr. B to take risks to increase his in-dependence and enhance his self-esteem.

Mrs. R's circumstances were quite different. She was an 83-year-old widow who had lived in the same house for nearly forty years. Her husband had died 12 years ago, and she was committed to remaining in her own home. As a retired school teacher, she was a bright and feisty woman, but her health was frail. Her vision had declined over the last three years, and she now had very little vision. After a fall that resulted in a broken hip, a long recovery, and a short stay in a nursing home, she was determined to go home and continue to live independently.

The rehabilitation teacher arranged for Mrs. R to receive Talking Books. She had been an avid reader, and this activity helped to fill long hours. It also kept her connected and gave her something to talk about. Mrs. R described the Talking Book program as a "Godsend." The rehabilitation teacher also taught Mrs. R braille, beginning with Grade 1 for labeling items and taking notes. Mrs. R enjoyed learning new skills and put her energy into learning Grade 2 braille. She also got out her old typewriter and began to relearn touch typing through free cor-respondence lessons from the Hadley School for the Blind.

Mrs. R had been an exceptional cook, but she was now fearful of burning or cutting herself. The rehabilitation teacher began by address-ing safety issues. She marked the oven and the range for the most common temperatures, and she encouraged Mrs. R to use a braille timer. She noted the importance of defining a "safe spot" near the range where she could set things if they got too hot. Mrs. R was encouraged to make the breads that she had always enjoyed, and she gained considerable pleasure in sharing her baked goods with friends and family.

Mrs. R and the rehabilitation teacher did a safety check throughout her home. They worked on eliminating glare and creating color con-trasts for safety. Mrs. R removed her unnecessary throw rugs. She decided to put a handrail on the basement stairway and to increase the lighting in the basement. She tried hard to eliminate her old habit of storing things on the basement steps.

The rehabilitation teacher was concerned about assuring that Mrs. R was eating well when she was alone. Mrs. R wouldn't have anything to do with Meals-on-Wheels, but she was willing to join a lifelong friend at a nutrition site that was only four blocks away. The agency O&M instructor taught Mrs. R the route to the meal site, and both the O&M specialist and the rehabilitation teacher conducted a brief training session with the staff of the aging agency to smooth the way.

These examples portray the range of services that rehabilitation teachers provide to older persons. As problem solvers, rehabilitation teachers carefully assess the consumer's circumstances and desires and, in conjunction with the older person, design strategies for responding to those needs.

Settings for Rehabilitation Teaching

Rehabilitation teachers work in a number of settings: state agencies for the blind, private nonprofit agencies, and the U.S. Department of Veterans Affairs (formerly the Veterans Administration). The services are itinerant (or field based) and center based. In residential programs, training may last from a few days to several weeks. These centers have specialized staff, including rehabilitation teachers, O&M specialists, recreation therapists, rehabilitation counselors, and manual arts instructors. Some programs are affiliated with hospitals and others with large rehabilitation facilities.

Rehabilitation teachers in residential programs often specialize in particular teaching areas. They may also have skills for working with special populations, for example, persons who are deaf and blind. The residential setting allows for several hours of training to be provided to clients each day. The team approach of the center allows teachers to combine their skills with other professionals to help clients reinforce skills development. In addition, the environment allows people who are blind and visually impaired to get together to review their training and share experiences.

Acton (1976) believed that the residential rehabilitation center was more efficient than the community-based model in helping clients achieve personal adjustment to vision loss. However, for the older visually impaired population the opposite may sometimes be true. Older visually impaired people may learn best in their own homes and communities and in the familiar environments where they will use the new skills.

With the funding of Title VII, Part C of the Rehabilitation Act, more agencies serving older visually impaired persons can provide rehabilitation teaching in the older person's home. Many clients still go to a community-based agency for blind persons for rehabilitation as well. Hensley (1987) reported the positive effects of successful daily living skills training on the anxiety and self-worth levels of 20 elderly persons in a community-based agency's day rehabilitation program. This option helps physically able older persons to get out into the community and meet other older people coping with vision loss while learning independent living skills.

Teaching in the field has different advantages. Although the contacts with clients may be limited because of caseload size and the logistics of caseload distribution, teachers can respond to the real and specific needs of older persons in their homes. Many field teachers also enjoy the independence and challenge of being the primary resource in a community.

By working in an individual's home, the field rehabilitation teacher is also in the best position to evaluate the older visually impaired person's physical environment and to suggest environmental modifications that maximize the person's functioning. The teacher can make practical suggestions about glare reduction, lighting improvements, the use of color contrast, organization of personal and household items, and adaptations of existing home appliances. Working with the client on practical applications helps make the most efficient use of the person's resources.

Rehabilitation teachers in the field often find the need to coordinate community resources, including visiting nurses and services from the aging network, such as Meals-on-Wheels and home health aides. As a consequence, rehabilitation teachers often provide in-service training to their colleagues in the human services to encourage older blind and visually impaired clients to remain involved in community activities. The example of Mrs. R illustrates how a rehabilitation teacher might use community resources.

Rehabilitation teachers in centers, community agencies, or the homes of older persons increasingly recognize that as clients gain skills, their increased independence may have a considerable impact on the family members. A study by Crews (1988) addressed the concerns of family members (spouses and adult children). In a sample of 43 families, 84 percent of spouses and 80 percent of adult children who had parents living with them reported that safety was an important or critical concern. In this study, it was clear that family members who had an older blind person residing with them reported serious concerns about skills (meal preparation, especially) and knowing "when," "how," and "how much" to help. Adult children who did not have a parent living with them did not report the same levels of stress. Only 55 percent indicated safety as a concern. Adult children and spouses reported significantly less concern after rehabilitation teachers had provided instruction. The concern for safety among spouses dropped from 84 percent to 52 percent, and for adult children who had a parent living with them, the level of concern dropped from 80 percent to 40 percent. For adult children who did not have a parent living with them, however, the level of concern dropped from 55 percent to 46 percent. Although one cannot attribute all this change to the rehabilitation teacher's activities, it clearly plays a role.

By contrast, Utrup (1980) wrote about an older man who returned home after receiving several weeks of training at a residential center. He demonstrated his new skills to his wife by preparing breakfast for both of them. His wife, however, had grown accustomed to her husband's dependence, and the man's newly gained independence upset the household's equilibrium. Utrup observed that "unfortunately, rehabilitation is sometimes viewed by the spouse as a challenge to their effectiveness as a dutiful husband or wife" (p. 103). In some instances, family members thrive on "taking care of" the visually impaired individual and are lost when the role of caregiver is no longer necessary in the same way. Rehabilitation teachers can help family members to deal with these dependence/independence issues.

Rehabilitation teachers increasingly need to understand the dynamics of families in order to involve family members in the rehabilitation process. Ponchillia (1984) discusses the issues surrounding the need for family involvement in rehabilitation center programs and suggests strategies for enhancing family support. Part of the dynamics of families have to do with roles. Rehabilitation teachers must recognize and facilitate the roles of family members. Allowing spouses and adult children to be actively involved in the rehabilitation process encourages individual family members to recognize the increased capacity that rehabilitation teaching may bring about. The older visually impaired person and his or her family members must be sensitive to the changes that are occurring.

Although it is important to recognize that older persons need rehabilitative services mostly in the form of independent living skills training, it is critical to remember that some older persons who lose their vision still want to remain in or reenter the work force and must have access to vocational rehabilitation services. The value of serving older people who wish to work is gaining increased attention, and certainly as the population continues to age, more older people who are visually impaired will remain in the work force for both economic and social reasons (Corthell, 1990).

Adaptive Techniques and Assistive Devices

One of the roles of the rehabilitation teacher is to introduce blind and visually impaired persons to the variety of adaptive techniques and assistive devices and to help them make selections. The rehabilitation teacher provides training in specific skills and in the use of adaptive devices and appliances. As the person's vision, needs, or life-style changes, it is frequently the rehabilitation teacher who helps the visually impaired person select new options. The following sections describe adaptive techniques and assistive devices that allow for greater independence when used by visually impaired persons.

COMMUNICATION SKILLS

Writing

Severe visual impairment often compromises a person's ability to use written communication skills. The skilled rehabilitation teacher helps clients assess their communication needs, level of useful vision, and general health before determining the most efficient and convenient methods of communication.

Written communication methods include braille, large-print handwriting, and typing. Any of these media can be adapted by visually impaired persons to fulfill the requirements of their daily activities, including writing checks, messages, letters, and shopping lists.

Braille

Braille is the most publicly recognized form of written communication for blind people, although less than 20 percent of legally blind people use Grade 2 braille. Braille is used for English and foreign languages, mathematics, computer and scientific notations, and music. It is written by hand with a slate and stylus, by a manual braillewriter, or by a computer.

The braille "cell" consists of six embossed dots. The configurations of the dots represent a letter, a word, a portion of a word, a number, a punctuation mark, a composition sign, or a symbol specific to the subject (such as music). Grade 1 braille consists of the alphabet, numbers, punctuation marks, and limited composition signs specific to braille. Grade 2 braille is more complex than Grade 1 and includes approximately 200 contractions—single symbols for commonly used combinations of letters, such as "ing," or whole words. Most reading materials are produced in Grade 2 braille. Many newly visually impaired older persons use jumbo-size braille rather than the standard size. Jumbo braille dots are larger, spaced farther apart, and easier to feel.

Braille is a useful communication tool for many older people. Because Grade 1 braille is relatively easy to learn, it should be introduced to older visually impaired people who are exploring alternatives to reading and writing print. Grade 1 braille is especially useful for such tasks as labeling, marking playing cards, writing telephone numbers and addresses, and keeping brief notes. Braille labels can also be used for marking stoves, clocks, timers, washers, dryers, and other appliances. Family members can learn to read and write Grade 1 braille visually. Their use and knowledge of braille can be helpful in incorporating the visually impaired person back into the household routine.

Large Print

Large print is a catchall term that encompasses a wide variety of print forms. Large print is not defined consistently. Thus, all large-print materials may not be equally useful to all readers.

Public libraries have large-print books, and commercial printing houses are increasing their publications of large-print titles. Most large-print material is published in 18-point type. This size type can be read by many visually impaired persons without using low vision devices or other adaptations.

The effective use of large print requires individualized training. The successful use of large print depends on the size of the print, print style, spacing of the letters and the lines, contrast, available lighting, angle at which the book or other material is being read, use of low vision devices, such as magnifiers and closed-circuit televisions (CCTVs), and the need and motivation of the reader.

Handwriting and Typing

Many visually impaired people have learned to use their remaining vision to accommodate a lifelong habit of handwriting. A rehabilitation teacher may recommend the use of a felt-tip marker or pen and a handwriting guide. Commercially available writing guides have designated writing spaces that allow a visually impaired person to write on a straight line. Tactual handwriting guides are available for writing signatures and checks and for addressing envelopes. These guides help individuals with all degrees of vision loss. Also useful for many visually impaired people is bold-lined paper. It is of standard weight and size with heavy black lines spaced farther apart than on conventional notebook paper.

Typing can also be used for writing personal correspondence, addressing envelopes, filling out checks, and preparing lists and messages for others. But many individuals cannot read what they have typed unless large-print elements or magnifiers are used. Nevertheless, many older people enjoy the challenge of learning to type and the knowledge that what they have typed can be easily read by others.

Computers

Personal computers are increasingly popular even among older people who did not grow up with computer technology. Although the technology continues to change rapidly, computers allow for voice output, production of large print, and braille. The quality of voice output has improved dramatically, and costs continue to decline. As computers become increasingly user friendly and as costs continue to decline, personal computers create significant options for independence.

Listening

Devices for listening provide visually impaired people access to printed material. Rehabilitation teachers offer instruction in listening skills, which can benefit blind and visually impaired persons who are unaccustomed to using listening as their primary method of learning.

Tape Recorders

Tape recorders are remarkably versatile devices but may seem too complicated to some older persons. Therefore, the rehabilitation teacher may need to help select the equipment and train the older person in its use. Many visually impaired persons use a standard two-track cassette recorder for personal correspondence and everyday use. Cassette recorders with advanced technology have four tracks, indexing capabilities, variable-speed adjustments, and compressed-speech capability. The use of compressed speech may require auditory training. It is often a preferred option for the visually impaired person who has been a rapid and avid reader.

The tape recorder can be used as a family message center, to store recipes, and to record business meetings. The National Library Service for the Blind and Physically Handicapped (NLS) of the Library of Congress provides a free state-of-the-art four-track cassette playback machine with rechargeable batteries to persons who use its services. With this machine, visually impaired, physically handicapped, and other print-handicapped persons who cannot read regular print can listen to recordings of books, magazines, and other reading materials available on loan through the NLS (see "Resources" for address). Further information about NLS and applications for its services are obtainable through state and local associations for the blind, public libraries, and state and regional libraries for the blind and physically handicapped.

Talking Book Machines
Talking Book machines are provided free by NLS to any blind, visually impaired, physically handicapped, or print-handicapped person. The machine, similar to a record player, uses Talking Book disks of books and magazines provided by NLS.

Listening to recordings played on a Talking Book machine requires more time than listening to those played on a cassette playback machine; Talking Book machines do not use variable speech speeds. Older clients who have difficulty adjusting to the four-track tape playback machine may prefer the disk player because it is more familiar and seems easier to operate.

NLS provides additional devices to make its machines accessible to physically handicapped persons. A remote on/off control is available, as are headphones with individually adjusted amplifiers and pillow speakers for persons who cannot use the headphones.

Devices for Reading Print
Over the years, research has been conducted on methods of making print accessible to blind people. Current computer technology, with outputs in braille, large print, and voice, continues to increase the accessibility of print for blind and visually impaired persons.

Kurzweil Reading Machine
The Kurzweil Reading Machine, housed in many libraries for public use, utilizes a computerized voice output to read a variety of printed materials. The Kurzweil Personal Reader, a compact version, is designed for individual purchase by the visually impaired person for home or

office use. The American Foundation for the Blind operates a loan program for the purchase of the personal reader.

Closed-Circuit Television

A CCTV has a television-type screen with a zoom lens that the reader can adjust. The magnification capabilities of CCTVs allow many people with low vision to read print. The reader can also adjust the light/dark contrast. A variety of CCTVs are on the market. The rehabilitation teacher can help the visually impaired person arrange for a demonstration of a CCTV.

Optacon

The Optacon, or the Optical to Tactile Converter, was developed by Telesensory, Inc. and allows readers to feel the shape of the print letters on the index finger through a series of retractable pins. The Optacon has a camera that picks up print contrasts on the page and converts the shape of the contrast to raised metal pins. As the reader moves the camera over the print, the pins imitate the letter and the reader feels raised letters pass under his or her index finger. The efficient use of the Optacon takes extensive instruction and practice. The reading speed is slow, but it can be useful to some blind persons.

DAILY LIVING SKILLS

Daily living skills, or activities of daily living (ADL), are the tasks and activities that a person carries out during the course of the day, excluding strictly vocational tasks. For the purposes of planning lessons in rehabilitation teaching, activities of daily living generally include the following broad categories—home management skills (meal preparation, housekeeping, labeling, shopping, doing laundry, handling household records, and general organizational techniques) and personal management skills (personal health care and hygiene, clothing care, eating techniques, grooming, and social skills). Home orientation and adaptive communication skills are necessary components of ADL skills.

On the basis of an evaluation and interview, the rehabilitation teacher develops an individualized teaching plan with the visually impaired person. The teacher and the consumer together determine the goals of the plan. Progress is continually evaluated, particularly for older people as they gain confidence in their abilities to teach themselves new techniques and to adapt their lifelong habits.

Survival skills—the solutions for basic needs (health, safety, and food preparation)—are always priorities in the teaching sequence. Because daily living activities are so extensive and people have such diversified daily routines, the teaching sequence varies from person to person. Two visually impaired people with the same rehabilitation teacher may learn different skills based on their needs, life-styles, motivation for learning, proficiency in the desired skills, and effectiveness of their current adaptations. The purpose of rehabilitation teaching is to create options by providing people with the skills and knowledge to make informed choices about their lives.

LEISURE-TIME ACTIVITIES

Older visually impaired persons may keenly feel their loss of vision in relation to leisure activities. Certainly, ADL skills are important, but if older people look forward to leisure time after retirement, they may feel cheated when reduced vision interferes with their recreational activities. It is important to consider leisure needs and to treat them seriously.

When the rehabilitation teacher evaluates an older person's life skills needs, it is essential to focus on the first part of the term—life. Life is more than the skills of daily functioning. It involves activities one can talk about, get dressed for, and look forward to. Individuals who have never had hobbies or whose favorite activities do not accommodate reduced vision present a challenge. Ludwig, Luxton, and Attmore (1988) offer ideas and resources for leisure activities that may be useful to older visually impaired persons, family members, and professionals.

Leisure activities can include anything, active or passive, that provides enjoyment for the participant. Activities can be performed by the individual or in a group, at home or in the community. They can be creative or aesthetic, social, intellectual, or physical. The rehabilitation teacher assists the older visually impaired person in exploring new and renewed leisure pursuits.

Current Issues

Since the 1980s, serious personnel shortages have affected this country's ability to meet the needs of the growing population of blind and visually impaired individuals. There is a tremendous need to recruit future rehabilitation teachers and O&M specialists into professional preparation programs. There is also a serious need to recruit members of minority groups to meet the needs of growing numbers of blind and visually impaired minority persons. Older black and Hispanic persons experience vision loss at a higher rate than the general population, but language and cultural barriers may prevent these older persons from seeking services. The availability of bilingual and bicultural professionals may help eliminate some of these barriers to service.

Most recently, paraprofessional rehabilitation teaching assistants are being trained to teach skills under the supervision of certified rehabilitation teachers. Minority recruitment efforts are also occurring in this area to improve service accessibility for minority persons.

One issue that needs attention is the fact that both rehabilitation teachers and O&M specialists are currently ineligible for third-party reimbursement, particularly through Medicare and Medicaid. If an older consumer falls and fractures her hip because she did not see the top of a flight of stairs, Medicare or Medicaid pays for her physical rehabilitation by physical and occupational therapists. But Medicare and Medicaid do not give reimbursement for rehabilitation services that teach safety techniques that have the potential to prevent falls. This issue requires continued legislative advocacy to establish third-party reimbursement for broader rehabilitation services.

The matter of licensure is critical in relation to eligibility for third-party payments. At present, there is no state or national mechanism for the licensing of the professional disciplines involved in the field of blindness rehabilitation. A committee of the Association for Education and Rehabilitation of the Blind and Visually Impaired, the primary professional organization in the field of blindness, is working to establish national licensing standards and to assist in determining the status of certified rehabilitation teachers for licensing eligibility. It is essential for professionals in the field of rehabilitation for persons who are blind and visually impaired to work to ensure that qualified persons deliver effective services nationwide.

References

Acton, J. J. (1976). Establishing and maintaining a therapeutic environment in a residential rehabilitation center for the blind. *The New Outlook for the Blind,* 70(4): 149-152.

Asenjo, J. A. (1975). *Rehabilitation teaching for the blind and visually impaired: The state of the art, 1975.* New York: American Foundation for the Blind.

Cosgrove, E. (1961). *Home teachers of the adult blind.* Washington, DC: American Association of Workers for the Blind.

Corthell, D. W. (Ed.). (1990). *Aging in America: Implications for vocational rehabilitation and independent living.* Seventeenth Institute on Rehabilitation Issues. Menomonie, WI: University of Wisconsin-Stout.

Crews, J. E. (1988). Family concerns and older people who are blind. Manuscript submitted for publication.

Crews, J. E. (1991). *The needs of older people who are blind in Michigan: A report to the Michigan State Legislature.* Lansing: Michigan Commission for the Blind.

Fenderson, D. A. (1986). Aging, disability and therapeutic optimism. In S. J. Brody & G. E. Ruff (Eds.), *Aging and rehabilitation: Advances in the state of the art* (pp. 3-12). New York: Springer.

Fulton, J. P., & Katz, S. (1986). Characteristics of the disabled elderly and implications for rehabilitation. In S. J. Brody & G. E. Ruff (Eds.), *Aging and rehabilitation: Advances in the state of the art* (pp. 36-46). New York: Springer.

Hensley, M. (1987). Rehabilitation in daily living skills: Effects on anxiety and self-worth in elderly blind persons. *Journal of Visual Impairment & Blindness,* 81, 330.

Koestler, F. (1976). *The unseen minority: A social history of blindness in the United States.* New York: David McKay.

Ludwig, I., Luxton., L., & Attmore, M. (1988). *Creative recreation for blind and visually impaired adults.* New York: American Foundation for the Blind.

Ponchillia, P. E. (1984). Family services: Role of the center-based teaching professional. *Journal of Visual Impairment & Blindness, 78:* 97-100.

Utrup, R. G. (1980). Rehabilitation teaching: Developing a professional character, confronting issues, and planning positively for the future. *AAWB Blindness Annual.* Alexandria, VA: American Association of Workers for the Blind.

Williams, T. F. (1984). *Rehabilitation in the aging.* New York: Raven.

CHAPTER 12

Orientation and Mobility Services for Older Persons

Steven J. LaGrow and Bruce B. Blasch

Most Americans live in apartments or single-family dwellings and move freely about their communities to meet their daily life needs. "Mobility," the ability to move about safely and efficiently on foot or by motor vehicle, underlies many of the activities that collectively permit independent living. These activities include going to work, shopping, seeing friends, participating in social and religious activities, and visiting doctors and other health care providers. Independent mobility is a vital ingredient in attaining personal independence and vocational success, and thus it is highly regarded by our mobile society (Foulke, 1971).

Many persons at some time in their lives become limited, if only temporarily, in the ability to move about. Mobility limitations may be caused by the onset of physical, sensory, or cognitive impairment or by a combination of these and other factors. Some limitations are amenable to medical treatment, which results in restoration of full independence. Limitations may also be remediated by training individuals in adaptive skills. Orientation and mobility training (or mobility training) for persons with visual impairment, in which work has been ongoing for approximately 35 years, is an example of training to remediate functional mobility limitations. Mobility instruction—helping visually impaired people develop or reestablish independent mobility—has focused increased attention on the centrality of mobility in human development (Welsh & Blasch, 1980).

The authors thank Drs. Richard Long, William De l'Aune, David Martino-Saltzman, and Betty Rose Connell for their contributions to this chapter.

The two skills—orientation and mobility—involve separate bodies of knowledge but are usually taught simultaneously. Orientation techniques teach travelers to utilize sensory information to establish their position in space in relation to the physical environment and thereby help them determine their position in relation to all significant objects in that environment (Hill & Ponder, 1976). When people are oriented, they know where they are, where they wish to go, and how to get there.

Mobility techniques for visually impaired individuals are designed to allow an individual to travel safely and independently from one point to another. They are more observable to others than are orientation techniques; mobility techniques generally rely on the use of long canes, sighted guides, electronic travel aids (ETAs), or dog guides.

Aging is likely to play a role in changes in an individual's pattern of mobility. The process of normal aging results in certain fairly predictable changes in one's physical status and probably brings changes in social and family roles as well. Examples of physical change are at least small declines in sensory ability (e.g., presbycusis, the gradual loss of hearing associated with aging) and in certain cognitive capabilities (e.g., problem-solving ability). Social and family role changes may be retirement, death of a spouse, loss of a social network, and initiation of live-in support. It is likely that type and degree of independent mobility maintained by an older person depend on a complex set of variables, including sensory and cognitive ability, personality characteristics, the local travel environment, and the traveler's social and family needs. Because people vary greatly in their abilities and needs for independent travel, a continuum of services is necessary to help persons attain skill in independent mobility.

Mobility instruction may include orienting individuals to the layout of the home or immediate environment and training in basic sighted guide, self-protective, or cane skills for travel needs that are limited to familiar, controlled environments. Other individuals need skills to travel independently in their own neighborhoods, to their places of employment, or to other familiar areas. Some need to develop generalization skills for unfamiliar environments and to incorporate a knowledge of public transportation into their mobility repertoire—for travel beyond reasonable walking range or for independent travel to all areas within or between cities. Instruction in orientation and mobility is typically provided by a mobility specialist. However, rehabilitation teachers may also provide orientation to the indoor environment (see Chapter 11).

The amount and type of instruction depend on the individual's specific travel requirements and learning style. University-trained mobility specialists generally provide center-based instruction in natural environments often near rehabilitation or training centers. The instruction, which uses individualized lessons, has a predetermined curriculum of broad skills and knowledge that can be generalized to all environments.

One view is that many older visually impaired persons expect fewer changes than younger persons do in their places of residence and travel habits and therefore require a curriculum of instruction different from that for younger visually impaired individuals. For the older person, a self-directed and individually designed approach may be most relevant (Ingalls, 1973; Welsh, 1980). The goals of older people, particularly those who live among a limited number of visually impaired individuals and whose travel may be limited to the home, neighborhood, nursing home, or other familiar areas, are often addressed by an itinerant instructor providing training for a specific environment.

Initially, travel goals may be limited to those specifically requested by an older person. The lessons, techniques, and goals should be structured to ensure success. If a person has some success, motivation to try more complex tasks and environments may follow. Success often encourages initial goals to expand as confidence grows.

Range of Needs

The mobility needs of older persons range from limited independence to unrestricted travel in unfamiliar environments. Some people want to go only from the front steps to the mailbox. Others maintain a full business schedule and social life and want to engage in unrestricted travel. The range of needs demonstrated by older people may be the same as that of younger persons (Ponchilla & Kaarlela, 1982; Senior Blind Program, 1981).

Unfortunately, only limited scientific study documents the degree to which personal factors (e.g., degree and duration of vision loss, health problems, amount of O&M training) and environmental factors (e.g., presence of sidewalks, availability of public transportation) affect independence in travel. Long, McNeal, and Griffin-Shirley (1990) at the Rehabilitation Research and Development Center of the Veterans Administration Medical Center in Atlanta, Georgia, completed in-depth, face-to-face interviews about travel habits and abilities with older and middle-aged blind and visually impaired persons and older persons with normal sight. Three-fourths of the 28 middle-aged blind individuals and the 28 older sighted individuals responded "yes" when asked if they had traveled outside their houses and yards by themselves in the past week. Only one-fourth of the older blind individuals responded affirmatively to this question. Of the older blind travelers, only 3 reported traveling independently to a destination; 6 others reported they walked for exercise in their immediate neighborhoods. The three groups did not differ on the reported number of destinations within walking distance of their residences. The mean for all groups was 3 destinations.

Another measure of independent mobility was the response to the question: "In the past year, how often on average have you traveled outside your house and yard by yourself?" Responses were given to a scale in which 1 represented "daily" and 5 "never." The mean response of the middle-aged blind individuals was 2.36 ($SD=1.4$); the mean response of older blind individuals was 3.65 ($SD=1.6$); and the mean response of older sighted individuals was 2.50 ($SD=1.4$) ($F=7.09$, $df=2.84$, $p=.001$). Analysis of variance revealed that older blind respondents differed from the two other groups.

A similar pattern of results was reported for satisfaction with independence in travel beyond one's home and yard. Older blind persons were significantly less satisfied than the other two groups. Thirty-six percent reported they were very dissatisfied with their levels of independence in travel; only 14 percent of persons in the other two groups gave a similar response.

The presence of sidewalks in front of or adjacent to one's residence was related to independence in travel among older persons ($\chi=5.06$,

$p=.02$). Duration of blindness was also related to frequency of independent travel in the past year among older individuals. Persons who had been blind for 10 or more years at the time of the interview reported greater frequency of independent travel than did those who had been blind for less than 10 years.

To determine whether limitations in independent travel related to limitations in travel performance, 14 young blind persons and 16 elderly blind persons who participated in the interview study were later videotaped as they walked an unfamiliar four-block route in a residential and small-business setting. Mobility performance was measured by reviewing the videotape and counting the frequency of the following behaviors (see Long, Rieser, & Hill [1990] for a description of this method): stopping, veering off the path, shorelining, contacting objects with a cane, intervention by the spotter, searching with the hand or foot, and contacting objects with the body.

Because these behaviors were not likely to have equal effects on safety in independent travel, different emphases were assigned to the seven behaviors by five mobility specialists. The specialists ranked the behaviors in the following order—from the most unsafe to the least unsafe—according to the potential threat of the behavior to safe and efficient travel:
1. intervention by the spotter
2. contacting objects with the body
3. veering off the path
4. searching with the hand or foot
5. contacting objects with a cane
6. stopping
7. shorelining.

The mean correlation of the specialists' ratings with each other was .522 ($SD=.49$).

Older and younger blind persons did not differ on total weighted mobility scores. The mean (SD) of the older group was 2.71 ($SD=2.50$); the mean of the younger group was 2.33 ($SD=1.99$). Older blind individuals had significantly more body contacts than younger blind persons; this behavior occurred approximately four times more often among older blind travelers. Younger blind people had significantly more cane contacts than older blind persons.

It appears that older people who are blind or visually impaired are at risk of being subject to significant limitations in independent mobility beyond their houses and yards. Brief periods of training for these older individuals in their home environments may result in significant increases in independent travel, with related increases in social stimulation and feelings of competence. Travel independence may be one factor allowing older blind persons to continue independent living arrangements, as the Senior Blind Program (1981) of the Michigan Commission for the Blind reported. Mobility specialists should consider giving older persons route training to destinations in the home community that are likely to be highly reinforcing or desirable. Although a program that serves older persons exclusively may concentrate on neighborhood instruction, practitioners should remember that some older blind individuals want and need the full range of O&M instruction.

Older persons may rely heavily on the assistance of individuals with whom they live to get around in the community. Thus, it is important to ensure that caregivers receive adequate training on the use of sighted guide techniques so they can guide the older person effectively and without risk of injury to themselves or the visually impaired person. Service delivery providers must be prepared to intervene at crisis points, such as the death of a spouse, so that older blind and visually impaired persons do not become isolated or institutionalized prematurely or unnecessarily. Mobility specialists need to develop modified instructional and travel techniques that accommodate the older person's physical condition and particular travel needs.

Range of Abilities

Several factors influence the newly blind or visually impaired person's potential for success in O&M. Newly visually impaired persons in the United States are most likely to be over age 75, have some remaining vision, and have concomitant physical or sensory impairments that may further complicate the performance of O&M tasks (Cruishank, 1978). Most complications result from reduction in the reception of information through sensory modalities, a decline in general health, and difficulties with memory and orientation.

SENSORY INFORMATION

Reduction in hearing or tactile sensitivity and deviations in balance, posture, and gait are common in older people (Welsh, 1980). Reduction in hearing, often the result of presbycusis, may be the most common secondary loss for older people (Welsh, 1980; Wiener, 1980). Reductions in tactile sensitivity accompanying diabetes and arthritis can minimize the amount of direct contact made between travelers and their environment. There has been limited research on the effects of the interaction among various limitations on independent mobility of elderly persons.

One concern for elderly people, in general, is fear of falling. Injuries from falls are a major health problem in the United States. Approximately one-third of all fatal falls are sustained by people over age 65 (Baker, O'Neil, & Karpf, 1984). Falls are a complex phenomenon, and a variety of environmentally and behaviorally based causes has been discussed (Connell, 1987). One contributing factor is the decrement in motor and physical ability that typically occurs with age. Maximum muscle strength declines 15 to 35 percent from age 20 to age 60, and maximum speed of movement declines by about 90 percent over the same period (Hadley, Radebaugh, & Suzeman, 1985).

Bone mass will also lessen, particularly among women. Although such changes can limit intense physical exertion, they normally do not affect everyday walking. However, these and other decreases in motor ability may combine with decrements in sensory and cognitive ability to create significant loss of functional capabilities, including mobility. The major importance of these facts involves the cyclical component of exercise, which stresses bone and muscle and builds strength. Lack of exercise allows physical loss to escalate and increases the probability of falling and hesitance to travel (Woollacott, Shumway-Cook, & Nashner, 1986).

A limited number of medical and epidemiological studies have focused on the environmental factors in falls by elderly persons. In a classic study of falls among elderly individuals living in a community, one-third of a large sample of falls were categorized as accidents resulting from missteps on stairs, trips and slips on level surfaces, and situations involving inadequate lighting (Sheldon, 1960). A recent case-controlled study of elderly fallers who lived in the community assessed the hazardousness of common residential design features and household objects, such as flooring, furniture, lighting, storage areas, stairways, and bathroom fixtures and furnishings (DeVito, 1987, 1988; Rodriguez, 1988). Another study found that falls occurred when there was a reduction in proprioception in conjunction with a dark environment, when an enduring or transient reduction in visual input occurred in conjunction with a trip hazard, or when both circumstances occurred (Tinetti, 1987). Collectively, these studies suggest that environmental factors may contribute to falls that occur in conjunction with seemingly safe as well as obviously hazardous conditions. Sometimes, difficulties obtaining adequate and accurate sensory input about physical surroundings play a role in falls; such difficulties may result from the situation-specific interaction between personal factors, such as sensory functioning, and environmental conditions, such as lighting (Owen, 1985; Tobias & Hoedler, 1981).

Concern about the possibility of a fall, particularly for the older person with a visual impairment, carries with it major implications for mobility specialists and training programs offered to elderly visually impaired persons. Deviations in balance, posture, and gait caused by inner ear problems, arthritis, general health problems, and a slow pace can affect an older person's ability to project straight lines, walk a straight line, and trust his or her estimate of distance traveled and the degree of turn (DiFrancesco-Aust, 1980; Fleharty, 1968; Kimbrough, 1966). Recognition of these problems is important because success in most mobility tasks is greatly dependent on walking a straight line and interpreting sensory clues (Shingledecker, 1983). Reduction in reception of information from any sense, especially hearing, can destroy the possibility of independent travel for a totally blind person. Fortunately, most older people have some degree of usable vision. Even the most limited vision, if used selectively, can compensate for other serious sensory losses (LaGrow, 1978). In general, use of vision is encouraged if vision is not relied on to the exclusion of the other senses.

Vision can also compensate for reductions in tactile sensitivity if it is sufficient for fine discrimination at moderate range (3 to 6 feet). Often other adaptations, including environmental interventions, are needed (Sicurella, 1977). If older people cannot safely identify stairways tactilely or visually in their own dwellings, the use of high-contrast materials in stairways or handrails that vary in height at obvious, abrupt increments may be useful. High-contrast materials aid visual reception, and abrupt increments in height signal the presence of steps.

HEALTH AND ENDURANCE

The older person's general health is important in mobility training. Chronic diseases from which many older persons suffer inhibit their ability to move. The Senior Blind Program (1981) reported that over 88 percent of its clients had undergone a stroke or had other health problems, mainly chronic diseases such as arthritis, diabetes, and cardiovascular disease.

Chronic health problems can reduce endurance and the ability to perform. Some problems dictate the time of day appropriate for O&M instruction. For example, diabetics often experience disorientation, difficulty in concentrating, susceptibility to diabetic reactions, and fluctuating visual ability in relation to the timing of meals and insulin intake. Other difficulties, such as those associated with cardiovascular disease, may dictate the length of lessons and the type of travel that is safe. Stroke patients or those with arthritis often need extensive adaptations to basic travel techniques. Instruction should follow consultation with the person's physician.

MEMORY AND ORIENTATION

Cognitive impairment has an effect on ability to travel in a complex environment. Research with blinded veterans has revealed no significant relationship between level of intellectual functioning as measured by the WAIS (Wechler Adult Intelligence Scale) IQ and mobility performance (De l'Aune & Needham, 1977). However, none of the subjects in this study exhibited significant cognitive dysfunction. A more sophisticated assessment of cognitive effort required by mobility tasks (sedentary tasks, sighted guide, and independent mobility) of differing degrees of difficulty through a secondary task methodology demonstrated a significant and reliable effect of cognitive impairment on ability to travel (Geruschat & De l'Aune, 1990).

Because the difficulty of mobility-related tasks increases with the presence of additional sensory and motor impairments, the cognitive capacity of multiply impaired clients can be expected to be taxed even more when presented with these tasks. These relationships are a matter of concern because of the increase of age-related cognitive dysfunctions and the corresponding aging of the visually impaired population.

Becoming lost or disoriented while attempting to move about in the familiar environments of everyday life is a major problem for many elderly persons. This possibility is also a constant source of anxiety for their spouses and caregivers (Martino-Saltzman, 1989). It is not unusual to hear about sighted elderly persons, longtime residents of a neighborhood, who suddenly find themselves unable to find their way home or who become afraid to leave their homes for fear of getting lost (Hiatt, 1985). A survey of 170 nursing homes revealed that such incidents characterized a significant proportion (approximately 25 to 50 percent) of the elderly population (not specifically visually impaired individuals) who were described as disoriented in their own buildings (Hiatt, 1985).

The term "wandering" has often been applied to such various behaviors as pacing, leaving a building or residence, and appearing confused (Martino-Saltzman, Blasch, Morris, & McNeal, 1991). Dementia with accompanying memory loss is probably the most frequently cited correlate of wandering. Being lost or disoriented—independent of a visual condition and of familiarity with a complex environment—may be interpreted as a sign of dementia in older people. Unfortunately, there has been little research or effort to differentiate between an elderly person's disoriented state or difficulty with orientation or way finding and dementia-related wandering behavior. At this point it may be difficult to determine if the elderly person with a visual impairment has difficulty with way finding or spatial orientation or has an age-related problem, such as dementia-related wandering.

A breakdown in the way-finding process may be the result of one or more factors. One may not acquire the necessary environmental information for the task because of failure to attend to appropriate visual cues or to store the appropriate data. One may have difficulty making the inferences necessary to extract the spatial layout of an area—knowledge essential for the efficient solution of some way-finding problems. One may learn the spatial layout but be unable to retrieve the information. Also, the knowledge of a route or layout may be adequate, but for some reason, orientation in the environment is impossible.

Maintaining orientation requires organization, memory, and the recall of numerous environmental clues received sequentially from different sensory systems (Hill & Ponder, 1976). Many memory problems are related to the information given. Sometimes, people provide more information than can be easily assimilated, deliver it in an unstructured manner, and fail to specify directions and exact location.

Older blind and visually impaired persons need an organizational and recall system to handle information received and need time for assimilation. Complex information should be broken into numerous chains of discrete information and stored mentally, in braille, or on an audiotape for review and recall. Complex environments must be broken down into logically contained sections that are taught successively. Therefore, after being exposed to the same route several times, one might learn to recognize a landmark at each decision point and associate the appropriate step in the way-finding process with that landmark (e.g., "I'm at the elevators, so I turn left"). Some individuals might commit the entire sequence of turns to memory (e.g., "At the next intersection I make a left, then a right at the cafeteria"). Or they might infer the location of each landmark in relation to every other landmark, mentally laying out the route.

Although sufficient for many way-finding situations, such strategies do not provide the flexibility to plan shortcuts or devise detours when obstacles force the person to deviate from a known path. There is also the question of whether persons who have not been able to develop an abstract level of environmental problem-solving and way-finding ability over several decades will be able to accomplish it in their sixth, seventh, or eighth decade.

A study of elderly persons who relocated to unfamiliar nursing homes produced important data (Pastalan & Bourestom, 1975). The mortality rate significantly increased in the month before and the three months following relocation. In addition, a reduced range of travel following relocation was one of the strongest predictors of mortality. Although several factors may account for the increased mortality rate, it is important to note that individuals who made three site visits to the new home as part of an orientation program before the move were at less risk for morbidity and mortality following the move. This finding seems to implicate disorientation in the new setting as a major contributor to decline in physical status. Weisman (1982) has suggested that elderly individuals may experience a sense of loss of perceived control when they are unable to find their way in an environment. In turn, this feeling can affect the disoriented person's sense of well-being. However, no research has examined the possible relationship between way-finding competence and sense of well-being.

Mobility instruction for the elderly person with a visual impairment must not only take into account the multitude of personal and environmental factors relating to mobility but must also encompass a number of options available to individuals who lack sufficient sensory, motor, or cognitive abilities, or a combination of these, when they undertake specific mobility tasks. These options include choosing simpler routes, asking for selective assistance, and traveling with a companion. Other options are training in O&M and in low vision, motor, or cognitive skills. Orthopedic canes, orthotics, and wheelchairs are options for individuals with motor impairments. Another option is to use sensory devices—the long cane, dog guide, or ETAs (i.e., the laser cane, Mowat Sensor, Sonicguide™, Russell Pathsounder, and POLARON)—and hearing devices. Each option attempts to alleviate a functional loss caused by the individual's impairment.

Orientation and Mobility Procedures

O&M training is sequential, individualized, success-based instruction. The skills taught usually include sighted guide, self-protective, trailing, and cane techniques. The skills are often presented in this order, although the sequence can vary, depending on individual needs or the demands of the environment. The environments of instruction are similarly sequenced, from controlled indoor environments to familiar outdoor environments to unfamiliar environments.

O&M instruction is deliberately sequenced to ensure success in each lesson. Each lesson has a definite starting and ending point (objective) and should be planned so the student will find the objective. Each route should be analyzed in advance to ensure that the skills to meet the objective are introduced and mastered before they are applied on the actual route. Given that many elderly persons may be affected by the sensory impairments and other factors discussed earlier, standard O&M techniques may have to be modified to take concomitant limitations into account. The following sections present the standard techniques and suggest modifications. The modifications are not intended to be all-inclusive or appropriate for every possible situation.

SIGHTED GUIDE TECHNIQUES

Sighted guides are probably the most common form of travel assistance used by elderly visually impaired persons. Some blind persons rely on them exclusively, but it is more common for a sighted guide to be used selectively to supplement the individual's primary travel device—a cane or a dog guide.

Sighted guide techniques allow two individuals to walk together in a safe, energy-efficient, and socially acceptable manner while enabling the blind person to participate actively in travel decisions. Established positions allow the blind traveler to interpret environmental information transmitted through the movements of the guide's body. Sighted guide techniques include the following procedures: (1) basic sighted guide, (2) reversing directions, (3) negotiating narrow passageways, (4) transferring sides, (5) negotiating doorways, (6) negotiating stairways, and (7) seating. (See appendix at the end of this chapter for step-by-step descriptions.)

These procedures and adaptations are not the only acceptable sighted guide techniques. Variations and adaptations can meet a person's special needs. The common denominator in all sighted guide techniques is that the traveler remains to the side and behind the guide so the traveler can interpret the guide's movements and anticipate the various demands of the environment. Typically, the guide pauses or stops before the negotiation of each new environmental event to indicate that a new demand is imminent.

Basic Sighted Guide

In the basic sighted guide technique, the visually impaired traveler may be positioned on either side of the guide. Preference for position may accommodate hearing loss in one ear or the need to carry an orthopedic cane in a particular hand. The guide always goes first; the traveler is never pushed or manipulated from behind. The blind person grasps the guide's arm just above or near the elbow with the thumb on the outside of the guide's arm and the fingers on the inside (see Figure 1). The traveler's arm is bent at about 90 degrees at the elbow, a position that helps maintain a constant distance between the traveler and the guide. The contact between the traveler and the guide provides the traveler with direct information from the guide, and the position of the hand on the back of the guide's arm prevents the traveler's hand from sliding forward and narrowing the distance between the traveler and the guide.

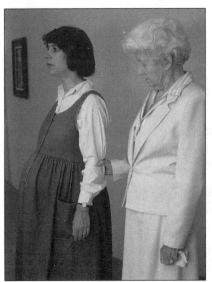

One extremely important factor for the guide to remember is that a curb, stairs, or any change of elevation should always be approached at a perpendicular angle. If the guide approaches at another angle, the traveler may reach the elevation change before the guide or after the anticipated time.

Figure 1: Basic sighted guide technique.

Rounded curbs and circular stairs present particular problems and should be approached and negotiated with care.

The basic sighted guide technique may be adapted in a number of ways to compensate for someone's reduced stability, speed, or range of movement or for the preference of guide or traveler (see Figure 2). These adaptations can be extremely useful to the older person but provide less forward protection and reduce possible reaction time.

Speed of travel should be adjusted to ensure a comfortable pace for the traveler. However, the guide should be aware that the person's ability to recognize

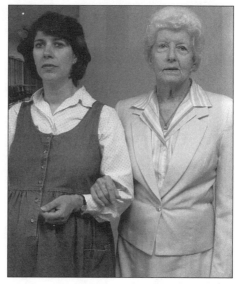

Figure 2: Adaptation of the basic sighted guide technique.

turns accurately is often dependent on the speed of travel and the sharpness of turn. The blind traveler may be unaware of changes in direction if the change is gradual (a sweeping turn) or broken into short segments or if the traveler has an inner-ear problem. Accuracy of recognition can be facilitated by adding a short pause before each turn and following the pause with a definite and pronounced change of direction.

Reversing Directions

In reversing directions, the guide and the traveler may make 180-degree turns with a simple pivot (see Figure 3 a-c). When this is done, the guide pivots around the traveler to avoid swinging him or her in space. However, a pivot of two bodies requires three full body widths. A reversing-directions procedure can be used to accomplish a 180-degree turn within the space presently occupied.

One way to accomplish a 180-degree turn, delineated in the appendix, allows the guide and the traveler to maintain contact and reverse

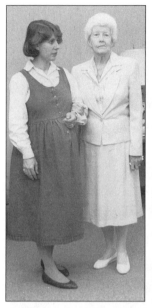 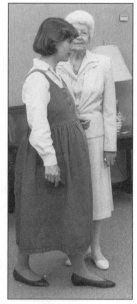 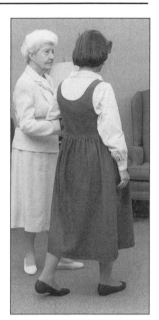

Figure 3 a, b, and c: Standard procedure for reversing directions.

directions in a minimum of space. This basic technique can be adapted to provide the traveler continuous physical support and additional stabilization while turning and can be completed within the space originally occupied by the two.

Negotiating Narrow Passageways

The technique for negotiating narrow passageways allows the guide and the traveler to move through an area, such as a doorway or an aisle, that could not be negotiated comfortably if they occupied their usual 1½ body-width space. This technique can be initiated and terminated solely through the movement of the guide's arm (see Figure 4). Therefore, conversation need not be interrupted. An adaptation of this technique may include providing a verbal clue for changing positions to allow the traveler to use both hands for stabilization against the guide's back or for gaining stability and contact.

Transferring Sides

The technique in which the traveler and the guide transfer sides allows the traveler to move behind the guide to establish the sighted guide position on the opposite side while maintaining continuous contact with the guide (see Figure 5). Either member of the tandem may enlist this technique with a verbal statement. The technique can be modified to allow traveler and guide to transfer sides without utilizing additional space or to allow the traveler to remain stationary while the guide sidesteps across or behind the traveler to the opposite side.

Negotiating Doorways

The techniques for negotiating doorways described in the appendix allow the traveler to be an active participant in traversing doorways. These techniques are initiated through nonverbal cues transmitted to the traveler through the movement of the guide's body. Techniques for handling doorways can easily be adapted for persons with reduced stability, speed of reaction, or strength (see Figure 6).

Handling the door provides additional participation for the traveler. However, doors can be negotiated without the traveler's active participation. If necessary, the traveler can simply follow the guide through the doorway. The guide, however, should always deal with the door's leading edge and release it cleanly to avoid turning his or her body and to prevent the door from closing on the traveler.

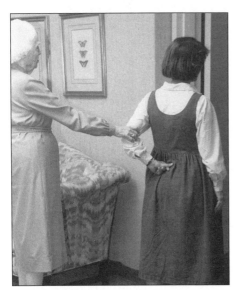 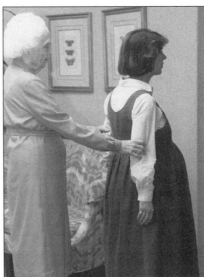

Figure 4: Negotiating a narrow passageway.   Figure 5: Transferring sides.

Negotiating Stairways

Ascending and descending stairways are often stressful for older blind persons. The techniques for negotiating stairways in the appendix follow the same principle used by sighted persons who rely on vision to identify only the first and last steps of a given stairwell and any changes in the pattern of steps within the stairwell. The traveler should be encouraged simply to follow the guide's lead. Those with low vision should not attempt to see each step as they ascend or descend (see Figure 7). Techniques for negotiating stairways can be adapted by adding verbal clues, allowing the traveler to use handrails, having the guide provide extra support, and having the guide carry the traveler's orthopedic cane, if one is used and the traveler prefers the handrail.

Seating

The technique for seating described in this chapter's appendix is a method for locating seats with a minimum of awkwardness. The primary emphasis is to facilitate ease in various seating situations while minimizing the guide's need for physical maneuvering of the traveler.

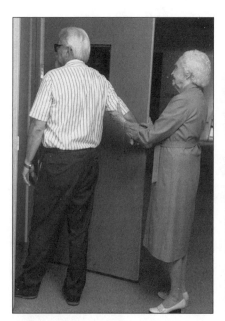

Figure 6: Negotiating a doorway.

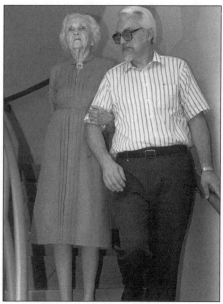

Figure 7: Descending a stairway.

Circumstances that arise from seating are potentially unsafe and are also highly awkward for blind and visually impaired persons.

SELF-PROTECTIVE TECHNIQUES

Self-protective techniques provide the traveler protection when traversing short distances in familiar, controlled environments (see appendix). The upper-hand and forearm and the lower-hand and forearm techniques are specifically tailored to meet the demands of this situation. The upper-hand and forearm technique should also be used any time the traveler extends his or her head beyond the body space presently occupied, such as when leaning forward to retrieve a dropped object, to protect the head or face from hitting obstacles in the environment.

Although self-protective techniques can be adapted for individuals, such as those with arthritis, who have difficulty maintaining the positions described, marked deviations typically result in a loss of protection and decreased reaction time. Those persons who use walkers or wheelchairs have little forward protection because both hands are usually occupied. Even for users of electric wheelchairs, which do not require both hands for control, forward protection from the hand or arm is negligible because of the person's seating arrangement. Three ETAs—the Russell Pathsounder, Mowat Sensor, and POLARON (see Figure 8 for the POLARON and Mowat Sensor)—provide adequate prewarning of objects ahead and can be used selectively with supportive devices and wheelchairs. These devices do not provide adequate information concerning the presence of downward steps or stairways and should be used only in controlled indoor environments or with other primary mobility devices, such as canes and dog guides.

The Russell Pathsounder, a battery-operated device that emits and receives ultrasonic signals, is worn around the neck or is mounted on a wheelchair or walker. It may be used with walkers, wheelchairs, and orthopedic canes to provide information about objects in the traveler's path, particularly when those objects extend above the level of the waist (Farmer, 1980). This device sends out ultrasonic sound over a cone-shaped area that roughly covers a person's projected line of travel from

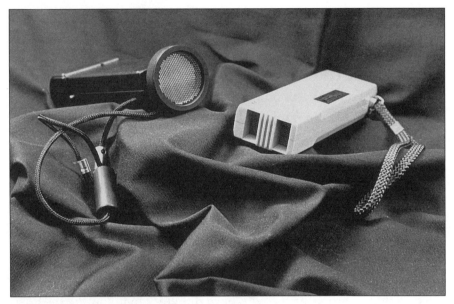

Figure 8: The POLARON and Mowat Sensor.

shoulder to shoulder. When an object is encountered, it reflects the emitted sound back to the receiver through a vibrator in the neck strap.

The Mowat Sensor, also a battery-operated device that emits ultrasonic sound (Mellor, 1981), is hand held and can be used to detect objects in the path of wheelchair users. This device is not recommended for use with walkers. The Mowat Sensor also provides information through vibration, and vibration speed can be used, for example, to estimate distance.

The POLARON may be either hand held or mounted on the neck and is battery operated. The POLARON's ultrasonic sonar system detects objects within selectable maximum ranges of 4, 8, or 16 feet. The user can also select a vibrotactile or audible warning signal at one of two volume levels.

TRAILING

Trailing techniques are used to find specific objectives along a wall, maintain a straight line of travel, and maintain contact with the environment while moving through space (see appendix). Trailing is often used in conjunction with the upper-hand and forearm or lower-hand

and forearm technique described in the appendix, depending on the location of objects from which protection is required. (During trailing, rings should be rotated and clasped in the palm of the hand to prevent damage.)

Trailing is highly efficient but slow. The traveler can locate doorways, intersecting hallways, and numerous landmarks while moving or can use the wall for support and as a place to rest while easily maintaining orientation. Trailing can be accomplished by hand, with the Mowat Sensor, POLARON, or Russell Pathsounder, or when using a long cane (see Figure 9). The cane expands the usefulness of the trailing technique into more complex, less controlled, or unfamiliar environments.

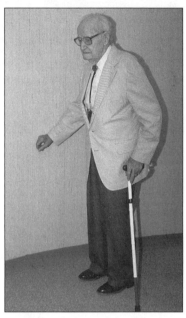

Figure 9: Trailing technique done with the hand, using a support cane.

CANE TECHNIQUES

The cane extends one's reach to explore the environment. The two basic canes are the long cane and the folding cane (see Figure 10). The long cane protects the individual from collision with objects in the path of travel and identifies significant changes in elevation and texture of the surface. The length of the cane is prescribed according to an individual's height, length of stride, and speed of travel. The cane is usually a long, hollow aluminum tube with a rubber grip and a nylon tip that conducts tactile information from the tip to the hand of the user.

The long cane is probably the most efficient mobility device yet devised (Farmer, 1980). Its length, when made use of in conjunction with systematic techniques for handling the cane, allows approximately 3 feet of warning for objects or drop-offs in a traveler's path and extends an individual's reach for exploration from 4 to 5 feet. The cane pro-

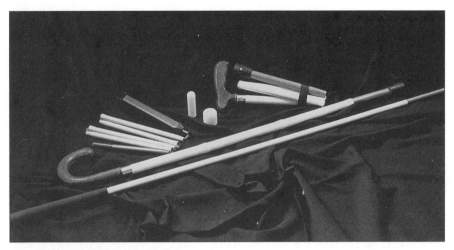

Figure 10: Different types of canes.

vides adequate protection for the lower body and provides information about the integrity of the surface to be stepped on. It does not,
however, protect the upper body.

Folding or collapsible canes are variations of the basic long cane. They
telescope or fold in on themselves for storage (Farmer, 1980). Although
they are used in the same manner as the long cane, they tend to be
less durable and often do not conduct tactile information from the tip
to the grip as effectively as does the long cane. Many travelers prefer
a long cane for extensive travel and a folding cane for social events
because it is easy to store.

The cane is usually modified only to adjust for a person's length of
stride or speed of travel. However, its length may also be extended if
it is to be used in conjunction with an orthopedic cane (see Figure 11)
or if the individual cannot keep his or her hand centered. Canes can
be adapted or redesigned for amputees and for persons with arthritis
in their hands or fingers who require bulkier grips (Farmer, 1980).

Diagonal Technique

The diagonal cane technique provides an independent means of travel
only within a familiar, controlled environment. It does not protect the
traveler's body from low objects on the grip side of the body, that is,

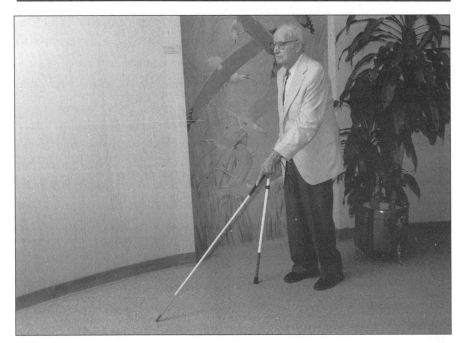

Figure 11: The long cane used in conjunction with an orthopedic cane.

the side of the body on which the cane is held. The cane can be held in either hand in front of and across the body for protection from objects in the direct line of travel. The traveler can "choke up" on the grip by sliding the grip hand down toward the cane's shaft to provide additional protection on the grip side. If the traveler has a hearing impairment, a Mowat Sensor can also be used for initial alignment, which involves positioning the side of the body against a flat surface, and to identify openings and intersecting hallways when the individual is not trailing.

Visually impaired persons with sufficient sight for safe travel who want to be recognized as having a severe visual impairment often prefer the diagonal technique. These persons may also require the cane for selective environmental exploration.

Touch Technique

The touch technique provides maximum protection and information from the cane and can be used in all environments. In this technique, the cane is used to check the environment in front of each foot before the person brings the foot forward. The cane is moved from side to side to describe a path through which the individual travels; it protects each side of the traveler equally while detecting low objects and drop-offs.

Instruction in the touch technique begins in a controlled indoor environment, where self-protection and diagonal techniques are used, and then proceeds into residential, semibusiness, and business environments. Visually impaired persons learn to cross quiet residential streets and traffic-light intersections in the busiest areas of town and to negotiate elevators, escalators, buses, subways, and trains.

Referrals

Independent travel techniques, including cane techniques, should be taught by certified university-trained O&M specialists. Others may provide instruction in the use of sighted guide and self-protective techniques in controlled indoor environments.

Referrals to specialists can be made by contacting state and private agencies that serve blind and visually impaired persons in the United States or Canada. The American Foundation for the Blind's *Directory of Services for Blind and Visually Impaired Persons in the United States* (1988) lists agencies that provide direct or consultative services for blind and visually impaired individuals. Dog guides are also highly efficient mobility tools. Referrals for dog guides can be made through mobility specialists or by contacting any of the dog guide schools listed in the *Directory of Services.*

Conclusion

Many older blind and visually impaired persons have health, physical, or sensory impairments requiring adaptations of standard orientation and mobility procedures. Appropriate mobility instruction should be tailored to meet the specific needs of the individual under instruction. No single adaptation is required by all older persons in order for them to become independent travelers, nor are all adaptations in this chapter relevant to older persons. Indeed, there are numerous research efforts under way to determine the most appropriate modifications to mobility training and the techniques necessary for the older person who is visually impaired. The needs of older travelers should not be over-simplified, although the needs of some older persons may be limited by the scope and complexity of the environment. Even limited travel may occur in extremely complex environments, and limitations accompanying the normal aging process can make negotiation of even the simplest of environments difficult for the visually impaired older person.

Mobility instruction should begin with a thorough examination of the older person's travel requirements. The assessment addresses stated travel needs, the environments of travel, and the relationship of the individual's physical and sensory abilities to these travel goals.

Travel goals should be enumerated and sequenced so that instruction is initially presented in a simple, nonthreatening environment and then in more complex areas. This sequencing is particularly important for many older persons who are hesitant to learn cane travel. Preferably, instruction should be conducted in the actual environment of need. The sequence of instruction should also be adjusted to ensure that prerequisite skills are introduced and mastered before they are needed for multipart tasks. The sequence of instruction should ensure a measure of success during each lesson and introduce orientation and mobility skills in a logical order.

Successful, safe, independent travel is a necessary part of each individual's life experience. The acquisition of travel skills contributes to the quality of a person's life. Therefore, the desire for independent travel, no matter how old the person, should not be dismissed as unworthy of professional attention. Total independence is as realistic for visually impaired older persons as it is for visually impaired travelers who are younger.

References

American Foundation for the Blind. (1988). *Directory of services for blind and visually impaired persons in the United States* (23rd ed.). New York: Author.

Baker, S. P., O'Neil, B., & Karpf, R. (1984). *The injury fact book*. Lexington, MA: Lexington Books.

Connell, B. R. (1987). Environmental and behavioral contributions to falls in the elderly. In D. Lawrence, R. Habe, A. Hacker, & D. Sherrod (Eds.), *People's Needs/Planet Management, Paths to Co-Existence* (Proceedings of the 18th Annual Environmental and Design Research Association Conference). Washington, DC: Environmental Design Research Association.

Cruishank, N. (1978). *The older blind person.* Paper presented at the Second National Conference on Aging and Blindness, Atlanta, GA.

De l'Aune, W., & Needham, W. (1977). Personality determiners of successful prosthetic and sensory aid use. In M. Cannon (Ed.), *Proceedings: The Fifth New England Bioengineering Conference* (pp. 111-115). New York: Pergamon.

DeVito, C. A. (1987). The Dade County study to assess falls among the elderly. In *Environmental risk factors for falls among the elderly.* 1987 Injury in America Conference, Atlanta, GA.

DeVito, C. A. (1988, September). *Falls and injuries.* Paper presented at the Frailty and Falls Injuries Conference, Bethesda, MD.

DiFrancesco-Aust, A. (1980). Kinesiology. In R. Welsh & B. Blasch (Eds.), *Foundations of orientation and mobility* (pp. 37-71). New York: American Foundation for the Blind.

Farmer, L. (1980). Mobility devices. In R. Welsh & B. Blasch (Eds.), *Foundations of orientation and mobility* (pp. 357-402). New York: American Foundation for the Blind.

Fleharty, D. (1968). *An analysis of relationship between walking speed and veering.* Unpublished manuscript, Western Michigan University, Department of Blind Rehabilitation, Kalamazoo.

Foulke, E. (1971). The perceptual basis for mobility. *American Foundation for the Blind Research Bulletin, 23:* 1-8.

Geruschat, D., & De l'Aune, W. (1990). Reliability and validity of O&M instructor observations. *Journal of Visual Impairment & Blindness, 83*(9): 457-460.

Hadley, E., Radebaugh, T. S., & Suzeman, R. (1985). Falls and gait disorders among the elderly. *Clinics in Geriatric Medicine, 1*(3): 497-500.

Hiatt, L. G. (1985). Wandering behavior of older people in nursing homes: A study of hyperactivity, disorientation, and the spatial environment. *Dissertation Abstracts International, 45,* (University Microfilms No. 86-01, 653).

Hill, E., & Ponder, P. (1976). *Orientation and mobility techniques: A guide for the practitioner.* New York: American Foundation for the Blind.

Ingalls, J. (1973). *A trainer's guide to andragogy.* Waltham, MA: Data Educational.

Kimbrough, J. (1966). *The effects of prescribed changes in individual characteristics of walking and standing on the veering tendency in blind persons.* Unpublished manuscript, Western Michigan University, Department of Blind Rehabilitation, Kalamazoo.

LaGrow, S. (1978). Preferred corner technique in low vision. *Long Cane News, 10:* 5-11.

Long, R. G., Rieser, J. J., & Hill, E. W. (1990). Mobility in individuals with moderate visual impairments. *Journal of Visual Impairment & Blindness, 84*(3): 111-118.

Long, R. G., McNeal, L. W., & Griffin-Shirley, N. (1990). *The effect of visual loss on mobility of elderly persons.* Final Report, National Institute on Disability and Rehabilitation Research Grant No. 133GH70038.

Martino-Saltzman, D. (1989). *Wandering behavior in nursing home residents and psychological correlates.* Unpublished doctoral dissertation, Georgia State University College of Arts and Sciences, Atlanta.

Martino-Saltzman, D., Blasch, B., Morris, R., & McNeal, L. (1991). Travel behavior of nursing home residents perceived as wanderers and non-wanderers. *The Gerontologist, 31*(5): 666-672.

Mellor, M. (1981). *Aids for the 80s: What they are and what they do.* New York: American Foundation for the Blind.

Owen, D. H. (1985). Maintaining posture and avoiding tripping: Optical information for detecting and controlling orientation and locomotion. *Clinics in Geriatric Medicine, 1:* 581-600.

Pastalan, L., & Bourestom, N. (1975). *Forced relocation: Setting, staff, and patient effects.* Final report to the Mental Health Services Development Branch, National Institute of Mental Health. Ann Arbor: The University of Michigan, Institute of Gerontology.

Ponchilla, P., & Kaarlela, R. (1982). *Factors influencing skill performance of blind adults.* Unpublished manuscript.

Rodriguez, J. (1988). *Assessment of environmental hazards.* Paper presented at the Frailty and Falls Injuries Conference, Bethesda, MD.

Senior Blind Program. (1981). *The first year, 1980-81.* Lansing: Michigan Commission for the Blind.

Sheldon, J. H. (1960). On the natural history of falls in old age. *British Medical Journal, 2:* 1685-1690.

Shingledecker, C. (1983). Measuring the mental effort of blind mobility. *Journal of Visual Impairment & Blindness, 77*(7): 334-339.

Sicurella, V. J. (1977). Color contrast as an aid for visually impaired persons. *Journal of Visual Impairment & Blindness, 71*(6): 252-257.

Tinetti, M. (1987, February). Chronic, acute and environmental risk factors for falls among community-living elderly. Paper presented at the 1987 Injury in America Conference, Atlanta, GA.

Tobias, J. S., & Hoedler, F. (1981). Visual perception of verticality and horizontality among elderly fallers. *Archives of Physical Medicine and Rehabilitation, 62:* 619-622.

Weisman, G. D. (1982). Wayfinding and architectural legibility: Design considerations in housing environments for the elderly. In L. S. Liben, A. N. Patterson, & N. Newcombe (Eds.), *Spatial representation across the life-span: Theory and application.* New York: Academic Press.

Welsh, R. (1980). Visually impaired older persons. In R. Welsh & B. Blasch (Eds.), *Foundations of orientation and mobility* (pp. 420-428). New York: American Foundation for the Blind.

Welsh, R., & Blasch, B. (1980). Introduction. In R. Welsh & B. Blasch (Eds.), *Foundations of orientation and mobility* (pp. 1-7). New York: American Foundation for the Blind.

Wiener, W. (1980). Audition. In R. Welsh & B. Blasch (Eds.), *Foundations of orientation and mobility* (pp. 115-185). New York: American Foundation for the Blind.

Woollacott, M. H., Shumway-Cook, A., & Nashner, L. (1986). Aging and postural control: Changes in sensory organization and muscular coordination. *International Journal of Aging and Human Development, 23*(2): 97-115.

APPENDIX: ORIENTATION AND MOBILITY (O&M) PROCEDURES

This section presents basic O&M procedures adapted from E. Hill and P. Ponder, *Orientation and mobility techniques: A guide for the practitioner* (New York: American Foundation for the Blind, 1976).

Sighted Guide Procedures

BASIC TECHNIQUES

The guide and the traveler face the same direction. The guide may establish contact with the traveler by placing the back of his or her hand against the traveler's arm. Physical contact between the guide and the traveler eliminates awkwardness. The guide should also verbally announce his or her intention to act as a guide. Once contact has been established, the traveler does the following:

1. Slides a hand up the guide's arm to just above the elbow.
2. Grasps the guide's arm with the thumb on the outside and fingers on the inside of the guide's arm.
3. Positions the upper arm close to the side and at vertical alignment with the upper body.
4. Flexes the lower arm to form a 90-degree angle at the elbow with the upper arm so that the lower arm is parallel with the floor.

REVERSING DIRECTIONS

To reverse directions, the following steps are used:

1. The guide and the traveler turn to face one another.
2. The guide may step back while turning to ensure that guide and traveler are in direct alignment.
3. The traveler turns to face the guide while maintaining contact with him or her.
4. The traveler reaches out with his or her free hand to grasp the guide's free arm.
5. The traveler releases the original grip when contact is established with the new guiding arm.
6. When the traveler establishes contact with the opposite arm of the guide, the traveler and the guide complete the 180-degree turn.
7. The guide may step forward while completing the last half of the turn to reestablish his or her position in front of the traveler.

NEGOTIATING NARROW PASSAGEWAYS

This technique can be initiated and terminated with the following nonverbal clues:

1. The guide signals that the narrow passageway technique is required by moving his or her arm back.
2. The guide's arm is hyperextended behind his or her body with the elbow aligned at the middle of the back.
3. The traveler responds by extending his or her arm and moving behind the guide.
4. The two travel in this manner, occupying only one body width, until the narrow passageway is traversed.
5. To resume the basic sighted guide position, the guide moves his or her arm forward to its normal position.

TRANSFERRING SIDES

When there is a need to transfer sides, the following nonverbal procedure is used:

1. The guide comes to a complete stop.
2. The traveler places the back of his or her free hand against the back of the guide's arm above the original grip.

3. The traveler's fingers are pointed toward the guide's opposite arm.

4. The traveler then releases the original grip and turns 90 degrees to face the opposite side of the guide.

5. The traveler trails across the guide's back until the guide's free arm is contacted.

6. Upon contacting the opposite arm, the traveler reestablishes his or her grip and turns to face forward, completing the transfer of sides.

NEGOTIATING DOORWAYS

When approaching doors that open on the side of the traveler, the following techniques can be initiated with nonverbal clues:

1. As the door is manipulated, the traveler moves behind the guide.

2. The traveler protects his or her body with the free hand by holding the arm out and forward at about rib height.

3. The elbow is crooked, bringing the upper arm across the body and out in front of it for protection.

4. The palm is rotated toward the door.

5. The hand is moved laterally toward the door until contact is made.

6. The traveler holds the door until he or she goes through the doorway.

7. The door is then released, and the traveler reassumes the basic sighted guide position.

When approaching doors that open on the opposite side of the traveler, the following techniques can be used:

1. When the traveler realizes the door is open but that the guide's arm is not being used, he or she moves laterally behind the guide.

2. Placing a free hand on the guide's arm, the traveler establishes a grip on the arm above the original grip.

3. The original grip is then released.

4. That hand is then used to reach across the guide's back while protecting the body as before.

5. When the door is contacted, it is held until both the traveler and the guide have gone through the doorway.

6. The traveler moves back behind the guide to reestablish his or her original grip and position.

These techniques can be used to negotiate doors that are closed as well. In this case, the traveler contacts the door, grasps the doorknob, and closes the door after going through the doorway.

NEGOTIATING STAIRWAYS

The techniques for descending and ascending stairs are similar. The traveler becomes aware that steps are to be negotiated through the upward or downward action of the guide's arm. For descending stairs, the following techniques are used:

1. The guide approaches the stairs directly, pausing at the top of the first step, with the toes aligned with the edge of the step.

2. As the guide begins to descend the stairs, his or her arm moves forward and then down.

3. The traveler shifts his or her weight back, slides a foot forward to the edge of the first step, and then follows the guide down.

4. The traveler remains one step above the guide as they descend, using a consistent and contralateral pace.

5. When the guide reaches the last step, he or she pauses, steps down, and then steps out.

6. The combined clues of the pause in the guide's pace and the forward movement of the guide's arm indicate to the traveler that there is one last step to be negotiated.

The techniques for ascending stairs is similar, except that the guide places his or her toes at the first riser and steps up. The traveler shifts his or her weight forward and follows.

SEATING

Seating is initiated as the guide approaches the desired chair, using the following techniques:

1. The guide stops approximately one-half step from the chair.

2. The guide informs the traveler of the chair's position and proximity.

3. The guide may reach out and contact the chair with his or her arm.
4. The traveler trails the guide's arm to the chair, examines the chair, and then turns and places the back of his or her legs next to the chair.
5. The traveler sits on the chair.

Self-Protective and Trailing Techniques

UPPER-HAND AND FOREARM TECHNIQUE

The upper-hand and forearm technique protects the upper body from overhangs and objects that extend vertically to the floor. This technique consists of the following steps:

1. The arm is flexed to shoulder height.
2. The forearm is flexed at the elbow to form an angle of approximately 130 degrees, providing forward protection and adequate reaction time.
3. The forearm is inwardly rotated so that the palm faces forward.
4. The fingers are extended.
5. The tips of the fingers are extended just beyond the opposite shoulder.

LOWER-HAND AND FOREARM TECHNIQUE

The lower-hand and forearm technique protects the pelvic area and helps the traveler locate low objects, such as desks, counters, and chairs. The following steps are used:

1. The arm is slightly flexed at the shoulder until the hand is 6 to 8 inches forward of the body.
2. The arm is positioned so that the hand is at the midline of the body.
3. The fingers are extended down and relaxed.

TRAILING

The trailing technique helps the traveler maintain a parallel line of travel and locate specific objectives. The following steps are used for trailing:

1. The traveler positions his or her body parallel to the trailing surface without exceeding a distance of 10 inches and faces the intended line of travel.
2. The trailing arm is extended at the shoulder until the hand is waist high on the trailing surface.
3. The hand is turned so that the side of the hand is in contact with the surface.
4. The fingers are curled to avoid jamming and to absorb contact.
5. The trailing hand is kept forward of the body to allow the traveler adequate reaction time.

CHAPTER 13

Issues in the Continuum of Long-Term Care

Alberta L. Orr

Only within the last three decades has the term "long-term care" come into being and been widely recognized. Even today the meaning of long-term care is commonly misunderstood and misinterpreted. The most frequent misinterpretation is that long-term care is synonymous with institutional care, primarily that given in a nursing home. But long-term care is more. As recently as the 1960s, those who were frail, disabled, or chronically ill were cared for at home, either by family members, friends, or neighbors. Only when care of a level caregivers could not provide was required was institutional care utilized, usually as a last resort.

Policymakers, health care and social service planners, and practitioners in the field of aging have defined and redefined long-term care. Long-term care is the range of health and social services provided over a sustained period of time, along a continuum, from community-based to residential care, that maximizes the older person's ability to live and function as independently as possible, while compensating for functional impairments and preventing further disability and dysfunction. The continuum of long-term care services ranges from a combination of community-based services to a variety of residential living and care options. Community-based services include those described in Chapter 9—door-to-door transportation, senior citizens centers, nutrition services, housekeeping, chore services, escort services, friendly visiting, telephone reassurance, home health care, and emergency response systems. These services, designed to help the older person remain at home, are frequently provided in conjunction with help from family caregivers. Adult day care, respite care services, and hospice care provide essential support to the family caregiver as well as additional care to the older person still able and choosing to remain at home.

When living independently is no longer an option for the older person, a range of living arrangements is still possible before care in a nursing home is needed. These living arrangements include shared housing, board and care, congregate housing, enriched housing, life care at home (LCAH), and continuing-care retirement communities (CCRCs). Nursing home care itself consists of three levels that reflect the extent of need for nursing care: custodial care, intermediate care, and skilled nursing care.

These options are available to the older blind or visually impaired person. However, for many older persons who lose their vision, and particularly for those who are newly visually impaired, rehabilitation services from an agency for blind persons are an essential part of an array of needed services. These rehabilitation services are part of the community-based long-term care continuum. Nevertheless, neither the blindness field nor the aging field has yet perceived or defined rehabilitation services as such. Considerable effort must take place at the federal, state, and local levels to change the perception and coordination of service delivery.

Long-term care issues have been paramount in the field of aging and among legislators and the older consumers of these services since the beginning of the 1980s. The issues are critical, complex, and even catastrophic. This chapter presents the current state of the continuum of long-term services and the importance of environmental and technological advances for maximum independence of consumers. Critical issues of caregiving—elder abuse, the cost and quality of services, and plans and methods of financing long-term care through public and private insurance—are described. Innovative long-term care options and future directions in meeting needs of older persons requiring long-term care are also discussed.

Community-Based Services

A variety of community-based services available to all persons 60 years of age and over and funded through the Older Americans Act (OAA) constitutes the beginning of the continuum of long-term care. These services technically are available to all elderly persons but are less accessible to many older persons with special needs. For example, service providers are frequently unfamiliar with older persons who are blind or visually impaired and how to serve them. They may be uncertain about how to meet the needs of these clients or may not know what those needs are. They may also be intimidated by the older person who is visually impaired and may think that the person can best be helped by service providers in the blindness system. Therefore, obtaining access to the community-based service delivery system may be a challenge to the older person who is visually impaired and to family members. (These services have been outlined by Dolsen in Chapter 9.) For these reasons and because of the steady growth in the older visually impaired population, service providers in the field of aging need to receive training about aging and vision loss.

The impact of vision loss may lead older persons to feel unable to do anything independently, especially to go outside their homes. They may begin to think of and describe themselves to others as "homebound." Fear of being unable to manage alone or to perform daily tasks independently leads older visually impaired persons, and often family members, to think a nursing home is the only answer. This thought occurs even if vision loss is the only presenting problem, because older visually impaired persons are frequently unfamiliar with the range of community-based services available or believe they are ineligible for these services.

Older visually impaired persons may need some assistance with activities of daily living in their homes and with getting outside their homes. This kind of assistance can prevent unnecessary, premature, and costly institutionalization. Rehabilitation services from an agency for blind persons can also enable older visually impaired individuals to regain the skills necessary to function as independently as possible, to continue to live alone in their homes, and to remain part of their communities. In 1988, the cost was over $6.9 billion to institutionalize the nation's elderly blind and severely visually impaired population. It is estimated that in 2020 it will cost $9.5 billion to provide nursing home care to the country's elderly blind population (Crews, 1988). Rehabilitation services, particularly those specified in Title VII, Part C of the Rehabilitation Act, providing for independent living skills training to older visually impaired persons, have the potential to reduce this cost while serving people more effectively, if they are funded at a level higher than the current one.

For elderly visually impaired individuals still physically able to get out of their homes, the senior citizens center can be a lifeline to community life, sighted neighbors, and activities that enhance morale and self-esteem. The key to attending senior citizens centers for older visually impaired persons may be door-to-door transportation available through the center or another community-based social service agency serving elderly people. Such transportation services enable older visually impaired persons to keep essential medical, social service, and legal appointments within the community. The other key element is an environment free of the attitudinal barriers that inhibit the successful integration of older visually impaired persons into center activities.

Nutrition services are essential for the older person who has difficulty seeing. Provided in a congregate setting, a hot meal with others has both nutritional and psychological value. Nutrition services also include home-delivered meals. Both can help the older visually impaired person who is no longer able to cook. Such services are particularly helpful as an interim service while the older visually impaired person learns safety techniques in cooking during the rehabilitation process. Older visually impaired persons may also benefit from chore services, such as those encompassing heavy house cleaning, minor home repairs, and yard work.

Some older visually impaired persons may not be able to go out of the house because they have not yet received orientation and mobility (O&M) training from an agency for blind persons or because they have other disabling conditions or illnesses hindering mobility. In either case, three services bring a part of the community to the older homebound visually impaired person—friendly visiting, telephone reassurance, and the help of a senior companion. These services frequently operate out of a senior citizens center, a social service agency, or a religious organization. Friendly visiting provides regular visits to the older person who is isolated and needs companionship. Visits are made by volunteers, often senior citizens themselves, who can sit and talk, listen, write letters, or do errands. Telephone reassurance from volunteers who make daily or regularly scheduled calls to the older person living alone ensures that the individual is well and provides emotional support and information about community events. If the older person does not answer the phone, neighbors, relatives, or the police are notified to investigate. Many older persons, including some older visually impaired persons who have chronic illnesses such as heart conditions, benefit from the installation of an emergency response system connected to a local police station or rescue squad for help during a medical emergency.

The term "home care" refers to a range of home health care services as well as the in-home supportive services just described. Included in these services are skilled nursing care and physical, occupational, and speech therapy. Personal care services, such as assistance with bathing, dressing, toileting, and help with medications, meal preparation, and housekeeping are available. Again, it is important to note that newly visually impaired persons may need some of this assistance; however, training is available to help them regain their independent living skills so that these services can be terminated.

Home health care services can make a tremendous difference in the life of an older person who is waiting for such training or is in the process of being trained. They are usually required when other conditions are also present. However, home health care, an effective alternative to institutional care for many older people, may be quite costly. Medicare coverage for home health care is limited in scope and duration. Long-term care insurance to meet these costs has been a pressing issue among policymakers since the 1980s.

ADULT DAY CARE

The older visually impaired person with additional physical disabilities who does not require 24-hour nursing care may benefit from attending an adult day care center. This arrangement can also provide relief for family caregivers. Adult day care centers emphasize rehabilitation and health care as well as social activities. Centers may offer a hot lunch, snacks, assistance with medication, personal care, and counseling.

Adult day care is a young and rapidly growing community-based long-term care service. The adult day care center provides environmental support for independent living for older visually impaired persons. According to the National Adult Care 1989 Census conducted by the National Institute of Adult Day Care of the National Council on the Aging (NCOA), approximately 2,100 centers in the country provide care to about 45,000 older and disabled adults in almost every state (NCOA, 1990). Three-quarters of these centers opened in the last 10 years. States with the largest number of centers are in the East, the Midwest, and the South, followed by the Middle Atlantic and the New England regions. Most of the centers are in small metropolitan areas (38 percent) and large rural areas (35 percent); 20 percent are in large urban areas and 7 percent in small rural areas. If adult day care is to be incorporated into national long-term care policy, centers must become available nationally. The infrastructure is finally taking form with centers in every state. At this time, however, there are no national regulations governing the operation of adult day care centers, and not all states require licensing. Therefore, the quality of service varies tremendously. NCOA publishes a directory of 847 centers that meet NCOA's standards. In 1987, the House of Representatives approved the creation of a new Title III, Part D of the OAA program providing in-home and adult day care services for frail elderly individuals, with adult care as its newest component. Adult day care will continue to expand in the next decade and will require standards for quality of care. Adult day care is an example of a respite model.

RESPITE CARE

Respite care provides relief for caregivers at home and can make a difference in the lives of older visually impaired persons and their families. In this form of care, the older person's needs are met by someone other than the primary caregiver for varying periods of time that can range from a few hours to several days. Respite care allows elderly persons to remain at home and to avoid nursing home placement, in spite of the need for 24-hour care. It is traditionally provided by professional staff and trained volunteers and usually sponsored by synagogues, churches, nursing homes, home health agencies, and volunteer organizations. Respite care enables caregivers who work full or part time to continue to do so. More models and methods for providing respite care are emerging.

HOSPICE CARE

Hospice care is an alternative form of medical and custodial care for the terminally ill patient. It is provided either in the patient's home or in a separate nonmedical setting. Its goal is to provide the patient with pain management, family involvement, and death with dignity. Hospice care benefits the older person and family members. Designed to serve terminally ill people of any age and their families, hospice care aims to alleviate pain and keep the patient comfortable rather than to provide active medical care. In this form of care, a team of doctors, nurses, social workers, clergy members, and volunteers provide physical, psychological, social, and spiritual care, often in the patient's home.

OTHER PROGRAMS

Innovative programs, such as the Senior Companion Programs, frequently sponsored by area agencies on aging (AAAs) or other service organizations, train healthy and active older persons to use their natural skills as caregivers within the long-term care continuum. Thus, they provide companionship, chore, and escort services to frail and homebound elderly individuals. These programs are a cost-effective service supporting the long-term care industry. The American Foundation for the Blind (AFB) initiated a senior companion demonstration project in 1989 to train older visually impaired persons as senior companions to other visually impaired older persons or other older frail or disabled persons. This model demonstrates that older visually impaired persons can be productive and contributing members of the community, not solely recipients of services.

The U.S. Department of Veterans Affairs (VA) also offers a range of long-term care services for veterans. Some of these services and programs relevant to the older visually impaired veteran are nursing home and domiciliary care, community nursing home care including community residential care, hospital-based home care, adult day health care, psychiatric day treatment centers, hospice care, and respite care.

The older visually impaired person and family members, with the assistance of a social worker at a community service agency for elderly persons, can create the most appropriate individualized package of community-based services to enable the older person to remain at home and function as independently as possible.

"Eldercare"

"Eldercare" is a concept of the 1990s that calls for national, state, and local coalitions to work toward coordinated service delivery for older persons who are most at risk—those who are frail, poor, isolated, female, and age 85 or over. In early 1991, the commissioner of the Administration on Aging (AOA) recommended a national "eldercare" campaign for older at-risk persons who need community-based care. The AOA urged the establishment of National Eldercare Institutes to address the problems of employment, housing, support services, long-term care, and other service needs. It will commit $15 million to a campaign in the 1990s that consists of three components—public awareness, expanded involvement by various agencies and organizations, and a demonstration project ("AOA to commit," 1991).

The public awareness campaign was designed to make every segment of society aware of the impact of the demographic changes taking place in this country and the availability of community-based and in-home services for older at-risk persons. The second component was designed to expand the involvement of a wide variety of agencies and organizations representing government, business, labor, and the voluntary, civic, and religious communities. This coordinated involvement is an essential element in an era of limited financial resources. A national demonstration project on coalition building focuses on older persons who are at risk because they do not have caregivers to provide needed assistance and support.

In 1990, the National Association of Area Agencies on Aging initiated a national survey of eldercare activities of the aging network to determine the extent to which employers provided services to employees with caregiving responsibilities, including seminars on issues related to aging, caregiver support groups, and information fairs at the work site about community-based services. The national focus on eldercare may help more older persons to continue in their own homes in the years to come.

Living Arrangements and Options for Housing

At the onset of severe vision loss, the older visually impaired person is confronted with the challenging question, "Will I be able to continue to live alone in my home?" For many, including those who are totally blind, living alone is possible. However, if it is not physically or psychologically possible for the individual to live independently, a continuum of options exists.

The older visually impaired person and family members may decide that the best option for the older person is to live with an adult child. If this arrangement is not desirable or feasible, nonfamilial living arrangements are also possible, including shared housing, board and care, congregate housing, and a CCRC. Every option is not necessarily available to older persons in their immediate communities, however.

Shared housing—home sharing or house sharing—involves two or more unrelated persons living together, each having his or her own bedroom and sharing such common areas as the living room, the kitchen, and the bathroom. Shared housing provides the benefits of living in a house or apartment with other persons—sharing rent, exchanging chore services and eating together, and experiencing increased physical and emotional safety. This arrangement can be made in the private home of another individual or in an agency-sponsored apartment.

If more assistance is needed, board and care homes, also referred to as sheltered housing, residential care facilities, and domiciliaries, provide rooms, meals, and some degree of personal assistance, including help with bathing, dressing, getting in and out of bed, taking medication, and arranging transportation to and from medical and social service appointments. Board and care homes may benefit the older visually impaired person who has limited family or other resources for daily assistance. The disadvantage of board and care homes in general is that quality and standards vary dramatically from home to home; not all states have specific licensing procedures for board and care. The VA operates some domiciliaries, but most are operated privately.

Congregate housing is another semi-independent living option for the older visually impaired person. In this form of housing, both private and communal living space and support services necessary to maintain an independent life-style are provided. Congregate housing facilities range in size from 35 to 300 units. Enriched housing developments, a form of congregate housing, provide meals and transportation. Arrangements for personal care assistance and housekeeping are optional. Many provide on-site medical services, such as those provided by a full- time nurse, and are closely linked to acute-care facilities. Increased availability of enriched housing could meet the needs of greater numbers of older persons. In the case of shared housing, some board and care homes, and congregate settings, the opportunity for the individual to bring personal possessions, including some furniture, to his or her own private room is helpful, especially psychologically, and assists in orientation to a new environment.

The last two decades have seen an increase in retirement communities, particularly in the southeastern and southwestern states. A special form of retirement community, the CCRC, often referred to as life care, offers the older person a lifelong housing option with a full range of health care and social services. Nursing care and a skilled nursing unit are built into CCRCs, so that residents can move to a higher level of care if health deteriorates and greater assistance is needed. Some CCRCs offer health care benefits built into the initial cost; others require payment for some health care services. All require a lump sum entrance fee and monthly fees and serve as a means of purchasing long-term care insurance within a residential setting. CCRCs are not readily available to most elderly people because they are costly. However, they are a developing option in the area of supportive housing and long-term care insurance that will continue to expand.

Residential Facilities

Nursing home care is frequently perceived by professional service providers in the field of aging as well as by family caregivers and older persons themselves as the end of the continuum of long-term care, the last resort. Nursing homes are perceived as separate from community-based services, but this perception needs to change. Nursing homes need to begin to function as part of the community's services and to be considered as such. Nursing home administrators are trying to bring the community into the nursing home and to enable residents who are able to go out into the community to do so—to participate in a senior citizens center, for example. This reinterpretation of nursing homes would allow the home to be viewed more positively within the continuum of long-term care and to be viewed as more than a last resort.

The most recent trend has been to continue to develop and expand community-based long-term care services, particularly home health care, to keep the majority of older persons in need of personal services and health care out of nursing homes. However, nursing homes remain the best solution for many older persons under many sets of circumstances. When caregiving becomes too burdensome or if health conditions require 24-hour skilled nursing, older persons and their families may consider placement. This is an extremely difficult decision for all families and particularly for the older person, who almost never wants this option. The decision to be placed in a nursing home should be made by the older person and family members whenever the older person is able to participate; family members or others should not decide on behalf of the older person.

The move to a nursing home is difficult for the older visually impaired person; it means adjusting to a new environment, which can threaten the person's self-confidence, feeling of autonomy, and independent mobility. This is particularly true for the ambulatory visually impaired resident. About 4 percent of nursing home residents are totally blind, and another 30 percent are severely visually impaired. The increase in admission of those 75 and over will increase the percentage of those residents who are visually impaired. Nursing home staff need to have in-service training opportunities to learn about vision loss and about helping residents to be as self-sufficient as possible.

There are three levels of nursing home care—custodial, intermediate, and skilled. Custodial care is designed to serve many who do not need the care of a practical nurse but who do need supervision and assistance with meals, personal hygiene, and daily activities. Intermediate care is suitable for older persons who do not require around-the-clock nursing care but who are unable to live alone. This level of care is referred to as "health related." Skilled nursing is for patients who need intensive care 24 hours a day, as well as supervision and treatment by a registered nurse under the direction of a physician. In general, the level of nursing home care required is determined by the older person's physical condition. The quality of care in nursing homes has been under close scrutiny since the 1980s to ensure proper care and treatment of patients.

Issues in Service and Care

ELDER ABUSE

During the past three decades, the public has become aware of the neglect or abuse of frail elderly persons, often perpetrated by people expected to lend them support and assistance, including family members, neighbors, and service providers in residential settings. Abuse exists in financial, psychological, and physical forms. It is estimated that 1 million older persons are abused each year ("National resource centers," 1991).

Family members, emotionally and financially burdened by caregiving for elderly relatives, may find themselves in abusive situations. Staff in long-term care facilities may also be abusive because they are burned out and frustrated by difficult or demanding situations. Elderly people who do not have the capacity to handle their personal and financial affairs can be helped by community guardianship programs, which provide competent and trustworthy persons to help them meet their obligations. But those who are at the mercy of abusive and exploitive family members or neighbors need much more help than a friendly manager can give. Through departments of social services or AAAs, most states provide protective services that empower professionals to intervene on behalf of vulnerable older persons.

In 1985, a group of social service professionals joined together to form the National Committee for the Prevention of Elder Abuse to advocate for legislation on the mandatory reporting of abuse and services to protect elderly people from abuse and to serve those who have been abused. The committee also focuses on research, public awareness, and training related to elder abuse.

To focus greater national attention on elder abuse issues, the U.S. Department of Health and Human Services established an Elder Abuse Task Force to develop a comprehensive strategy of prevention, investigation, reporting, and follow-up. The National Aging Resource Center on Elder Abuse and the National Center for State Long-Term Care Ombudsman Resources have written issue papers on the topic to assist the task force. They identify five issues: (1) self-neglect, (2) mandatory reporting of abuse (in eight states reporting by professionals is still voluntary), (3) definitions (from state to state, definitions of physical abuse, neglect, and exploitation differ), (4) poor coordination of the agencies involved with elder abuse, manifested at the state, federal, and local levels, and (5) the availability of resources ("National resource centers," 1991).

Prevention is the most important factor regarding institutional abuse. Because the variables most closely connected to physical abuse are staff-patient conflict and burnout, the nurse's aide training requirements included in the Omnibus Budget Reconciliation Act of 1987 began to address these issues. The 1990 legislation of this act mandates that nursing home residents understand and exercise their rights in many areas, including the area of abuse.

Of particular significance are the issues of physical and psychological abuse, physical restraint, and overmedication. Far too frequently, older persons are restrained in beds, wheelchairs, or gerichairs, supposedly for safety but largely because there are insufficient staff to help older residents walk and exercise in order to retain an appearance of physical autonomy, as well as self-esteem. These issues are particularly important for older visually impaired and blind nursing home residents, who are frequently left in isolation because of a lack of understanding of their social and psychological needs. A statewide study conducted by geriatric specialists at Yale University found that 66 percent of elderly patients in 12 facilities were regularly restrained in chairs or beds. Although restraints are frequently used to prevent falls, distressed residents who try to get out of the restraints injure themselves ("Nursing home elders tied," 1991).

The project "Free to Be in Vermont," sponsored by the Kendal Corporation, addresses the issue of restraint. The project is based in six nursing homes and provides in-service training for caregivers. It also publishes a quarterly newsletter, *Untie the Elderly,* and a manual on alternatives to restraints. A survey of Vermont's 50 nursing homes reveals a 50 percent decrease in the use of mechanical restraints (Downs, 1990).

Current nursing home reform guidelines prohibit the use of restraints or tranquilizing medications unless prescribed by a physician for a specific medical problem. For abusive caregivers, support groups exist that can help people learn from others in similar circumstances and handle the issues surrounding the burden of providing care. Concern about elder abuse will continue as the number of frail elderly persons continues to grow.

ENVIRONMENTAL DESIGN

Environments are central to the independent functioning, dignity, and well-being of elderly persons. Planning for environmental design cannot be reduced to considering whether green is a restful color or whether braille markings should be placed near elevator buttons. The vision, hearing, mobility, agility, and endurance problems of older persons must be considered. The effort spent moving through or spending time in unfriendly environments can be exhausting, overwhelming, and inhibiting to the older person. A basic understanding of the impact of the physical and psychological environment on older people can help planners and service providers create user-friendly environments for the elderly population. Such an understanding can also help family members, community-based service providers, and older persons themselves create environments that facilitate independent functioning.

Environment in this context and environmental design go beyond the physical environment to include psychological, social, phenomenological, and cultural factors (Hiatt, 1985; Lawton, 1979, 1985). Examples of environmental attributes of particular interest to the fields of aging and blindness are the following:

- *Physical features.* Physical factors include size and configuration or shape, solid and void areas, paths, lighting levels, acoustical properties, aromas, and textures and their distinctiveness.
- *Psychological attributes.* The concept of psychological attributes is related to people's individualized reactions to the environment, including preferences or images of how environments look or ought to look.
- *Social properties.* Social attributes refer to the impact of people—their numbers, roles, and mix—and the effects of density or crowding on the environment.
- *Cultural attributes.* Cultural attributes are norms, codes, regulations, traditions, and patterns of use that develop over time. Making changes in the environment requires a clear understanding of existing cultural attributes (Hiatt, 1985; Parr, 1980).

Environments and their design are especially important to older people for the following reasons: They communicate information and expectations, can contribute to unnecessary disability or injury and inhibit functioning, can further interfere with the decreased mobility experienced by many older persons or facilitate the person's remaining capability for mobility, can compensate for lost or diminished functioning, and can serve as tools to prompt memory and aid activities of daily living. Both community-based and residential settings as well as the home can be modified to enhance functioning when there is some knowledge of both the inhibiting and facilitating factors for older people in general and special populations in particular.

The majority of older people are affected by conditions that influence the quality of their perception of visual detail, particularly their ability to distinguish between figure and background (Faye, 1984; Rosenbloom, 1982). However, through increases in lighting levels to 50 to 100 foot candles for close-up tasks, contrast sensitivity is often facilitated (Fozard, Wolf, Bell, McFarland, & Podolsky, 1977; Hiatt, 1987). By improving the visual qualities of the environment, the options for persons with low vision are improved and the likelihood of independence is increased (Hiatt, 1986). This is particularly important, because as a result of diminished vision, an older person's patterns of behavior may change—he or she may do less reading (Berkowitz, Hiatt, De Toledo, Shapiro, & Lurie, 1979), may engage in fewer activities that require close work (Silver, Gould, Irvine, & Cullinan, 1978), and may be limited in movement (Hiatt, 1988; Fozard, 1980).

Rehabilitation teachers, O&M specialists, and occupational therapists are extremely adept at identifying features of the natural environment and incorporating them into their teaching. A familiar environment— places, furnishings, and arrangements—can serve as a learning tool that can provide a sense of security and allow the individual to focus on new information or skills.

Rehabilitation professionals, like designers, may think in terms of gradients of difficulty and select learning environments as a context of training so that an individual has a good measure of stimulation but does not experience overload. Objects in the environment may be meaningful to older people from lifelong experience and therefore useful in activities, such as way finding and reminiscence. The rehabilitation teacher can also provide consultation to those planning and designing environments for older persons.

Features of the environment may contribute to an older person's natural skills of orienteering and wayfinding. Orienteering refers to the mental understanding of one's whereabouts; way finding expresses the practical skills of getting from place to place. Environmental features may also influence the person's awareness of the debilitating effects of a condition. Noisy surroundings not only increase physical stress but may also decrease the individual's attention span, making for forgetfulness and irritability (Cohen & Eisdorfer, 1979; Fozard, 1980; McCartney, 1979). They are also an inhibiting environment for the older hearing impaired person. The reduction of background noise has the potential to improve the older person's speech, comprehension, and attentiveness. Nursing homes and retirement communities are increasingly using carpeting to absorb noise and add to the homelike atmosphere of communal living arrangements (Pease, 1986).

The greatest challenge for the next generation of architects, environmental planners, and interior designers is to develop an environmental system of caring in which older persons can continue to live independently or maximize independent functioning with the help of technology that addresses increased and changing needs. Service providers in the fields of aging and blindness should learn about environmental factors that facilitate independence for older visually impaired people and help older persons and family members make minor adjustments to the home environment.

FAMILY CAREGIVING

For centuries, family members, primarily women, have served as caregivers to those of all ages who are physically or mentally impaired, as well as to elderly members of the family. Such caregiving was carried out without question, without thinking about options or alternatives, and as a result of personal ethics, religious thinking, and a desire to care for a parent.

For every older person in a nursing home, there are now four in the community receiving help from an informal system of unpaid family caregivers (Glasse, 1987). However, the dramatic growth of the presence of women in the workplace and prevailing changes in geographic proximity to aging parents have changed the ability of many persons to provide care 24 hours a day without outside support or services. In spite of these changes, the largest portion of long-term care in this country is provided by family caregivers. One reason is that the cost of home health care is covered only minimally by Medicare; another reason is the astronomic cost of nursing home care.

Family caregiving has become a critical issue over the last two decades because of the increasing numbers of older Americans, particularly those 85 and over. And older people in their sixties, seventies, and eighties themselves are called on to provide assistance to older relatives and friends.

The rhetoric of many policymakers in this country, in an era of a decreasing federal budget for health care services, is that the best place for those who need care is with their families. The further implication is that caregiving is an obligation that is taken lightly, assumed at little personal and financial cost to the caregiver, and met gladly with no reservations. This is frequently not the case.

During the 1980s, many studies found that working women, despite their employment, continued to meet their caregiving responsibilities. But the studies revealed that the combination of demands can result in the need for many women to leave their jobs. Gibeau and Anastas (1989) interviewed women working full time and found, on the average, that the women gave approximately 16 hours a week to caregiving, almost the equivalent of a half-time job itself.

A look at family caregivers nationwide reveals an exhausting image:

- Many caregivers are on duty 16 hours a day (Olsen, 1986).
- In 9 out of 10 cases, female caregivers are also employed outside the home (Friss, 1987).
- Caregivers who are employed rely less on paid help, spend more time giving care than they do on their jobs, and give care to more functionally impaired relatives (Perry, 1987).
- Those who work at a job for fewer than 20 hours a week have more stress and a greater burden than those who work longer hours, because they are juggling major portions of both tasks (Olsen, 1986).
- Some have been giving care for over 30 years at great personal sacrifice (Olsen, 1986).
- Caregiving interferes with the personal life of the caregiver, particularly when the older relative comes to live with the caregiver and her family (Olsen, 1986).
- The stresses and strains of the overburdened caregiver have the potential to result in abuse and neglect, as witnessed in this country (Ambrogi, 1987).

In spite of the strain, many caregivers and their older relatives opt for family caregiving because they are fearful of strangers providing care in the home. This fear is largely the result of the abuse that exists in the home care system. Although caregivers receive satisfaction in caring for a loved one and opt to do so over placing the person in a nursing home, they do so at a cost policymakers are beginning to recognize.

Gerontological researchers have examined and reexamined some critical questions related to family caregiving. What is the social and psychological impact on the caregiver? How much income is lost by caregivers who must leave the workplace or reduce their hours of employment? How does the tremendous time commitment to the ill or impaired older person affect job performance? How do family caregivers who are elderly themselves respond to their role as caregiver, and at what cost to their own health and psychological well-being do they do so? What leads caregivers and their older impaired relatives to seek nursing home placements? One longitudinal study at Michigan State University hopes to determine whether the increasing impact of the burden of care, the deteriorating health of the patient, or both lead to greater use of services within the community as well as to increased placement in nursing homes (Olsen, 1986). The results of the study will have a significant impact on the direction that long-term care policies will take in this country.

Service providers to the elderly population and agencies with a range of community-based services have identified and responded to the need for support for family caregivers by establishing support groups. Many caregivers feel burdened and isolated from the rest of the world. Some have no opportunity to talk about their feelings, to think creatively about modifications to their current pattern of caregiving, or to learn about additional resources of service and support within the local community. Support groups for caregivers are designed to meet these needs. Sometimes only within this context can a caregiver get in touch with some of what an older relative is experiencing as a result of needing help. And, most important, the caregiver may be able to express intense, conflicting feelings and needs.

The older visually impaired person, like other older people with various impairments and needs for assistance, suffers from two overwhelming fears related to receiving care—the fear of loss of personal autonomy and the fear that the already busy and soon overburdened caregiver will resent the time spent in giving care and will eventually resent him or her. These fears and feelings of guilt remain unspoken while the older person lives with the threat that a once positive relationship or a relationship already fraught with strain will be destroyed. Caregivers, too, are unable to speak to their older relatives about their own concerns. Families in these circumstances may benefit tremendously from the services of a social worker who can support each person through experiencing these feelings and enable everyone to talk and listen to the others.

Policymakers must begin to listen to the calls for help from elderly individuals and family caregivers and create an effective national long-term care policy that benefits the entire family unit. With demands on families escalating, national policies can no longer afford to force families to assume the role of caregiver solely because long-term care, especially long-term home health care, is too costly.

Demographics of Long-Term Care

The percentage of older persons residing in nursing homes (5 percent) as compared to those living in the community (95 percent) has remained constant over the last 10 years. Although the percentage of those over 65 in nursing homes remains at 5 percent, the number of residents in nursing homes increased by 17 percent from 1977 to 1987 and approached a total of 1.5 million older persons (National Center for Health Statistics, 1987). The number of older persons requiring care at various intermittent points along a continuum is growing rapidly. Eighty-five percent of those 65 and over living outside a nursing home have at least one chronic condition—arthritis, hypertension, hearing impairment, arteriosclerosis, or visual impairment (Blake, 1984).

One perspective on long-term care and health care in this country is that the issues involved greatly affect women—middle-aged and older women, especially women 85 years and over. Some pertinent statistics follow (Perry, 1987):

- Women make up nearly 60 percent of the elderly population in the United States.
- The most likely candidates for nursing home care are older women over 80 who live alone.
- One-fourth of women who live beyond 85 will spend some time in a nursing home, and an even larger number will need help with personal care or other in-home services.
- Older women 85 and over outnumber men in this cohort 3 to 1.
- The rate of poverty among older women in general and women in the over-85 age group in particular is twice that among older men.
- Fifty percent of older women have incomes of $6,000 or less, only about $500 above the poverty level.
- Three-fourths of older women are poor, giving them a poverty rate that in 1985 was nearly twice what it was among men (Porter & Greenstein, 1987).
- Women 85 and over spend 42 percent of their incomes on out-of-pocket health care costs.
- Seventy percent of those providing care are women.

The old-old—those age 85 and over—are the fastest growing portion of the population and are at the greatest risk of being in need of health care, social services, and caregiving by friends and family; they are also being asked to give care to other elderly persons. This population is at the greatest risk of having multiple chronic conditions. Elderly persons in need of care have from one to six chronic conditions, such as stroke, heart disease, and Alzheimer's disease. Although they have lower incomes than those in the 65-74 age group, their Medicare expenses are 77 percent higher. Out-of-pocket health care costs approximate 16 percent of the income of elderly people, higher than what it was before Medicare was established (Perry, 1987).

The National Center for Health Statistics conducted a national nursing home survey in 1985. Its results, released during 1987, include the following data and demographics:

- There are 1.6 million nursing home beds, a 22 percent increase in facilities since 1977.
- Almost half (49.3 percent) of the residents live in facilities operated by profit-making chains.

- Eighty-eight percent of the nursing home population are over the age of 65; 75 percent of the population are women.
- Women are twice as likely as men to be in a nursing home (6 percent of elderly females over 85, compared with 3 percent of elderly males). One in four women but only one in seven men lives in a nursing home.
- Twenty-six percent of nursing home residents are severely visually impaired.
- Elderly black persons are more likely to have conditions that hinder their performance of the activities of daily living, but they are less likely than are white persons to be in nursing homes.
- In 1985, nursing home residents were more dependent on assistance for activities of daily living than were residents in a 1977 study.
- Sixty-three percent of residents were significantly disoriented or memory impaired.
- Forty-two percent of the women and 36 percent of the men were on Medicaid, although about half of the residents of nursing homes paid privately for their first month of nursing home care.
- Black residents were almost twice as likely to be on Medicaid (70 percent) as were white residents (38 percent).

In addition, a recent report on nursing home admissions and deaths outlined the following (Kemper & Murtaugh, 1991):

- Forty-three percent of all Americans who turned 65 in 1990 will spend time in nursing homes before they die, and more than 900,000 of the 2.2 million who turned 65 are likely to enter nursing homes at least once.
- Almost 200,000 will spend more than five years in nursing homes.
- Nearly two-thirds of nursing home residents will be women.
- Whites will continue to use nursing homes more than blacks.
- Nearly one-third of those over 65 in 1990 will spend at least three months in nursing homes, 25 percent will spend a year in nursing homes, and 9 percent will spend five years ("Forty-three percent of elderly," 1991).

These statistics only begin to suggest the need for innovative long-term care programs as well as a national policy to meet the costs of long-term care in this country.

Quality of Life

The recent emphasis on and expansion of community-based care are the result of humanitarianism and the need for cost containment. Community-based care is humanitarian because it enables the older person to remain in familiar surroundings, is the least disruptive to the person's established life, and creates the opportunity for choice in regard to options for care. It was generally believed that providing care in the home would be less costly than residential nursing home care and would reduce Medicaid costs. However, it is not clear whether nursing home care or home and community-based care is more cost-effective; larger numbers of older persons are remaining at home and require increasing hours of home care, which increases Medicaid costs for this form of care.

HOME HEALTH CARE

Home health care is a burgeoning service along the continuum of long-term care. Its availability, quality, and cost have become crucial issues in Congress. The 1980s saw a dramatic growth in the home health care industry, primarily among profit-making companies determined to tap the lucrative Medicare market. Payments from Medicare are the lifeline of the home health care industry; 80 to 90 percent of those served are age 65 and older. Agencies vary greatly in quality of service, and even the Health Care Financing Administration (HCFA) indicates that consumers cannot assume that a Medicare-certified agency's services and personnel meet any standards and provide the highest quality care. Considerable abuse exists within the system. The abuse is twofold—financial abuse by agencies of the Medicare system and poor care for patients who depend on home health care for survival. Many home health care aides fail to perform their tasks fully, and a lack of proper supervision of aides by agencies makes home care patients vulnerable to substandard practices. Unfortunately, those most vulnerable and dependent on the home health aide are fearful of reporting the poor care they are receiving, especially if it is the only care available to them. Instead, they withstand the neglect they experience. The future of home health care requires stricter federal and state regulation of the system to ensure quality and cost-effectiveness.

NURSING HOME CARE: THE NEED FOR REFORM

For the 5 percent of the population over 65 residing in nursing homes, a report by the Institute of Medicine (1986) concluded that the quality of life in many nursing homes is unsatisfactory and that patients are not getting the quality and quantity of care medically and psychologically indicated. The National Citizens Committee for Nursing Home Reform (NCCNHR), which has continually called for high-quality care, is strongly urging more effective government regulation of nursing homes based on the findings of that report. Twenty organizations coordinated by the NCCNHR, called the "Campaign for Quality Care in Nursing Homes," addressed key nursing home reform issues in the late 1980s.

In general, insufficient numbers of nurses are available in nursing homes, with regulations allowing one licensed practical nurse to cover an intermediate-care facility for as long as 16 hours. Nursing homes discriminate in their admissions procedures, preferring private-pay patients over those requiring public support. Thus, the poorest older persons, those most needing intensive health care services, have the least access to quality care.

Advocacy efforts calling for nursing home reform resulted in the Nursing Home Reform Amendments in the 1987 Omnibus Budget Reconciliation Act. The 1990 Budget Reconciliation Act made technical additions to the 1987 act. These additions related to nurse's aide training, competency evaluations, annual resident review, staffing ratios, resident assessment, and other key regulations.

The OAA as amended in 1978 mandated a long-term care ombudsman program in every state, which was charged with the following activities to ensure the health, safety, welfare, and rights of residents of long-term care facilities (Evren, 1987):

- Investigating complaints regarding administrative action that may adversely affect a patient's well-being,
- Monitoring the development and implementation of federal, state, and local laws, regulations, and policies regarding long-term care facilities,
- Providing information to public agencies regarding the problems of facility residents,

- Training volunteers and promoting the involvement of citizens organizations in the ombudsman program, and
- Carrying out other activities as the U.S. commissioner on aging deems appropriate.

The 1990 Budget Reconciliation Act included $2.4 million in new funds for the ombudsman programs for fiscal year 1991. Under this program, if family members and older persons experience difficulties and concerns within a nursing home, they should contact the nursing home administrator. When further help is needed, they should contact their state ombudsman.

Institutionalization of an older physically and perhaps mentally frail person against his or her will is of critical concern in this country and was identified by ombudsmen nationwide as an area for change (Evren, 1987). Family members unable or unwilling to care for an older relative sometimes arrange placement without consulting the older person. Such unauthorized decisions place the older frail person out of control of his or her own life.

Ombudsman programs throughout the country indicate that the number of undesired placements varies from state to state and is determined by such factors as preplacement screening, availability of community resources, cultural norms, geographic differences in care, and availability of nursing home beds. Preplacement screening enables the wishes of the elderly person to be ascertained and may allow the individual to obtain his or her expressed choice for care. The ombudsman program calls for prescreening interviews.

Quality of Care

The staff of most nursing homes have had little or no training about vision loss and are therefore ill-prepared to handle the many issues of visually impaired residents. On admission to a nursing home, patients receive an ophthalmological evaluation. Beyond an eye exam every one to two years, little is done in day-to-day care to detect gradual vision loss. There is a growing need for in-service training regarding vision loss among residents so that staff can help visually impaired residents be as independent as possible and early signs of vision loss can be detected. A curriculum on aging and vision loss for nursing home staff has been prepared by the Pennsylvania College of Optometry, and a training video has been prepared for nursing home staff by the Rehabilitation Research and Development Center of the Veterans Administration Medical Center of Atlanta. AFB, in cooperation with the Delta Gamma Foundation, prepared in-service training materials to be used with nursing home staff by Delta Gamma sorority alumnae volunteers. The most recent curriculum is being developed by AFB to train nurse's aides and other nonprofessional staff who are the primary hands-on caregivers in nursing homes and retirement centers.

The Impact of Diagnosis-Related Groups

In the late 1980s, an examination of patients admitted to nursing homes, particularly for short-term care, revealed the presence of younger patients with a variety of medical problems requiring additional skilled care after transfer from acute-care hospitals. Their presence was largely the result of the diagnosis-related group (DRG) system created by the federal government in an era of fiscal constraint. The system was an attempt to control escalating health care expenditures as part of Medicare cost-containment efforts. Under this system, Medicare reimbursement to a hospital is through a prospective, predetermined, fixed payment based on diagnosis, rather than on actual services needed or performed or time spent in the hospital. Patients are assigned a given DRG category based on age, sex, and discharge status, and a standard reimbursement for a disease is made, irrespective of the extent of the patient's needs. It is in a hospital's best interest to discharge an elderly patient to a nursing home early and to retain the reimbursement for that diagnosis to compensate for another patient who must remain beyond the allowable DRG-identified discharge time. Although the intention of policymakers is to create a system that will cap rising hospital costs by reducing unnecessary services, the fear of professional service providers is that this intention motivates hospitals to skimp on services and exert pressure for early discharge at the expense of sound medical care. A system to decrease spending and cap costs may in fact be jeopardizing the health of older persons requiring acute care in hospitals as well as in nursing homes.

In light of the impact of the use of DRGs, hospital discharge planners and the aging services network need better coordination and educational materials to ensure continuity of care for older patients, according to the Long-Term Care National Resource Center at the University of California at Los Angeles and the University of Southern California ("Aging network and discharge planners," 1991). This is an area requiring considerable strengthening so that older persons may receive the posthospitalization care they need, whether the discharge is to the home or a long-term care facility.

Overall, issues relating to the quality of long-term care services, at home and in nursing homes, are many and varied. They call for stricter regulations to ensure quality care now and in the future, and they suggest the extent of the problem facing legislators, planners, and service providers to the elderly population today.

Who Pays for Long-Term Care?

Older Americans are well aware that home health care and nursing home care costs are astronomical and, for most, beyond their ability to pay out of pocket. However, when asked directly who pays for these costs, most are unable to produce an answer that approaches accuracy.

According to a one-year study by the Commonwealth Fund Commission on Elderly People Living Alone (Commonwealth Fund, 1987), two-thirds of America's elderly population are either uncertain, confused, or misinformed about meeting long-term care costs. Twenty-eight percent were not sure who pays for long-term care, 23 percent believed that some type of private health insurance would cover the costs, and 15 percent indicated that Medicare would pay. Still others thought their savings, family funds and assets, or Medicaid would meet the cost of long-term care (Gordon, 1986; Tell, Batten, Cohen, & Larson, 1986). Other polls indicate that large numbers of older persons have no financial plan to pay for long-term care and that this unprepared state results from ignorance about their own current coverage and the major misperception that their current insurance, even if it is only Medicare, will pay for nursing home costs.

ISSUES IN FINANCING

In 1987, the cost of long-term care was estimated at $38 billion a year (National Health Council, 1987). In times of deficit reduction and federal budget restraint, it is difficult to envision a national policy that will meet the costs of long-term nursing home care, the principal source of catastrophic out-of-pocket expenses for elderly people (Rice & Gabel, 1986). Meeting those costs has created worry and alarm among elderly individuals and their families in the 1980s and into the 1990s. Designing mechanisms to respond to this situation is a highly complex problem facing legislators in the United States. Although limited solutions are proposed at the federal level to address the cost of nursing home stays, nothing proposed thus far will effectively meet the costs of long-term care outside the nursing home. Service providers to elderly people have not advanced any creative solutions for elderly clients requiring nursing home care. The majority of older persons in this category will eventually use up their assets (or "spend down") so they can eventually qualify for Medicaid coverage. At the same time, spouses of elderly nursing home residents struggle against personal impoverishment to ensure quality care for their loved ones.

Currently, patients pay about half of long-term care expenses. Medicaid pays much of the other half, with Medicare and private insurance contributing approximately 3 percent. Despite the substantial improvements in income status and health care coverage of elderly persons over the last 20 years, older people spend approximately 16 percent of their income on health care. Per capita out-of-pocket health expenses for each older person, 65 and older, not including long-term nursing home care, exceeded $1,000 in 1984, more than three times that spent before Medicare. Even adding payments from Medicaid and "medigap" insurance designed to pay for services not reimbursed by Medicare, one-fourth of the total acute-care bill is paid out of pocket by elderly persons (Waldo, Levit, & Lazenby, 1986).

In 1991, older persons paid $29.90 per month for Medicare Part B premiums, and the cost is projected to rise to $46.10 by 1995. This increase is the result of annual federal budget crises. The current proposal for Medicare cuts calls for $43.8 billion over five years from 1991 to 1995. The Medicare deductible will also increase from $75 to $100. Older persons currently seek out private medigap insurance coverage to meet costs not covered by Medicare. Because of the scramble for private insurance coverage among the elderly population, state insurance commissioners have identified nine private health insurance policies to supplement Medicare coverage. These nine policies offer a range of coverage from basic hospital and physician deductibles to health care at home, prescription drugs, and preventive screenings.

Both public insurance and the private market need to respond to the long-term health care financing crisis. Current policies are minimal and ineffective. Medicare covers the cost of all services in a skilled nursing facility for the first 20 days; coverage continues from day 21 through 100, but at some cost to the individual. Termination of benefits does not necessarily coincide with the end of the patient's need for service. What ends is the narrowly defined need for skilled nursing care on which current coverage depends. Medicaid is basically responsible for the bulk of public financing of long-term care, but its protection is limited. Eligibility depends on a person's resources, and the nature and availability of benefits depend on the state's willingness and ability to pay. Medicaid's connection to poverty is also a major psychological dilemma for many older persons.

At the federal and state levels and within the private insurance market, solutions to the need for long-term care coverage are presented continually. All agree that a catastrophic insurance benefit is essential for the nation's elderly population. The U.S. Bipartisan Commission on Comprehensive Health Care (renamed the Pepper Commission), directed by P.L. 100-360, declared that the health care system was at a grave point. The commission's recommendations include a five-point program on health coverage and a long-term care reform plan. The long-term care reform plan calls for the establishment of government or social insurance to keep resources intact for severely disabled people at home (or with the potential to return home after a short nursing home stay), with family and community-based care available and affordable, and for the provision of a "floor" of protection against impoverishment for all those seeking broader protection.

In this era of fiscal restraint, private options have also been essential complements to public plans. The reverse annuity mortgage plan, which enables the older person to convert the equity in his or her home to liquid assets while continuing to live there, has been proposed to pay for services. Such an alternative can, however, be viewed as counter to the protection of elderly individuals against catastrophe because it waters down the need for public coverage.

Long-term care retirement communities, CCRCs, and social health maintenance organizations (SHMOs) are widely recognized examples of private arrangements. Research at Brandeis University interested in expanding the concept of life care into a less expensive version developed an LCAH model that provides comprehensive long-term care services and insurance to middle-income elderly individuals who remain at home (Tell, Cohen, Larson, & Batten, 1987). LCAH is a hybrid program combining elements of the CCRC program and the SHMO and bringing together financial security and health services with the freedom and independence of living at home and within the broader community. The difficulty is that these long-term care insurance options are not readily available to elderly persons of all incomes. However, they may meet the financial needs of middle-income older persons.

THE STATES' RESPONSE

To encourage private insurers in the long-term care insurance business and to establish standards to protect consumers, the National Association of Insurance Commissioners adopted a model for states to follow in drafting legislation in 1986. The model defined "long-term care" as coverage for at least 12 consecutive months for one or more medically necessary diagnostic, preventive, therapeutic, rehabilitative, maintenance, or personal care services provided in a setting other than an acute-care unit of a hospital. States need to provide an incentive to insurance companies to offer the insurance. And, even more important, states must protect consumers against inadequate policies. Consumers, who often do not know which coverage even begins to meet the cost of long-term care, need to be educated about long-term care insurance products.

Fourteen states have enacted laws addressing long-term care insurance issues. Six have ordered studies on ways to promote the development of long-term care policies. Another eight have set standards for policies or mandated coverage under health insurance policies. Some states have responded because they hope such policies will curb their skyrocketing Medicaid outlays. However, studies from the Brookings Institution indicate that Medicaid expenses will be eased only marginally by new expansion of private long-term care insurance (Hanley, 1987).

PRIVATE INSURANCE
Private long-term care insurance is tremendously controversial. Some believe that only broad, federally sponsored social insurance for long-term care can—or should—meet the costs of such care. Others support the role of privately developed and financed long-term care insurance.

The private long-term care insurance market has been in existence only since 1982. Because the purchase of long-term nursing home care insurance is not a viable option for the majority of older Americans, its success has been limited. However, the prospect that Medicare coverage for long-term care will not be available in the near future has spurred the private health insurance industry to enter what it believes will be a $20 billion market by the year 2020. Although it is estimated that only 25 to 30 percent of the nation's elderly population will be able to afford private insurance in 2020, one study indicates that real income of people 65 and over will double by then. This study projects that long-term care insurance will pay for as much as 11.3 percent of nursing home costs by 2020, compared to the less than 3 percent it covers now ("Aetna offers," 1987).

Many insurance companies already sell nursing home insurance policies, others are preparing to test the market, and many cover only nursing home care. Fewer than 300,000 older persons in this country can afford to purchase long-term care insurance (Klein, 1987). Nevertheless, an estimated 200,000 individual long-term care insurance policies are in effect nationwide. Until now, though, the primary mechanism for people to buy insurance has been through an employer, enabling them to take advantage of group rates. Aetna offered the first group long-term care insurance policy when it agreed to underwrite such a policy for the state of Alaska, which mandated an optional long-term care benefit for its retired state employees in 1986. Given that paying for long-term care in the future is becoming an anxiety-producing concern for older employees and that providing care to an impaired family member often places an employee under severe emotional and financial stress, long-term care coverage is an issue employers will need to address.

Because of the complexity and enormity of meeting the cost of long-term care, coverage for such care is a patchwork of public and private noncomprehensive benefits even when combined. Private insurance offering long-term care coverage is a partial solution at present and does not preclude the need for a larger public sector role.

Summary

Issues related to the cost, quality, and financing of long-term care dominate the field of aging today. Innovative long-term care programs designs across the United States are attempts to close the gaps in care. Creativity is needed nationwide in both planning and implementing service options, as well as in financing these service models. A focus on the poorest elderly population is also essential to ensure equitable service options across income levels. All older Americans should be assured of equal access to high-quality care, choice in regard to forms of care, and the highest level of independence achievable to improve their quality of life.

As policymakers attempt to create solutions for the 1990s, they do so knowing the need for care will increase and the need to finance such care will grow exponentially. In the year 2020, the baby boom generation will be caught up in its own years of degenerative illness. The United States will experience an unprecedented wave of pressure to limit health care costs, both for acute-care and chronic-care services and insurance. Older Americans, many of them with varying degrees of disabilities and chronic illnesses, will look to the future with hope for longer and healthier lives; humane, high-quality and comprehensive care; and public insurance coverage to meet the costs.

References

Aetna offers first group long-term insurance policy. (1987). *Older Americans Report*, p. 1.

Aging network and discharge planners need better coordination. (1991). *Older Americans Report*, p. 95.

Ambrogi, D. M. (1987). Conflicts (and solutions) in family caregiving. *The Aging Connection, 8:* 7.

AOA to commit $15 million on national elder care campaign. (1991, February 15). *Older Americans Report*, p. 63.

Berkowitz, M., Hiatt, L. G., De Toledo, P., Shapiro, J., & Lurie, M. (1979). *Reading with print limitations: The role of health care institutions in satisfying the reading needs of residents with print limitations* (Vol. 3). New York: American Foundation for the Blind.

Blake, R. (1984). What disables American elderly? *Generations, 7*(4): 6-9.

Cohen, D., & Eisdorfer, C. (1979). Cognitive theory and assessment of change in the elderly. In A. Raskin & L. Jarvik (Eds.), *Psychiatric symptoms and cognitive loss in the elderly* (pp. 273-282). New York: Halsted.

Commonwealth Fund Commission on Elderly People Living Alone. (1987). *Old, alone and poor: A plan for reducing poverty among elderly people living alone.* Baltimore: Author.

Crews, J. E. (1988). No one left to push: The public policy of aging and blindness. *Journal of Educational Gerontology, 14*(3): 399-409.

Downs, M. (1990). Free to be in Vermont. *Untie the Elderly, 2*(3): 1.

Evren, L. T. (1987). Long-term care ombudsman: National survey of their views. *Generations, 11*(4): 43-46.

Faye, E. (1984). Visual rehabilitation in the geriatric population. In E. E. Faye (Ed.), *Clinical low vision* (2nd ed., pp. 123-126). Boston: Little, Brown.

Forty-three percent of elderly will need nursing homes. (1991). *Older Americans Report*, p. 83.

Fozard, J. (1980). The time for remembering. In L. W. Poon (Ed.), *Aging in the 1980s* (pp. 497-534). Washington, DC: American Psychological Association.

Fozard, J., Wolf, E., Bell, B., McFarland, R. A., & Podolsky, S. (1977). Visual perception and communication. In J. E. Birren & K. W. Schaie (Eds.), *Handbook of the psychology of aging*, pp. 497-534. New York: Van Nostrand Reinhold.

Friss, L. (1987). Caregivers who also work outside the home. *The Connection, 8*(1): 10.

Gibeau, J. L., & Anastas, J. W. (1989). Breadwinners and caregivers: Interviews with working women. *Journal of Gerontological Social Work, 14*(1): 19-40.

Glasse, L. (1987, March). *Caregivers—Unpaid workers in the health care system.* Paper presented to the National Voluntary Organization for Independent Living for the Aging at the meeting of the National Council on the Aging, Chicago, IL.

Gordon, N. (1986, March). *Statement before the Subcommittee on Health and the Environment, Committee on Energy and Commerce.* Washington, DC: Congressional Budget Office, U.S. House of Representatives.

Hanley, R. J. (1987, March). *The catastrophic costs of long-term care: How many, how much, and for whom?* Paper presented at the meeting of the American Society on Aging, Salt Lake City, UT.

Hiatt, L. G. (1985). Understanding the physical environment. *Pride Institute Journal of Long-Term Home Health Care, 4*(2): 12-22.

Hiatt, L. G. (1986). The vision care professional and institutional settings. In A. A. Rosenbloom & M. W. Morgan (Eds.), *Vision and aging: General and clinical perspectives* (pp. 231-242). New York: Professional/Capital Cities.

Hiatt, L. G. (1987). Designing for the vision and hearing impairments of the elderly. In V. Regnier & J. Pynoos (Eds.), *Housing the aged: Design directives and policy considerations* (pp. 341-372). New York: Elsevier.

Hiatt, L. G. (1988). Mobility and independence in long-term care: Implications for technology and environmental design. In G. Lesnoff-Caravagla (Ed.), *Aging in a technological society* (pp. 58-64). New York: Human Sciences.

Institute of Medicine (IOM) Committee on Nursing Home Regulation. (1986). *Improving the quality of care in nursing homes.* Washington, DC: National Academy Press.

Kemper, P., & Murtaugh, C. M. (1991). Lifetime use of nursing home care. *New England Journal of Medicine, 324*(9): 595-600.

Klein, D. A. (1987). The private side of long-term care insurance. *The Aging Connection, 8*(2): 4.

Lawton, M. P. (1979). Introduction: A background for the environmental study of aging. In T. O. Byerts, S. C. Howell, & L. A. Pastalan (Eds.), *Environmental Context of Aging* (pp. xiii-xxiv). New York: Garland.

Lawton, M. P. (1985). An introduction and overview to environment. *Pride Institute Journal of Long-Term Home Health Care, 4*(2): 1-11.

McCartney, J. (1979). Hearing problems: Speech and language problems associated with hearing loss and aural rehabilitation. In M. V. Jones (Ed.), *Speech and language problems of the aging.* Springfield, IL: Charles C Thomas.

National Center for Health Statistics. (1987). *1985 National nursing home survey.* Washington, DC: Author.

National Council on the Aging. (1990). ADC growth uncommon but impressive. *Networks, 2*(4): 9.

National Health Council (1987, November). *Washington Report,* p. 14.

"National resource centers identify key issues for HHS Task Force." (1991). *Network News, 8*(9): 4.

Nursing home elders tied, drugged. (1991, February/March). *Aging Today,* p. 4.

Olsen, E. A. (1986) Family caregiving: Current research and future policy. *The Aging Connection, 7*(5): 8-9.

Parr, J. (1980). The interaction of persons and living environments. In L. Poon (Ed.), *Aging in the 1980s.* Washington, DC: American Psychological Association.

Pease, J. A. (1986) Carpeting. *Generations. 11*(1): 41-44.

Perry, M. J. (1987). Women, ageism and health care. *The Aging Connection, 8*(2): 11.

Porter, K., & Greenstein, R. (1987). *On the other side of easy street: Myths and facts about the economics of old age.* Washington, DC: Villers Foundation.

Rice, T., & Gabel, J. (1986, Fall). Protecting the elderly against high health care costs. *Health Affairs,* p. 38.

Rosenbloom, A. A. (1982). Care of elderly people with low vision. *Journal of Visual Impairment & Blindness, 76*(6): 209-212.

Silver, J. H., Gould, E. S., Irvine, D., & Cullinan, T. R. (1978). Visual acuity at home and in eye clinics. *Transactions of the Ophthalmological Societies of the United Kingdom, 98* (Part 2): 252-257.

Tell, E., Batten J., Cohen M., & Larson M. (1986). *The market potential for long-term care finance and delivery options. Results of a telephone survey.* Unpublished manuscript, Brandeis University, Heller Graduate School, Health Policy Center, Waltham, MA.

Tell, E., Cohen M., Larson, M., & Batten, H. L. (1987). Assessing the elderly's preference for lifecare retirement options. *The Gerontologist, 27*(4): 503-509.

Waldo, D., Levit, K., & Lazenby, J. (1986). National health expenditures, 1985. *Health Care Financing Review, 8*(1): 1-22.

Meeting the Challenge

CHAPTER 14

Self-Help, Empowerment, and Advocacy

Anne Yeadon

The 1980s and early 1990s have been characterized by dramatic decreases in the funding of social programs coupled with a rapid increase in the number of elderly people whose needs and developing political power foreshadowed significant changes in the rehabilitation service field. Although demands are put forth for more equitable capital support of programs for elderly people, there are also promising trends in the development of self-help and other nontraditional support systems aimed at maximizing the personal freedom, initiative, and independence of elderly persons with disabilities. The challenges facing policymakers and personnel in the fields of aging and blindness include (1) recognizing the limitations of currently fragmented and poorly funded programs and refining self-help processes, materials, and mutual-support networks; (2) collaborating in the empowerment of previously dependent elderly clients; (3) coordinating community resources and the efforts of service providers and of older persons with disabilities; and (4) initiating new legislation and regulations reflecting all these changes in the system.

The Current System

Older visually impaired people, whether 55 or 105 years of age, male or female, working or nonworking, or living at home or in a long-term care facility, have a right to rehabilitation services. Few would argue with such a general statement. The debate centers on how such services should be delivered, in what form, by whom, at what cost, with what frequency, and with what degree of quality control and self-management by clients. Expertise in rehabilitation, whether in rehabilitation teaching, orientation and mobility (O&M) instruction, low vision services, communications, technological devices, or recreation and health care, has become increasingly sophisticated since World War II. However, many older people do not know services exist, do not know they are eligible for them, choose not to utilize such services, or, most important, do not have access to them. Most have made the necessary adaptations to their life-styles the hard way by their own initiative and determination and the informal assistance of family members. Some have felt unable to function independently at all and are unnecessarily dependent on family members or caregivers for assistance in daily activities.

Needs change with increasing years. Services for the elderly population must be timely, flexible, and relevant in order to be responsive to these changing needs. However, the medical model of a continuum of care, rather than a model of social and community-based support systems, has dominated the field. The alternatives of in-home care and day care, which have expanded during the last decade, have been used to a limited extent even though many residents of nursing homes or other long-term care facilities could have their needs met in the community if community-based support services were more widely available and affordable.

As professionals, what is our responsibility to older visually impaired persons, who often have multiple disabilities? How can we provide this population with a continuum of rehabilitation services from which they may choose? If private agencies do not receive third-party reimbursements to cover the costs of rehabilitation, how are such services to be financed?

Today's formal rehabilitation system offers inadequate and fragmented services to elderly disabled people. Lack of funds is usually cited as the cause of the problem. But even if adequate resources were available, the traditional system of delivering services through agencies for the blind is not the only way to meet the changing and wide-ranging needs of this population. The service delivery system in the field of aging must be collaboratively utilized as well. No matter what services are offered and by whom, a key factor is the general context within which problems and needs are perceived and remediated. What philosophy and assumptions are at the heart of any service that is provided?

Despite the move away from the Victorian do-goodism of the early 1900s, some service providers (teachers, senior citizens center personnel, and health care providers, for example) too often tend to promote and administer services that "take care of" rather than promote independent thinking and functioning of older persons with disabilities. If these impaired individuals, for example, elderly widows who live alone, are considered by many to be socially and personally vulnerable, then the concept of protecting them has a greater emotional appeal than that of enabling them to continue to be involved in community life. According to this conception, responding in any other way might be heartless and uncaring. Invariably, though, such charitable attitudes lead to misguided actions, especially in relation to blind and visually impaired persons and their potential for independence and productive activity. Furthermore, assumptions that promote dependence, that reduce pride and dignity, and that exclude individuals from decision making are antithetical to the entire rehabilitation process.

Older persons who are undergoing a major life change, whether loss of vision or loss of a spouse, invariably benefit if those around them help create a dignified and empathic environment for change and adjustment to that change. For recently visually impaired individuals, service providers can create such an environment by simply coordinating their clients' abilities to help themselves through use of basic adult learning principles that stimulate independent adult thinking and ensure the older person's participation in decision making.

Principles of Adult Learning

There are practical differences between the teaching and learning processes for adults and those for children. Pedagogy places the teacher in a directing role. "Andragogy," the process of adult learning, acknowledges the benefits of using the extensive life experiences of individuals, their tried and tested coping mechanisms, and their mature levels of independence in decision making. Andragogy promotes the qualities described in the discussion that follows; these qualities are particularly important in the working relationship between the older visually impaired person and the professionals involved in the rehabilitation process.

SELF-CONCEPT

Adults usually object to being placed in situations that violate their mature self-concepts. They do not like to be talked down to or treated with an apparent lack of respect. They certainly do not like being regarded as children. Yet adults often enter new situations, such as a rehabilitation program, expecting to be educated without regard to their life experiences and knowledge, to be told what to do, and to leave decision making to the professionals. In many instances, service providers do little to correct these expectations and often reinforce them.

Service providers often assume pedagogical attitudes toward elderly blind clients. For example, they use a person's first name without asking permission, speak slowly and assume that the person does not understand, lead the person around by the hand, and address him or her through a third person. These "Does he take sugar?" tendencies invariably erode the dignity and self-worth of mature and relatively independent individuals, foster the state of dependence, and frustrate their effective adaptation. The challenge is obvious—to encourage the full use of adult learning principles that enhance and stimulate each person's self-concept, self-help abilities, and responsibilities for making decisions and achieving goals.

PARTNERSHIP IN LEARNING

The life experiences of each older visually impaired person are a rich resource for self-motivated learning. Principles of adult education place the individual and the service provider in mutual and interchangeable positions of teacher and learner.

The role of a service provider is primarily that of facilitator. Generally, adults know whether they feel comfortable tackling situations in a particular way and when they feel safe and capable of handling a specific task without assistance. The challenge is for the service provider and the client to capitalize on the client's abilities, knowledge, familiarity, confidence, support mechanisms, and lifetime of common sense. Ideally, the relationship is characterized by each person's feeling respect for the other's knowledge, abilities, and experiences—a partnership in progressive adaptation to changing conditions. Professionals with an open ear can learn much from the older visually impaired person in a process that facilitates independent living skills.

READINESS TO LEARN

Pedagogy emphasizes sequential learning; andragogy utilizes selective learning based on an individual's perceptions of his or her problems and needs. When disabled persons identify a special area of need or interest, that point in time can be viewed as a "teachable moment," a time when these persons themselves decide what they need or want on the basis of their perceptions of the demands of the particular situation. When such a teachable moment arises, the service provider or informal helper can assume the role of "resource facilitator," the partner in a joint problem-solving process that melds professional techniques with an understanding of adult learning processes.

Lack of motivation is likely when the older visually impaired person is presented with learning situations and tasks that he or she considers irrelevant to immediate and individual needs. Therefore, older visually impaired persons should always be encouraged to set the direction for and be the motivating force behind the planning of goals and specific learning activities. This concept leads to the key element of adult learning and effective rehabilitation participation: Service providers must actively involve older persons in setting individualized goals and curriculum content. The providers must be willing to listen, abandon the role of director, explore innovative options for resolving problems, and spend time exploring the questions before rushing to predetermined solutions.

PROBLEM-CENTERED LEARNING

Adult learning principles emphasize problem-centered rather than subject-centered learning. For example, Cantor (1975) found that when older people cease to work, have limited incomes, and grow more frail, they frequently become homebound. In many cases, their mobility needs are less extensive and more general than those of younger clients. Under these circumstances, it may appear that they require fewer comprehensive courses on O&M instruction. But the opportunity for such instruction may be the one factor that liberates them from their homebound status. Frequently, if other disabilities are not present, being homebound is more a matter of perception than a reality for the older person.

Although it must not be assumed that older individuals cannot benefit from subject-centered courses, the key question is: What are their individual identifiable needs in relation to their specific situations? The answer establishes the framework for the formulation of goals and for direct problem-centered education, which leads to immediate improvements in adaptation and adjustment.

Self-Help Options

The rehabilitation service delivery system is frequently characterized and described by fragmented research, inadequate training procedures, lack of quality control and monitoring, gross underfunding, and non-integrated services. Therefore, the needs of entire groups of visually impaired people—most notably elderly persons, multiply disabled persons, and residents of long-term care facilities—have not received the full attention they deserve. This situation is often exacerbated by elderly people themselves, who, in the face of societal apathy, cannot or do not actively seek help and are only sporadically referred to the blind rehabilitation system by such specialists as ophthalmologists and optometrists or other health care professionals. As a result, many older visually impaired persons experience a notorious five-year gap between the onset of visual impairment and referral for rehabilitation services (Anarem Systems Research Corporation, 1978). Because any significant increase in the funding of traditional rehabilitation services is unlikely in the immediate future in spite of strong legislative advocacy, one must assume that the formal system will not be able to meet the needs of the growing number of older visually impaired persons.

Although current advocates call for an enormous increase in Title VII, Part C funds so that every state has $225,000 on top of the additional funds based on the density of the population of older persons, the current era of fiscal restraint does not promise the necessary $26 million needed nationwide. For this reason, it is helpful to explore a wide range of less traditional self-help options while continuing to advocate for increased allocations for independent living programs.

Self-help groups are developing throughout the nation to fulfill needs that are not met and to some extent cannot be met by the traditional agencies. The support received and the social interaction of participants can play a crucial role in the rehabilitation process (Mummah, 1975). Toseland and Hacker (1982) concluded that social workers and other human service professionals are important in supporting, maintaining, and initiating self-help groups and that most self-help leaders do not discourage the involvement of the professional.

The concept of self-help is not new. Today, an estimated 15 million individuals seek pragmatic help and emotional support from such informal mechanisms as Neurotics Anonymous, Mended Hearts (for heart surgery patients), Alcoholics Anonymous, Parents Anonymous (for parents of abused children), Widow-to-Widow programs, and Make It Today (for cancer patients) (Gartner & Reissman, 1977).

The primary strategies for the empowerment of clients and for self-help include the integration of the concepts of self-study, informational programs on radio and cable television, how-to publications, correspondence courses, telephone reassurance programs, peer-group support systems, and informal support groups of family members and friends who serve as caregivers. Such strategies supplement the direct one-to-one involvement of human service professionals, such as social workers, rehabilitation teachers, and O&M specialists, and actively promote basic adult learning principles. These methods encourage older people to participate as equals in the rehabilitation process and urge self-direction and the pragmatic utilization of life experiences and common sense. In addition, the therapeutic potential of the self-help approach is its ability to encourage people to overcome their sense of powerlessness and to use their strengths to resolve problems through the support of others in similar circumstances (Suler, 1984).

Gartner (Gartner & Reissman, 1977), cofounder of the National Self-Help Clearing House in New York City, described the role of a self-help group as bringing peers together to provide mutual assistance and to satisfy a common need. People identify with a reliable support network and accept the role of helper. Each member gains through this mutual-aid group model.

SELF-HELP GROUPS FOR VISUALLY IMPAIRED PEOPLE

Increasing numbers of peer-support and self-help groups for blind and visually impaired older persons have been documented by Orr (1990) in a review of innovative aspects of service delivery to this population. Peer-support groups were the most frequently reported innovative component of a rehabilitation agency's service to older visually impaired persons. One of the primary reasons for this frequency is the limited or zero cost of offering this service to clients and the enormous possible benefit for older people who might otherwise be isolated. The service may require the use of agency or community space and only an hour a week of a staff person's time until an indigenous leader emerges. Increasingly, agencies for blind persons are working cooperatively with agencies for elderly persons, particularly senior citizens centers, when establishing peer-support groups. Many self-help groups for visually impaired older persons are held in senior centers rather than agencies for blind persons to facilitate the older person's integration into center and community life.

The Vision Foundation, founded in 1970, is a consumer-based service in Boston that sponsors a dozen self-help groups (Winer, 1982). A typical vision support group involves 8 to 15 people with various degrees of vision loss who meet regularly at a convenient location. The discussions tend to center on such questions as, "Can anyone understand how I really feel?" "How are others with similar problems coping?" "How can I reach out for professional help when I have been self-sufficient for 60 or more years?" "Isn't rehabilitation for those who are totally blind?" "Is rehabilitation assistance like welfare?" "Is it just for those who can be trained to work?" "Should I go into a nursing home?" and "How will I ever be able to live independently?"

The agency's support groups rarely rely on a professional counselor, but the value of the group meetings through the personal contacts is immeasurable. This approach reflects Suler's (1984) characterization of a self-help group as combining egalitarianism, grass-roots decision making, and the ability to change oneself by one's own efforts.

VISIONS/Services for the Blind and Visually Impaired in New York City initiated a model of service delivery for older visually impaired persons in the late 1960s. The model brought groups of older visually impaired persons to a local senior center to help them get integrated into the activities of the center and the community. A key component was a support group meeting in the morning, before center activities began. The support groups helped the members deal with issues related to vision loss and being visually impaired in a sighted setting, as well as the psychosocial aspects of the aging process (Orr, 1985).

A more formal approach of the Senior Blind Program at the Michigan State Commission for the Blind is through a mutual self-help group for elderly blind persons working in conjunction with a rehabilitation professional (Byers-Lang, 1984). This program uses volunteer peer counselors over age 55 who are legally blind who work under the professional guidance and supervision of a rehabilitation teacher. The rehabilitation teacher provides training in adjustment-related skills and coordination of efforts among agencies, other professionals, and basic counseling services (Byers-Lang, 1984). After a six-month training program, the volunteer peer workers are expected to demonstrate a knowledge of counseling in terms of understanding and applying the skills of listening, facilitating, and general helping behavior. The monthly group meetings are managed by the peer counselors and may include films and lectures on eye diseases, low vision, audiology, devices and appliances, Library of Congress services, Talking Books, and labeling and shopping techniques. This program brings together rehabilitation teachers and service providers from Michigan-area agencies on aging who promote the self-help groups by providing radio announcements, features in local newspapers, staff involvement at meetings, and the peer counselors who serve as role models. These individuals pool their skills, energy, and time to provide emotional support and pragmatic help to newly visually impaired older people.

In addition to the replication of ideas and materials from such programs as the Vision Foundation and the Senior Blind Program, one tool that may be useful in establishing self-help groups is the American Foundation for the Blind's *What Are Friends For?*, a self-help/peer discussion program in which older persons work together to identify needs, modify physical and social environments, and compensate for the loss of one sense through better use of another. Additional materials can be obtained from the Self-Help Clearing House in New York City, which also provides information on local chapters and regional self-help clearinghouses, and from the U.S. Department of Health and Human Services (1980).

SELF-STUDY

Closely related to the concept of self-help is that of private and individual self-study. Here the degree of professional input can also vary tremendously. Self-help publications in the form of hints and how-to booklets, resource-access manuals, and other initiative-oriented products are increasingly available and can be used by older persons at their own pace and time, with or without help from family members or friends. Self-study publications often help dispel the myths and stereotypes of what it means to be old and blind.

Roberts (1984) has emphasized the importance of positive biographies, autobiographies, and fictional works about blind people in his writings. These books can be useful tools to complement rehabilitation. A relevant biography often enhances the individual's adjustment to blindness. The reader may be relieved to learn that another blind person also felt isolated, helpless, and misunderstood by loved ones during the early stages of adjustment.

VISIONS/Services for the Blind and Visually Impaired, previously known as the Center for Independent Living, developed consumer self-study kits on sensory development, housekeeping skills, basic indoor mobility, and personal management. These kits are an effective alternative for those highly motivated older visually impaired persons who choose not to or are unable to attend a center-based rehabilitation facility because of poor health, multiple disabilities, a reluctance to leave their homes, or a desire to work independently at home rather than with a rehabilitation teacher at home. Each kit contains a large-print book and six cassette tapes in a format that gives clients an opportunity to gain a measure of control over their learning situation by using precise self-evaluation criteria for determining whether they have mastered a task.

The kits can be used by older people in the privacy of their own homes and at their own learning pace, with or without the help of family members or friends. They can also be used by professional rehabilitation teachers as backup material for homework purposes and by husband-and-wife teams working together. In addition, they have been aired on radio in rural settings, where services are sparse and older individuals are especially isolated.

For many years, the Hadley School for the Blind in Winnetka, Illinois, has provided students with general educational materials for use at home. The school has shown that the use of such materials, along with an 800 information and counseling telephone number, is a cost-effective means of personalized study. As a result of follow-up studies, Marshall (1979) of the Hadley School concluded that:

- Home study is convenient, flexible, and relatively inexpensive. It is not contingent on the students' physical presence or particular time schedule.
- Home study delivers motivation in a manner different from resident study but does so with a high degree of consistency.
- Home study measures the learning experience at frequent intervals, never allowing students to progress substantially without checking their understanding. Misunderstandings are discussed in writing, and "correct" responses are provided. No "learning gap" occurs in home study. After receiving "grades," students review any part of the curriculum for which a perfect score has not been achieved.
- Home study is personal, applied education. It is designed for immediate use and direct application and is totally practical.

The combination of self-study kits for use at home with access to a teacher via an 800 telephone number appears to offer the best of both worlds for some visually impaired persons. It allows independent study and immediate personalized professional feedback on progress that motivates clients to continue to learn additional skills.

Other self-study publications provide clear, basic descriptions of specific eye diseases and disorders and step-by-step ways of tackling everyday tasks (such as how to pour a cup of coffee without relying entirely on remaining vision and without scalding oneself). They are useful not only for familiarizing older people and their informal support groups with available services and resources but also for stimulating and encouraging them to reach out for self-help and professional services. However, a far broader range of easy-to-use self-help materials for visually impaired consumers is still urgently needed; and more effective access, independent utilization, and dissemination methods must be devised.

GROUP THERAPY BY TELEPHONE

The written or taped word may be helpful to some older visually impaired persons, but others need a more personalized approach. The telephone can play a vital role in the rehabilitation process, especially for older multiply disabled persons who are homebound, people who live in isolated rural areas, and those who are not ready for face-to-face contact. A study conducted by the U.S. Veterans Administration in Washington State (Evans & Jauregy, 1982) examined the benefits of a short-term outreach program of group telephone therapy for elderly visually impaired veterans. It found group therapy useful in helping clients learn to cope with conflicts in interpersonal relations, feelings of agitation and depression, social withdrawal and inactivity, mismanagement of personal and family affairs, and a reported sense of loneliness.

The program involved groups of three clients plus a counselor who were scheduled for eight weekly one-hour telephone conference calls. Nondirective counseling was abandoned in favor of more aggressive, cognitive behavioral techniques. Evans and Jauregy (1982) noted that clients were better able to articulate the practical needs that would improve their quality of life and to handle the fears of continued visual deterioration with support from friends and family.

EDUCATION PROGRAMS VIA RADIO

Opportunities for self-help and self-study are as limitless as the human imagination. The use of the radio is an open-entry option in rehabilitation in which the older person is invisible to peers or professionals. Radio education programs that offer hints for dealing with vision problems and descriptions of available rehabilitation services enable older visually impaired persons to select what they need from their own problem-centered perspective and feel a sense of control over their learning. In addition, such an open-entry system eliminates the red tape of bureaucracies and the perceived stigma of being labeled legally blind.

An interesting experiment in public education via the radio was the Center for Independent Living's radio drama series, "Martha Tobias," initially aired in 1984 in New York City and disseminated through National Radio Reading Services. The series depicted an older woman in the early stages of visual loss. Each program was a 15-minute drama followed by an in-studio panel discussion of consumers and professionals. The series was designed to create an interest in and understanding of visual impairment and to explore the myths and prejudices related to aging and vision loss.

Changes in Formal Support Systems

At the opposite end of the self-help spectrum is political lobbying, which, as the Gray Panthers have shown, is an effective force that should not be ignored. Ideally, the older population will ultimately demand changes in the inadequate rehabilitation service system. So far, however, fiery political rhetoric and well-intentioned commitments to the problems of such forgotten groups as older visually impaired people have not eliminated the bureaucratic tangles and hurdles that continue to plague the effective delivery of services.

Year after year, the use of definitions related to occupation and economic status as a basis for analyzing problems and determining action has contributed directly to a massive cover-up of the problem of continuing to use legal blindness as the criterion for eligibility for rehabilitation. For example, many older people are functionally visually impaired but not legally blind. The answers to such apparently straightforward questions as "How blind is blind?" and "How many elderly people are there with disabilities?" obviously depend on how the terms are defined and who defines them. In many states, an individual must be legally blind to receive rehabilitation services. Even though the older person may be functionally impaired, unable to cook safely or travel independently, and, therefore, at risk of personal injury, the legal definition of blindness is still used as a primary criterion for determining eligibility for comprehensive rehabilitation services.

And then comes the second catch—rehabilitation services have historically been vocationally oriented. Only one piece of legislation, Title VII, Part C, specifically targets independent living skills training to older visually impaired persons in their own homes and communities. Only 28 states received Title VII, Part C funds in 1990 at a rate of approximately $200,000 per state. This minimal allocation continued in 1991. That amount does not allow all eligible older visually impaired persons in a state to receive the rehabilitation services they deserve. Although vocational rehabilitation also includes rehabilitation for "homemaker" status (that is, persons who are heads of households or who have major responsibilities in their homes or who live alone and can perform all aspects of household management), older persons are frequently given lower priority for receiving these services or are ineligible for them. They are also typically assigned lower priority to receive vocational rehabilitation services to help them obtain remunerative employment, in spite of the growing numbers of older persons interested in remaining in or reentering the work force.

Is there an unspoken hope here that a confusing numbers game of measurements of visual acuity and an emphasis on the economically nonproductive nature of elderly citizens will eventually cause most of those in need of services to allow themselves to depend on others for assistance in daily activities or to be absorbed into long-term care institutions and nursing homes? The costs in terms of massive institutional funding, the waste of human resources, and the diminution of human values are far greater than our society can bear and will increase alarmingly as the elderly population expands. Rehabilitation, though, is a cost-effective, humanitarian alternative.

Options must be explored for a highly flexible system of community-based services that are efficient and cost-effective. New and innovative sources of financial support for adaptive equipment, transportation, home medical visits, part-time nursing care, in-home rehabilitation services, and low vision devices (not currently covered by Medicare or Medicaid) must be explored. Less costly options to institutionalization must be designed.

Long-Term Residential Care

Another system ripe for overhaul is that of long-term residential care. The traditional attitudes of providers that encourage dependence not only perpetuate the institutionalized climate of most facilities but eliminate the last semblances of independence, self-respect, and personal initiative in elderly people. Although dramatic new medical developments may, within a decade or two, substantially change society's perception and experience of aging, the rapidly increasing size of the over-85 population will tend to maintain the demand for long-term care facilities at least in the foreseeable future. Hence, improvements and changes must be made within the system as well as options outside the nursing home system. Emphasis must be placed on new and innovative living options, an improved climate for the care of patients by staff members who are trained to maximize each resident's potential for independence and dignity, and improved linkages among institutions, all external providers of care, and informal community groups. In-service training and workshops on special topics should be conducted by rehabilitation teachers and O&M specialists for the staffs of all institutions that serve visually disabled and multiply impaired residents. In addition, the environments of such institutions should be revitalized to facilitate spatial orientation and mobility and to encourage the functional independence of residents.

Such a framework for a new era of long-term residential care will be based not on the old attitude that facilities are repositories but on a fresh recognition of the potential for living of residents who choose such options. It will encourage a more balanced provision of rehabilitation and medical services and stimulate residents' participation in monitoring their own care and perhaps in managing the facility.

Senior Citizens Centers

Thousands of senior citizens centers across the country provide invaluable socialization and support services to older visually impaired people. Such services often include hot meals, personal counseling, recreational activities, help with entitlements, counseling, assistance with housing problems, crisis intervention, and specialized services for frail, disabled, or special-needs groups. Many centers offer Meals-on-Wheels to the homebound and provide home health care and home care through home-health aides, home attendants, housekeepers, and volunteer visitors and senior companions. Senior centers are in a prime position to provide resources and referrals to elderly people who experience functional difficulties because of visual impairment. Although service providers in senior centers do not always have as much information about services for visually impaired persons as they need, the framework exists as a basis for further expansion and improvements through in-service training.

The key elements are cooperation and coordination not only among the networks of agencies, centers, and facilities but among members of the various professional disciplines who serve the elderly population. Whenever possible, "segregated" facilities, such as senior citizens centers, long-term care facilities, agencies for visually impaired and blind persons, optometric centers, and adult education centers, must recognize the benefits of networking, of sharing activities and personnel, and of introducing those they serve to other vital resources, including sources of information and support mechanisms.

Rehabilitation personnel particularly must leave the confines of the specialized environments of agencies for visually impaired and blind persons and reach out to other service providers in settings where older people choose to spend their leisure time. They need to be accessible and visible to their potential clients by working in local senior citizens centers, storefront agencies, and local health services facilities. Local adult education programs can also play a vital role by familiarizing families and informal care groups with the normal aging process, the concepts of the rehabilitation model versus the medical care model of service delivery, and specific in-home strategies for self-help and nondependent adjustment to disabilities.

The integration of professional service agencies with social support facilities and senior citizens centers has the potential to provide the basis of major improvements in the roles and effectiveness of both groups. Together, these agencies and centers could implement volunteer buddy outreach networks to respond to the varied needs of at-risk groups, primarily homebound multiply disabled persons and those over age 85 who live alone. Self-help groups can be initiated for older disabled individuals and members of their informal support groups. Emergency and protective care systems, such as telephone reassurance services, friendly visiting, crime prevention, emergency in-home alarm systems, parent abuse and neglect services, information and referral networks, and crisis intervention counseling, can be developed, ideally by providers of services to elderly persons and those serving visually impaired persons working in partnership. Together, these professionals would have the influence to alert local community leaders to potential sources of funding (private, state, and federal) and to convince elected officials that the problems of elderly people, especially the visually impaired or otherwise disabled, require immediate attention, particularly in the area of improved rehabilitation services.

Conclusion

Stereotyped images that correlate aging with senility and retirement with lethargic and homebound nonproductivity do little to increase the self-respect of elderly people or encourage them to draw attention to their concerns and promote their interests and independence. Inevitably, images become reality; as the independence and social value of elderly people decrease, their need for institutional and other supports increases, and the financial burden they pose to family and society rises dramatically.

The informal care group of family, friends, and neighbors was the primary support network for ailing individuals in the community long before the advent of social service systems and their trained professionals. However, as the extended family and the informal system weakened, isolation became a primary social problem, and tax disincentives and publicly funded care systems that increase general dependence exacerbated the decline of family and community initiatives. It is ironic that the overall direct and indirect costs of perpetuating this syndrome of dependence are far higher than the costs that would be produced by a total overhaul of current practices and the development of strategies to promote independence, self-help, and personal dignity among older people. Such a reversal of attitudes and policies requires the combined efforts of consumers, informal care groups, and formal service agencies working to create opportunities for rehabilitation for all elderly persons and particularly those with disabilities.

If the needs of this forgotten majority are to be adequately met, efforts must be made at the local, state, and national levels to restimulate grass-roots support. The reluctance of elderly visually impaired people to accept existing minimal formal services may suggest that informal systems coupled with self-help materials and strategies might be an alternative means of serving some individuals. Contemporary societal trends encourage a wider variety of life-styles, open-access systems, informal networks, and easier life change potentials. Elderly people are becoming more aware of their ability to control their own situations, and they resent the intrusion of service systems that create dependence.

In such a climate of rapid social change, the informal network could be much more important. In preparation for such changes, professionals need to broaden their perspectives, increase their networking abilities, and cross professional boundaries to work alongside other service providers whose activities complement the rehabilitation process. They must expand their outreach activities by developing and implementing public education strategies via the printed and spoken word and through cable television and radio. They must become skilled in presenting simple, straightforward descriptions of the smorgasbord of services available to older visually impaired individuals, in helping older persons choose what is most relevant to their personal needs, and in creating a continuum of rehabilitation services that utilize both formal and informal resources. The use of radio education, the preparation of hints and how-to booklets, and the establishment of self-help groups and peer-helping-peer systems are all vital options in the expanding field of nontraditional services.

In the near future it is unlikely that personnel or economic resources will be sufficient for each older visually impaired person to receive needed rehabilitation services. Therefore, professionals must be innovative. They must disseminate information through a host of new and effective methods based on sharing knowledge, lessening the barriers between service providers and clients, and trusting older people to accept responsibility for their learning. Professionals must advance the principles of self-help and adult learning and become actively involved in lobbying for services for older people. Even though they may be behind the scenes, professionals have crucial roles as liaisons between the traditional and nontraditional systems—improving the legislative and community framework of the formal care system, serving as consultants and advisers in planning and implementing programs and services, and initiating and developing new and cost-effective programs that enable elderly consumers to decide their needs for rehabilitation.

The future looks promising if consumers and professionals in the fields of aging and rehabilitation pursue goals and work as partners in teaching and learning to increase the independence, life satisfaction, and dignity of all older visually impaired persons. There is no doubt that increased longevity, improved health care, and a debunking of the myths of the inevitable traumas of aging have heightened the potential power of elderly people and led them to expect improved services. We need more changes responsive to the growing and diversifying needs of older visually impaired persons. The ideas and opportunities are in place. Genuine intent and strong efforts are needed.

References

Anarem Systems Research Corporation. (1978). *Evaluation study of the New York Infirmary/Center for Independent Living.* New York: Center for Independent Living.

Byers-Lang, R. (1984). Network builders for elderly persons. *Journal of Visual Impairment & Blindness,* 78(5): 193-197.

Cantor, M. H. (1975). *The formal and informal support system of older New Yorkers.* Paper presented at the Symposium on Aging. The city: A viable environment for the elderly?, Jerusalem.

Evans, R. L., & Jauregy, B. M. (1982). Phone therapy outreach for blind elderly. *The Gerontologist, 22:* 32-35.

Gartner, A., & Reissman, F. (1977). *Self-help in the human services.* San Francisco: Jossey-Bass.

Marshall, C. (1979). *The Effectiveness of Home Study.* Chicago: La Salle Extension University.

Mummah, H. R. (1975). Group work with aged blind Japanese in the nursing home and in the community. *New Outlook for the Blind, 69*(4): 160-167.

Orr, A. L. (1985). Dealing with the death of a group member: Visually impaired elderly in the community (p. 315-332). In A. Gitterman & L. Shulman (Eds.), *Mutual Aid Groups and the Life Cycle.* Itasca, IL: Peacock.

Orr, A. L. (1990). *Innovative models of service delivery to older blind and visually impaired persons.* Unpublished paper.

Roberts, A. L. (1984). Bibliotherapy: A technique for counseling blind people. *Journal of Visual Impairment & Blindness, 78*(5): 197-199.

Suler, J. (1984). The role of ideology in self-help groups. *Social Policy, 14:* 29-36.

Toseland, R. W., & Hacker, L. (1982). Self-help groups and professional involvement. *Social Work, 27:* 341-347.

U.S. Department of Health and Human Services. (1980). *A guide to medical self-care and self-help groups for the elderly.* Washington, DC: U.S. Government Printing Office.

Winer, M. (1982). Self-help programs for people with sight loss. *Journal of Visual Impairment & Blindness, 76*(10): 393-397.

CHAPTER 15

The Future of Collaborative Planning and Service Delivery

Alberta L. Orr

As previous chapters in this book have indicated, an increasing number of older persons experience vision loss each decade, and concurrently, a growing percentage of the population of blind persons is age 65 and over. As a result, service providers in the fields of aging and blindness encounter older visually impaired persons who need services from both service delivery systems. To provide comprehensive programs to this special population, each service provider must understand

- what the older visually impaired person needs,
- how the older visually impaired person fits into the service delivery system,
- what services are available through the "other" service delivery system,
- how to make referrals to that system,
- how to establish a cooperative working relationship with an agency or agencies in the other system,
- how to plan collaboratively for this rapidly growing population and its changing and diverse needs, and
- how to deliver coordinated services.

In the 1990s, too few collaborative models exist between the aging and blindness fields. Many factors inhibit the establishment of working relationships between the two systems. A primary reason is that service providers in both fields frequently lack a working knowledge of the other service delivery system. Before effective collaborative planning and service delivery can occur, factors inhibiting the conceptualization and implementation of collaborative efforts must be understood and overcome. This chapter outlines the barriers to collaborative service delivery, reviews existing examples of collaborative efforts between the systems, suggests possibilities for further networking, and calls for formal mechanisms for coordinated planning and programming to grow out of federal, state, and locally initiated efforts.

Before a service provider can understand the role and function of the "other" service delivery system working on behalf of an older visually impaired client, it is important for that service provider to understand his or her own role and responsibility toward the client. Questions accompanying the increase in the population of older persons experiencing vision loss have been: "To whom does this older visually impaired person belong?" "Whose responsibility is she?" "Is the older visually impaired person primarily a client of the blindness agency and secondarily a client of an aging organization, or vice versa?"

An older person who is visually impaired needs to be viewed holistically rather than categorically; that is, he or she must be seen first and foremost as an individual rather than as someone who is defined by age, disability, or any other single characteristic. To which service delivery system does an older visually impaired person belong? The answer is to both. What the older visually impaired person needs first or most or concurrently is based on individual experiences of aging and sensory impairment. What he or she needs is also based on his or her perceived or expressed need or that of a family member, if the older person is less able to determine this independently. The primary goals related to collaborative planning and service delivery are that the older visually impaired person is aware that services are available from both systems, that he or she has access to them, that he or she has options, and that he or she receives coordinated comprehensive services as needed.

Older visually impaired persons represent a special population in both service delivery systems. Service providers in both systems have not been accustomed to serving this group. They have also had limited opportunities for education or training regarding the needs and issues of this population. Some have a limited understanding that it is their responsibility to serve older visually impaired persons. Many service providers believe that older visually impaired clients must belong to the other service delivery system by virtue of disability or age.

It is common for a social worker at an agency for elderly people to refer a visually impaired person to a blindness agency for home care or housekeeping services on the belief that these services must be available through the blindness system. However, the blindness agency will inform the client that these services are not available through the blindness system because the need for these services is based on generic functional limitations, not on blindness specifically. The client is referred back to the aging network, frequently through the area agency on aging (AAA). The frustrated client may just stop there and not pursue services, believing that assistance is unavailable or just too difficult to obtain. This older visually impaired client then "falls between the cracks" of both systems, while service providers from both systems feel they have each referred the client appropriately and that he or she will receive the help needed.

It is important to note that one of the primary reasons why service providers in aging may make such a referral to the blindness system is the scarcity of these services to meet the growing demand. They hope that if the service is available through the disability network, then it will lessen the burden on the aging network. However, if the agencies in the two systems worked together in a referral and service delivery process, the likelihood of the client's failing to receive any services at all would be greatly diminished. The prevailing lack of knowledge regarding roles, responsibilities, and how other systems work sets up barriers to working together. Collaboration on the delivery of services has tremendous potential toward the amelioration of this problem. Although there are examples of collaborative planning and service provision throughout the country for this special population, many more are needed, and information about successful models must be disseminated to educate others.

Barriers to Collaborative Service Delivery

A variety of barriers may prevent or impede the blind and visually impaired older population from utilizing the services of the aging system.

These barriers may be psychological or environmental. The community-based aging system has historically used a prevention model and has primarily served well elderly persons. Although the focus has shifted to include impaired elderly individuals, many at-risk groups remain underserved. The special populations of older persons that have been prioritized are those with the greatest political clout and those for which special funds exist, such as Alzheimer's patients and the developmentally disabled elderly population. Blind and visually impaired older persons, in particular, have not been a service priority of the aging field at the national or federal level.

Negative attitudes or intimidation on the part of staff members of agencies for the elderly population are also key barriers to service delivery. Many staff members assume that visually impaired clients require too much assistance to be integrated successfully into their agency's operation. Others believe that they are not adequately prepared to serve these clients and that too many additional staff hours will be necessary. Some staff also feel threatened by the notion that blind clients, particularly in senior citizens centers, are too great an insurance risk, believing that blind people will have more falls and greater injuries that will result in higher insurance premiums. Finally, many agency personnel simply believe that blind persons are incompetent and dependent (Hill & Harley, 1984; Horowitz & Cassels, 1985; New York Association for the Blind, 1985).

A statewide survey of the AAAs and agencies for blind persons was conducted in Pennsylvania to identify unmet service needs, facilitators, and barriers to service delivery to blind and visually impaired elderly persons (Biegel, Petchers, Snyder, & Beisgin, 1989). Survey results reflect the need for improved understanding of the requirements, resources, and areas of expertise of each system, with better communications between the systems being particularly important. The survey presents several strategies for ongoing interaction between the two networks.

One approach is to hold a series of statewide or regional workshops to bring together workers in the aging and blindness networks. Another more comprehensive strategy for state units on aging and state blindness agencies is to explore the feasibility of state and local agreements to enhance service delivery. The approach should be formal and contractual. Such a mechanism exists in Florida, for example, between the Florida Department of Aging and the Florida State Division of Blind Services. The two agencies developed a comprehensive cooperative agreement spelling out referral procedures and training sessions for state liaison personnel in a basic philosophy regarding cooperative service delivery. These agreements serve the following purposes: (1) to identify blind and visually impaired elderly persons as a high-priority service population, (2) to coordinate planning and efficient use of resources, (3) to improve understanding of the roles and responsibilities of each service system, and (4) to identify areas of agency-to-agency strengths, weaknesses, expertise, and resources in each system.

The state unit on aging can also encourage joint activities at the local level between the aging and blindness systems, such as contractual relationships, needs assessments, service planning, in-service training, joint projects and services, shared staff, and advocacy and outreach activities. These contractual interdepartmental agreements often serve as a stimulus and incentive for such activities. Discretionary funds from state offices on aging and blindness can fund innovative local model projects. Conversely, local agencies that fail to meet interagency requirements mandated by the state agreement could be penalized.

One potential problem that threatens long-term success in interagency efforts is the difference in how the aging and blindness systems perceive the relative importance of blind and visually impaired elderly persons as clients. As documented in the Pennsylvania survey, the majority of clients of agencies for the blind are elderly, although only a small percentage of clients at the AAAs are blind and visually impaired. The study documented 6 percent in this latter category, although the national average of older visually impaired persons is between 10 and 12 percent of the aging population. Therefore, the service needs of blind and visually impaired clients are frequently too far down on the list of priorities for agencies in the aging network, if only because of the small number of older visually impaired persons known to agencies in this system. Little or no thought is given to the potential number of older visually impaired persons not identified by the agency.

Another problem relates to the conflicting demands on aging agencies to prioritize services for a number of at-risk populations, including mentally ill persons, deaf persons, and persons with developmental disabilities or Alzheimer's disease. Service providers in the aging network find it difficult to respond to these competing requests because of limited fiscal resources to serve all elderly persons.

One essential element is accurate data gathered through improved data collection strategies to determine the number of older blind and visually impaired persons in the country in order to document the need for services from the aging network. Data from the U.S. Bureau of the Census more than likely represent a serious undercount of the real number of older blind and visually impaired persons. States vary widely in data collection mechanisms, but statewide registries of all low vision and blind persons would help provide better data for the planning of needed service programs. Data collection strategies should also establish more unified, universally agreed on definitions of blindness and visual impairment. The most appropriate descriptions of vision loss among older persons are "severe visual impairment," or difficulty reading newspaper print, and "low vision," or vision loss severe enough to interfere with the activities of daily living. State-level demographic surveys of the elderly population should also include questions about blindness and visual impairment if the field hopes to have an accurate picture of the numbers of persons needing services.

Collaborative Efforts at the Federal, State, and Local Levels

Most examples of effective collaboration between the aging and the blindness fields are observable on the local level. They are usually the result of the efforts of a creative worker in the blindness or the aging field who seeks services for a visually impaired elderly client that are more comprehensive than are those available from one service network. This individual effort may lead to an agency-to-agency effort to coordinate services so that future clients have easy access to both service systems. As each of the agency's staff members learns more about the workings of both service delivery systems, clients obtain improved access to needed services.

It is even more important for the need for collaborative service delivery to be recognized at the federal level. Although the Older Americans Act (OAA) technically makes service providers in the field of aging responsible for serving all older persons, it does not specifically mandate targeted service delivery to the older visually impaired population. At the time of the reauthorization of the OAA of 1988, advocates for the older blind and visually impaired population prepared appropriate language to be incorporated into the legislation. The result, however, was simply a list of the disabled and special populations of older persons, including the visually impaired elderly population that were to be served, unaccompanied by prescriptions or mandates for the delivery of services. It is to be hoped that future reauthorization will target services for special populations among elderly persons.

Administration on Aging Priority: Collaboration Between the Aging and Blindness Networks

A major incentive for agencies to implement a new service model is the funding available to do so. One way to establish the visually impaired population as a service priority at the federal level would be the formulation by the Administration on Aging (AOA) of a priority area to fund demonstration projects that would establish models of collaborative planning and service delivery between agencies for the elderly and for the visually impaired. The models could be statewide or regional demonstration models that could be replicated in other parts of the country. The American Foundation for the Blind has prepared the framework for such a priority area and submitted it to AOA for consideration in the next round of funding through its Coordinated Discretionary Grants Program. The priority area is under consideration for a future request for proposals.

Precedents exist in federal funding from AOA for collaboration between the two service fields. One such collaborative effort exists in the area of services to developmentally disabled older persons. A large number of developmentally disabled persons are "aging in place" in the homes of their families. They, too, need to be integrated into the mainstream of aging services. In 1990, an AOA priority area called for proposals to develop AOA/Administration on Developmental Disabilities state and local planning linkages to improve services to older persons with developmental disabilities.

In the late 1980s and early 1990s, AOA developed many memoranda of understanding between AOA and other federal agencies. As another strategy, AOA might develop a memorandum of understanding or a cooperative agreement with the Rehabilitation Services Administration (RSA) to create models to serve older visually impaired persons through collaborative planning. Such an agreement at the federal level would filter down to the state agencies and the localities on behalf of this population.

There are structural parallels between the aging and the blindness fields beginning at the federal level (AOA and RSA) that can serve as central points for collaborative planning. Each state has a state unit on aging as well as a state rehabilitation agency. Each state, however, does not have a separate rehabilitation agency that serves blind persons; some state rehabilitation agencies for the blind are absorbed within a general vocational rehabilitation agency. Nevertheless, 37 states have a separate state agency for the blind that could establish state-level linkages with the aging network calling for collaborative relationships at the state and local levels. Even those state blindness services that are part of generic vocational rehabilitation agencies can enter this type of relationship. Local agencies for elderly people can work either with the local office of the state agency for the blind or a private, nonprofit agency serving blind persons.

Collaborative Agreements Among National Organizations

Collaborative efforts and agreements are also important among national organizations in the blindness and aging fields. In 1988, the National Association of State Units on Aging and the National Council of State Agencies for the Blind established a memorandum of understanding because of their mutual advocacy and programmatic mission to enhance the independence, dignity, and well-being of the nation's older persons who are blind or visually impaired. The national associations agreed to work collaboratively at the national and state levels for policies and programs to protect the rights and benefits of all vulnerable older persons; enhance the development of a responsive, community-based, long-term care system for all vulnerable older persons; work toward the enhancement of a health care system that protects and maximizes the remaining vision of its clients; and expand opportunities for continued meaningful participation in all aspects of society by all older persons, including blind and visually impaired persons.

The organizations agreed to accomplish their advocacy goals cooperatively through the following activities:

1. developing effective public education campaigns to increase the level of awareness of the needs of the elderly blind and visually impaired population;
2. initiating joint efforts to ensure appropriate access to services, entitlements, and benefits by older visually impaired persons;
3. formulating and implementing professional development and training efforts between the two networks on both the state and national levels;
4. collecting and exchanging model state policies and regulations and best practice programmatic information to serve the needs of elderly blind and visually impaired persons.

In the early 1990s, however, many public and private service providers at the state and local levels still do not know enough about what they regard as the "other" service delivery system. A great deal more collaborative planning and service delivery must take place to implement written collaborative agreements and thereby make proposals for coordinated service delivery a reality.

Impact of Funding

Today, service providers in both fields struggle to be proactive in the development of innovative models of programs and services. Many continue simply to react to crises or to demands created by the proliferating needs of older people. One thing is certain in both fields. New funding opportunities for innovative service delivery or for the delivery of services to special populations drive directors of agencies to develop creative service models and to apply for funds to initiate these models.

A recent review of the blindness service delivery system was conducted to determine the level of collaboration and to identify new service delivery models (Orr, 1990). Survey questionnaires were sent to 283 blindness rehabilitation agencies throughout the country. Forty percent responded (113 agencies). Twenty-three of the respondents reported some collaboration with the aging field. Twelve of the 23 respondents reported providing an aspect of service to older blind and visually impaired persons through special project funds from the local AAA. These funds usually paid for a needs assessment of the older blind and visually impaired population; in-service training between the two service delivery fields; or a service such as a peer support group for older visually impaired persons at a local aging organization, such as a senior citizens center, rather than an agency for the blind. The key to further success in current projects is the dissemination of information about these collaborative efforts so they can be replicated and modified appropriately in other states and cities.

The idea suggested earlier for AOA to fund collaborative demonstration programs could be set up so that funds would be awarded only to those organizations successfully showing clear mechanisms for collaboration between the aging and blindness systems. Another strategy at the national level might be to require that all state blindness agencies funded by Title VII, Part C demonstrate how they will collaborate with state and local agencies for elderly people. A similar mechanism could be established within the OAA to mandate that state units on aging and AAAs show how they work with state and local agencies for blind persons on behalf of blind and visually impaired elderly clients. Another possibility is for the OAA to mandate that state and area plans include strategies for service delivery to the visually impaired elderly population with input from blindness agencies and visually impaired consumers.

Although collaborative efforts should be initiated from both fields, it may be easier for the initiative to come from the blindness field because the aging field is confronted by so many special populations with special needs, each clamoring for targeted services and integration into the mainstream of aging services. Directors and key staff of agencies for blind persons must join a local interagency council or group addressing the needs of older persons so they can become more closely associated with the aging service organizations and key service providers. These interagency networks are almost always present in the local community or county and represent service providers in the field of aging and ancillary services. Some interorganizational groups represent the aging and disability network at large, but far too frequently the blindness system is not represented. Through joint participation in these groups, service providers learn more about each organization and about accessing services and work toward collaborative efforts to maximize existing resources, particularly during tough fiscal times.

In this era of fiscal constraint, service providers across disciplines throughout the country continually seek ways to improve and expand services by maximizing resources. Increasing needs for services emerge for many subgroups of the overall population. In light of the current and projected number of older persons living longer and experiencing multiple problems, it is becoming increasingly difficult to serve these clients without cross-disciplinary efforts across many systems. It is to be hoped that collaborative efforts described in this chapter will inspire service providers at all levels to "think collaboration" and then to implement collaborative service delivery models.

References

Biegel, D. E., Petchers, M. K., Snyder, A., & Beisgin, B. (1989). Unmet needs and barriers to service delivery for the blind and visually impaired elderly. *The Gerontologist, 29*(1): 86-91.

Hill, M. M., & Harley, R. K. (1984). Orientation and mobility for aged visually impaired persons. *Journal of Visual Impairment & Blindness, 78*(2): 49-54.

Horowitz, A., & Cassels, I. (1985). *Vision education and outreach: Identifying and serving the visually impaired elderly.* New York: New York Association for the Blind.

New York Association for the Blind, National Center for Vision and Aging. (1985). *Vision impairment and aging: Targeting resources for consumers, clinicians and the aging network.* New York: Author.

Orr, A. L. (1990). *Innovative models of service delivery to older blind and visually impaired persons.* Unpublished paper.

Epilogue

Alberta L. Orr

In the coming decades, publicly funded programs and organizations will not be able to meet the needs of all older persons. Partnerships between public and private efforts within service delivery systems and across systems are needed, especially during these times of fiscal scarcity, to meet the increasing demand for services caused by the surging growth of the older population. The private sector's involvement in providing services to the elderly population is expanding rapidly. The U.S. Administration on Aging is calling for increased partnerships in the aging field; the blindness field must follow suit. Developments in the housing, health care, technology, insurance, and travel industries are giving rise to a plethora of services and products designed for the older consumer through the private arena. The growth of professional specializations such as geriatric case management and elder law and of new consumer products designed to facilitate the independent living of an increasingly frail and disabled older population illustrates the private sector's involvement with older consumers. The vast diversity of the older population and of the older visually impaired population will demand public-private partnerships within the blindness field and among the blindness and aging and ancillary fields. As we move toward the 21st century, we must work as agents for change to create a political and legislative agenda that will result in improved service planning and delivery on behalf of older persons who are visually impaired.

   In the decades to come, the demographics of aging must increasingly dictate public policy on behalf of the older population and the older disabled population; in many cases, new legislation will be called for, particularly during the cyclical reauthorization years of the primary federal legislation relating to aging and to blindness, the Older Americans Act and the Rehabilitation Act, respectively. In many other instances, changes in societal awareness and values will be the necessary element in forcing service delivery systems to become more accessible to all older persons and to those special populations, such as elderly visually impaired persons, who are at the greatest risk of losing their independence and experiencing a decline in quality of life unnecessarily. Whether in the area of legislative advocacy, public education, or service delivery, we will all have much to do.

RESOURCES

Services for blind and visually impaired people vary widely across the country, but assistance and information are available from a great number of sources. All states have departments of rehabilitation or commissions for the blind that can provide information on available services, including rehabilitation and independent living skills training, orientation and mobility (O&M) services, and low vision services and vision screening. In addition, each state has a state agency, department, or office responsible for state programs for older people funded by the Older Americans Act, and each county or group of counties has an area agency on aging (AAA) that will know about the availability of such programs as home-delivered meals, door-to-door transportation and escort services, and other services for elderly persons. Listings for these agencies can be found in the state and county government sections of local telephone directories.

Low vision evaluations are essential for helping people determine how to use their remaining vision to maximum advantage. Evaluations are available from low vision services, which can be found in such settings as hospitals, departments of ophthalmology at medical schools, and agencies for blind and visually impaired persons and which can also be obtained from some private practitioners. State and local agencies for blind and visually impaired persons can provide further information on sources of low vision services, as can the American Foundation for the Blind (AFB), whose address and telephone number are listed in the resource entries that follow.

Information and assistance are also available in regard to specific activities and areas. For example, the Library of Congress National Library Service (NLS) for the Blind and Physically Handicapped lends books on cassette and disk and in braille free of charge through a network of regional and subregional libraries across the country; information on how to enroll in this program can be obtained from NLS, which is listed in this resource section, or from local libraries. A great variety of large-print books and audiocassettes is also available commercially, and *The Complete Directory of Large Print Books and Serials* and *Words on Cassette*, both published by the R.R. Bowker Company in New Providence, New Jersey, provide a comprehensive listing.

Additional information about visual impairment and living with visual impairment can be obtained from a large variety of resources. Many organizations on the national, state, and local levels provide information, assistance, and referrals; operate toll-free hotlines; and publish materials that are valuable sources of information for visually impaired people and their families. AFB acts as a national clearing-house for information about blindness and visual impairment and operates a toll-free national hotline. The services of national and regional consultants are also available from AFB. Many of the other organizations listed in this section can also be contacted for general information about visual impairment or for specific information about a particular eye condition and relevant services. A complete listing of local, state, and national agencies and organizations serving blind and visually impaired persons is included in the *Directory of Services for Blind and Visually Impaired Persons in the United States and Canada,* published by AFB.

National Organizations in the Blindness Field

American Council of the Blind
1155 15th Street, N.W., Suite 720
Washington, DC 20005
(202) 467-5081 or (800) 424-8666

The American Council of the Blind (ACB) is a consumer organization that acts as a national clearinghouse for information. It also provides referrals, legal assistance and representation, consumer advocacy support, and consultative and advisory services to individuals, organizations, and agencies.

American Diabetes Association
National Service Center
P.O. Box 25757
1600 Duke Street
Alexandria, VA 22313
(703) 549-1500

The American Diabetes Association (ADA) provides information on diabetes, and conducts public and professional education programs, and publishes a variety of materials on diabetes.

American Foundation for the Blind
11 Penn Plaza, Suite 300
New York, NY 10001
(212) 502-7600 or (800) 232-5463 (Hotline)

The American Foundation for the Blind (AFB) provides a wide variety of services for blind and visually impaired persons and their families, professionals, and organizations and agencies. In addition to promoting the development of services, advocating for legislation, and conducting informational and educational programs, AFB operates the M.C. Migel Memorial Library, a special reference library on blindness. It publishes books, monographs, pamphlets, and periodicals in print and in recorded and braille formats and provides information about the latest technology available for blind and visually impaired persons through its National Technology Center. It also manufactures Talking Books and operates a toll-free information hotline. AFB maintains the following offices across the country as well as a governmental relations group in Washington, DC.

Governmental Relations Group
820 1st Street, N.E.
Suite 400
Washington, DC 20002
(202) 408-0200

AFB Midwest
401 North Michigan Avenue
Suite 308
Chicago, IL 60611
(312) 245-9961

AFB Southeast
100 Peachtree Street
Suite 620
Atlanta, GA 30303
(404) 525-2303

AFB Southwest
260 Treadway Plaza
Exchange Park
Dallas, TX 75235
(214) 352-7222

AFB West
111 Pine Street
Suite 725
San Francisco, CA 94111
(415) 392-4845

American Printing House for the Blind
1839 Frankfort Avenue
Louisville, KY 40206
(502) 895-2405

The American Printing House for the Blind (APH) administers an annual appropriation from Congress to provide textbooks and educational aids for legally blind students. In addition, it publishes braille and recorded editions of Reader's Digest *and recorded editions of* Newsweek *for persons of all ages.*

Association for Education and Rehabilitation of the Blind and Visually Impaired
206 North Washington Street, Suite 320
Alexandria, VA 22314
(703) 548-1884

The Association for Education and Rehabilitation of the Blind and Visually Impaired (AER) is a professional membership organization that promotes all phases of education and work for blind and visually impaired persons of all ages. AER conducts conferences, publishes newsletters and a journal, and operates a reference information center. It also certifies rehabilitation teachers, O&M specialists, and classroom teachers.

Association for Macular Diseases
210 East 64th Street
New York, NY 10021
(212) 605-3719

The Association for Macular Diseases is an information service for people with macular diseases. It publishes a quarterly newsletter, maintains a hotline for its members, and conducts nationwide educational seminars on macular degeneration for the public.

Association of Radio Reading Services
c/o Elizabeth Young
WUSS Radio Reading Services
University of South Florida
WRB209
Tampa, FL 33620
(813) 974-4193

The Association of Radio Reading Services is a membership organization of radio reading services across the country, which broadcast parts or entire issues of local newspapers every day. The association provides information on services and broadcasts.

Audio Description, Inc.
The Metropolitan Washington Ear
35 University Boulevard East
Silver Spring, MD 20901
(301) 681-6636

The Metropolitan Washington Ear publishes a newsletter for individuals interested in audiodescription, the narration of visual aspects of live performances in theaters and of selected television programs. It also provides information on radio reading services throughout the country.

Blinded Veterans Association
477 H Street, N.W.
Washington, DC 20001-2694
(202) 371-8880

The Blinded Veterans Association (BVA) provides support and assistance to blind veterans to enable them to take advantage of rehabilitation and vocational training benefits, job placement services, and other aid from federal, state, and local resources.

Blind Rehabilitation Service
U.S. Department of Veterans Affairs
810 Vermont Avenue, N.W.

Washington, DC 20420
(202) 233-3232

The Blind Rehabilitation Service oversees programs for blinded veterans within the U.S. Department of Veterans Affairs. It operates Blind Rehabilitation Centers across the country that offer instruction in the use of specialized electronic travel aids, reading machines, and other technological devices.

Choice Magazine Listening
P.O. Box 10
Port Washington, NY 11050
(516) 883-8280

Choice Magazine *records a bimonthly anthology of selected articles, fiction, and poetry from current periodicals that is distributed by individual subscription or free of charge on cassette tape through the regional library system of the Library of Congress National Library Service for the Blind and Physically Handicapped.*

Descriptive Video Service
WGBH-TV
125 Western Avenue
Boston, MA 02134
(617) 492-2777

Descriptive Video Service (DVS) publishes a newsletter and provides information for individuals interested in descriptive video services available in theaters and on selected television programs.

Foundation for Glaucoma Research
490 Post Street, Suite 1042
San Francisco, CA 94102
(415) 986-3162

The Foundation for Glaucoma Research supports preventive efforts through research and education to eliminate blindness caused by glaucoma. It conducts professional and public education through publications, lectures, and conferences.

Hadley School for the Blind
700 Elm Street
Winnetka, IL 60093
(708) 446-8111

The Hadley School for the Blind offers 125 correspondence courses in braille and on cassette for legally blind persons. Courses include special programs on independent living for older blind and visually impaired persons.

Howe Press
Perkins School for the Blind
175 North Beacon Street
Watertown, MA 02172
(617) 924-3490

The Howe Press manufactures and sells materials and equipment for reproducing materials in braille, including the Perkins Brailler, slates and styli, handwriting aids, braille games and paper, and drawing supplies.

In Touch Networks
15 West 65th Street
New York, NY 10023
(212) 769-6270

In Touch Networks maintains a volunteer reading service that allows blind and physically impaired people to listen to readings of articles from more than 100 newspapers and magazines via closed-circuit radio.

Library of Congress
National Library Service for the
Blind and Physically Handicapped
1291 Taylor Street, N.W.
Washington, DC 20542
(202) 707-5100 or (800) 424-9100

The National Library Service (NLS) for the Blind and Physically Handicapped conducts a national program to distribute free reading materials in braille and on recorded disks and cassettes to visually impaired and physically disabled persons who cannot utilize ordinary printed materials.

Matilda Ziegler Magazine for the Blind
20 West 17th Street
New York, NY 10011
(212) 242-0263

The Matilda Ziegler Magazine for the Blind *is published in braille and on disk. It is a free monthly general-interest periodical sent to any visually impaired person requesting it.*

National Association for Visually Handicapped
22 West 21st Street
New York, NY 10010
(212) 889-3141

The National Association for Visually Handicapped (NAVH) produces and distributes large-print reading materials to schools, libraries, senior citizens centers, hospitals, and individuals on request; assists libraries and senior centers in establishing large-print libraries; acts as an information clearinghouse and referral center regarding resources available to persons with low vision; produces and distributes information about limited vision and low vision devices; and sells large-print books, magnifiers, and other low vision aids.

National Eye Institute
9000 Rockville Pike
Building 31, Room 6A03
Bethesda, MD 20892
(301) 496-2234

The National Eye Institute conducts and funds research on the eye and visual disorders and publishes materials on visual impairment.

National Federation of the Blind
1800 Johnson Street
Baltimore, MD 21230
(301) 659-9314

The National Federation of the Blind (NFB) is a consumer organization that works to improve the social and economic opportunities of blind and visually impaired persons. It monitors all legislation affecting blind people, evaluates programs, assists in promoting needed services, funds scholarships for blind persons, conducts a public education program, and maintains affiliates in all states and the District of Columbia.

National Society to Prevent Blindness
500 East Remington Road
Schaumburg, IL 60173
(312) 843-2020

The National Society to Prevent Blindness (NSPB) conducts a program of public and professional education, research, and industrial and community services to prevent blindness.

Newspapers for the Blind
5508 Calkins Road
Flint, MI 48532
(313) 230-8866

Newspapers for the Blind reads issues of local newspapers over the telephone to subscribers and provides information on the availability of such services.

Recording for the Blind
20 Roszel Road
Princeton, NJ 08540
(609) 452-0606

Recording for the Blind (RFB) lends tape-recorded textbooks and other educational materials at no charge to visually, perceptually, and physically impaired students and professionals who pay an annual membership fee. Recording is done in a network of studios across the country.

RP Foundation Fighting Blindness
(National Retinitis Pigmentosa Foundation)
1401 Mt. Royal Avenue
Baltimore, MD 21217
(301) 255-9400

The RP Foundation Fighting Blindness conducts public education programs and supports research related to the cause, prevention, and treatment of retinitis pigmentosa. It maintains a network of affiliates across the country and conducts workshops as well as referral and donor programs.

Social Security Administration
U.S. Department of Health and Human Services
6401 Security Boulevard
Baltimore, MD 21235
(301) 965-1234

The Social Security Administration (SSA) oversees old age, survivors, and disability insurance programs under the provisions of the Social Security Act, including the Supplemental Security Income (SSI) program for aged, blind, and disabled persons. It maintains a network of offices across the country and publishes a variety of materials on social security benefits.

Taping for the Blind
3935 Essex Lane
Houston, TX 77027
(713) 622-2767

Taping for the Blind records reading materials on cassette for use by visually and physically impaired persons.

Organizations in the Aging Network

Administration on Aging
U.S. Department of Health and Human Services
300 Independence Avenue, S.W.
North Building, Room 4760
Washington, DC 20201
(202) 245-0724

The Administration on Aging (AOA) administers programs for older people funded under the Older Americans Act of 1965. It develops programs to pro-

mote the economic welfare and personal independence of older people and provides funds, advice, and assistance to promote the development of state-administered, community-based social services for older people.

American Association of Retired Persons
1909 K Street, N.W.
Washington, DC 20049
(202) 872-4700

A membership organization for older persons, the American Association of Retired Persons (AARP) offers a wide range of community services and educational programs, publishes a variety of pamphlets and magazines, and engages in advocacy efforts. It assists consumers, family members, and professionals with myriad issues related to aging.

National Association of Area Agencies on Aging
1112 15th Street, N.W., Suite 100
Washington, DC 20036
(202) 296-8130

The National Association of Area Agencies on Aging (NAAAA) provides referrals to local agencies.

National Council on the Aging
409 Third Avenue, S.W., Suite 200
Washington, DC 20024
(202) 479-1200

The National Council on the Aging (NCOA) represents professionals who provide direct services to elderly persons. It acts as a national information and consultation center and engages in a wide variety of activities to promote concern for older persons and their needs.

In addition, the following organizations can provide information on specific health and physical conditions associated with aging.

Alzheimer's Association
70 East Lake Street
Chicago, IL 60601
(312) 853-3060

American Heart Association
7320 Greenville Avenue
Dallas, TX 75231
(214) 750-5397

Arthritis Foundation
1314 Spring Street, N.W.
Atlanta, GA 30309
(404) 872-7100

Continence Restored
785 Park Avenue
New York, NY 10021
(212) 879-3131

Huntington's Disease Society of America
140 West 22nd Street
Sixth Floor
New York, NY 10011
(212) 242-1968

Medic Alert Foundation
P.O. Box 1009
Turlock, CA 95381-1009
(209) 668-3333

National Diabetes Information Clearinghouse
Box NDIC
Bethesda, MD 20892
(301) 468-2162

National Hearing Aid Society
20361 Middlebelt Street
Livonia, MI 48152
(313) 478-2610

National High Blood Pressure Information Center
4733 Bethesda Avenue
Bethesda, MD 20814
(301) 951-3260

National Institute of Neurological Disorders and Stroke Information Office
9000 Rockville Pike
Building 31, Room 8A06
Bethesda, MD 20892
(301) 496-5751

National Osteoporosis Foundation
1625 Eye Street, N.W., Suite 822

Washington, DC 20006
(202) 223-2226

National Stroke Association
200 East Hampden Avenue, Suite 240
Englewood, CO 80110
(303) 762-9922

Self-Help for Hard of Hearing People
7800 Wisconsin Avenue
Bethesda, MD 20814
(301) 657-2248 or (301) 657-2249 (TDD)

United Parkinson Foundation
360 West Superior Street
Chicago, IL 60610
(312) 664-2344

The following national organizations can assist professionals and family members with issues and resources related to long-term care needs.

American Association of Homes for the Aged (AAHA)
1129 20th Street, N.W., Suite 400
Washington, D.C. 20036
(202) 296-5960

American Health Care Association
1201 L Street, N.W.
Washington, DC 20005
(202) 842-4444

Foundation for Hospice & Home Care
519 C Street
Washington, DC 20002
(202) 547-7424

National Association for Home Care
519 C Street, N.E.
Washington, DC 20815
(202) 986-8741

National Association of Residential Care Facilities
1205 West Main Street, Suite 209
Richmond, VA 23220
(804) 355-3265

National Citizens Coalition for Nursing Home Reform
1424 16th Street, N.W., Suite 12
Washington, D.C. 20005
(202) 797-0657

National Hospice Organization
1901 North Fort Myer Drive, Suite 307
Arlington, VA 22209
(703) 243-5900

National Institute of Adult Day Care (**NIAD;** component of **NCOA**)
c/o New Horizons at Choate
21 Warren Avenue
Woburn, MA 01810
(617) 932-0800

National Institute on Community-Based Long Term Care
c/o Health Services Program
University of Kansas
110 Watkins Home
Lawrence, KS 66043

National Voluntary Organization for Independent Living for the Aging
c/o American College of International Physicians
5530 Wisconsin Avenue, N.W., Suite 1149
Washington, D.C. 20815
(202) 986-8741

The following organizations can provide assistance related to legal issues and the elderly.

American Bar Association Commission on the Legal Problems of the Elderly
1800 M Street, N.W.
Second Floor, South Lobby
Washington, DC 20036
(202) 331-2297

Legal Council for the Elderly
1909 K Street, N.W.
Washington, DC 20049
(202) 662-4933

Legal Services for the Elderly
132 West 43rd Street
Third Floor
New York, NY 10036
(212) 391-0120

The following organizations conduct research related to the elderly.

Alliance for Aging Research
2021 K Street, N.W., Suite 305
Washington, DC 20006
(202) 293-2856

American Federation for Aging Research
725 Park Avenue
New York, NY 10021
(212) 570-2090

National Center for Health Statistics
3700 East-West Highway
Hyattsville, MD 20782
(301) 436-8500

National Institute on Aging
Public Information Office
9000 Rockville Pike
Federal Building, Room 6C12
Bethesda, MD 20892
(301) 496-1752

Office of Disease Prevention and Health Promotion
330 C Street, S.W.
Mary Switzer Building, Room 2132
Washington, DC 20201
(202) 472-5660

The following are organizations related to volunteer and leisure activities.

Elder Craftsmen
135 East 65th Street
New York, NY 10021
(212) 861-5260

Elderhostel
80 Boylston Street, Suite 400
Boston, MA 02116
(617) 426-8056

National Association of Home Builders
Special Committee on Senior Housing
15th and M Streets, N.W.
Washington, DC 20005

National Retiree Volunteer Center
607 Marquette Avenue, #10
Minneapolis, MN 55402
(612) 341-2689

National Senior Sports Association
10560 Main Street, Suite 205
Fairfax, VA 22030
(703) 385-7540

Retired Senior Volunteer Program
c/o ACTION
806 Connecticut Avenue, N.W.
Washington, DC 20525
(202) 634-9353

The organizations below provide supportive assistance for adult children and other caregivers of the elderly population.

Children of Aging Parents
2761 Trenton Road
Levittown, PA 19056
(215) 945-6900

Concerned Relatives of Nursing Home Patients
3130 Mayfield Road
Cleveland Heights, OH 44118
(216) 321-0403

Selected Readings

American Foundation for the Blind. (1985). *Aging and vision: Making the most of impaired vision.* New York. Author.

American Foundation for the Blind. (1987). *Low vision questions and answers.* New York: Author.

American Foundation for the Blind. (1988). *Directory of services for blind and visually impaired persons in the United States, 23rd edition.* New York: Author.

Aston, S. J., DeSylvia, D., & Mancil, G. (1990). *Optometric gerontology: A resource manual.* Rockville, MD: Association of Schools and Colleges of Optometry.

Atchley, R.C. (1988). *Social forces and aging.* Belmont, CA: Washington Publishing.

Bailey, I. L., & Hall, A. (1990). *Visual impairment: An overview.* New York: American Foundation for the Blind.

Beliveau, M., Yeadon, A., & Aston S. (1986). *Innovative curriculum development research: To develop in-service training curriculum for providers of long-term care to elderly blind/visually impaired.* (Final Report. Innovation Grant No. G008535147). Washington, DC: National Institute of Handicapped Research.

Bond, J., & Coleman, P. (1990). *Aging in Society: An introduction to social gerontology.* Newbury, CA: Sage.

Bytheway, B. (Ed.). (1989). *Becoming and being old: Sociological approaches to later life.* Newbury, CA: Sage.

Dickman, I. R. (1983). *Making life more livable.* New York: American Foundation for the Blind.

Dychtwald, K. (1989). *Age wave: The challenges and opportunities of an aging America.* New York: St. Martin's Press.

Frengley, J. D., Murray, P., & Wykle, M.L. (1990). *Practicing rehabilitation with geriatric clients.* New York. Springer.

Harel, Z. (1990). *The vulnerable aged: People, services and policies.* New York: Springer.

Harris, L., & Associates (1987). *Problems facing elderly Americans living alone: A national survey.* New York: Commonwealth Fund Commission on Elderly People Living Alone.

Hiatt, L. G., et al. (1982). *What are friends for? Self help groups for persons with sensory loss.* New York: American Foundation for the Blind.

Hilton J. C. (1989). *Strategies for identifying blind and visually impaired nursing home residents.* New York: American Foundation for the Blind and the Delta Gamma Foundation.

Horowitz, A. (1988). *The prevalence and consequences of visual impairment among nursing home residents.* New York: Lighthouse for the Blind.

Jose, R. T. (1985). *Understanding low vision.* New York: American Foundation for the Blind.

Ludwig, I., Luxton, L., & Attmore, M. (1988). *Creative recreation for blind and visually impaired adults.* New York: American Foundation for the Blind.

Mace, N. L., & Rabins, P.V. (1990). *The 36-hour day: A family guide to caring for persons with Alzheimer's disease, related dementing illness, and memory loss in later life.* Baltimore: Johns Hopkins University Press.

Ringgold, N. P. (1991). *Out of the corner of my eye: Living with vision loss in later life.* New York: American Foundation for the Blind.

Rosenbloom, A. A., & Morgan, M. W. (Eds.). (1986). *Vision and aging: General and clinical perspectives.* New York: Professional Press Books.

Ross, M. A. (1984). *Fitness for the aging adult with visual impairment: An exercise and resource manual.* New York: American Foundation for the Blind.

ABOUT THE AUTHORS

Harold L. Bate is professor of audiology at the Department of Speech Pathology and Audiology, Western Michigan University at Kalamazoo.

Bruce B. Blasch is associate director of the Rehabilitation Research and Development Center, VA Medical Center, in Decatur, Georgia.

John E. Crews is health research scientist at the Rehabilitation Research and Development Center, VA Medical Center, in Decatur, Georgia, and was, at the time of writing, program manager at the Independent Living Rehabilitation Program, Michigan Commission for the Blind, in Saginaw.

Robert L. Dolsen is executive director of Region IV Area Agency on Aging in St. Joseph, Michigan, and a member of the board of the Michigan Association of Area Agencies on Aging.

Jon Hendricks is professor and chairman of the Department of Sociology, Oregon State University in Corvallis.

Randall T. Jose is clinical director of the Lighthouse of Houston/University of Houston Vision Rehabilitation Clinic and associate professor, College of Optometry/University of Houston in Houston, Texas.

Steven J. LaGrow is professor and head of rehabilitation studies at the Department of Psychology, Massey University in Palmerston North, New Zealand, and the president of the Orientation and Mobility Instructors Association of Australasia.

Lynne Luxton is doctoral candidate in the Department of Special Education, Teachers College, Columbia University, New York, New York, and was, at the time of writing, national consultant on rehabilitation teaching at the American Foundation for the Blind.

Raymond C. Mastalish is retired executive director of the National Association of Area Agencies on Aging and former assistant to the commissioner, U.S. Administration on Aging.

Robert B. Mitchell is associate professor at the Department of Biology, Pennsylvania State University in University Park.

Alberta L. Orr is national program associate specializing in aging at the American Foundation for the Blind, New York, New York, and former executive director of the East Bronx Council on Aging. The author of a wide range of articles, position papers, and government reports on the subject of aging, she is a 1991 recipient of the Volunteerism in Action Award from the National Council on the Aging.

Alfred A. Rosenbloom is director of low vision services at the Chicago Lighthouse for the Blind and adjunct professor at the College of Optometry/University of Houston. He is a member of the board of directors of the National Accreditation Council for Agencies Serving the Blind and Visually Handicapped and also a member of the board of trustees of the American Foundation for the Blind.

Anne Yeadon is founder and executive director of AWARE (Associates for World Action in Rehabilitation and Education), a recently formed organization in Mohegan Lake, New York, serving blind and visually impaired populations in developing nations and hard-to-reach groups in the United States and other industrialized nations.

Steven H. Zarit is professor of human development at the Department of Human Development and Family Studies and assistant director for research and training of the Gerontology Center, Pennsylvania State University in University Park.

The mission of the American Foundation for the Blind (AFB) is to enable persons who are blind or visually impaired to achieve equality of access and opportunity that will ensure freedom of choice in their lives. AFB accomplishes this mission by taking a national leadership role in the development and implementation of public policy and legislation, informational and educational programs, diversified products, and quality services. Among the services it delivers, AFB maintains a national hotline to provide information and assistance to callers. The hotline number is 1-800-232-5463; it is in operation Mondays through Fridays, 8:30 a.m. to 4:30 p.m. EST or EDT.